Genetic Secrets

Genetic Secrets

Protecting Privacy and

Confidentiality in the

Genetic Era

edited by Mark A. Rothstein

Yale University Press

New Haven and London

Printed in the United States of America.

Library of Congress Cataloging-in-Publication Data

Genetic secrets : protecting privacy and confidentiality in the
genetic era / edited by Mark A. Rothstein.
p.   cm.
Includes bibliographical references and index.
ISBN 0-300-07251-1 (cloth : alk. paper)
      0-300-08063-8 (pbk. : alk. paper)
1. Medical genetics—Moral and ethical aspects.   2. Medical genetics—Law and
legislation.   3. Medical records—Law and legislation.   4. Privacy, Right of.
5. Confidential communications—Physicians.   6. Medical records—Access
control.   I. Rothstein, Mark A.
RB155.G398   1997
323.44'8—dc21   97-28439

A catalogue record for this book is available from the British Library.

The paper in this book meets the guidelines for permanence and durability of the Committee on Production Guidelines for Book Longevity of the Council on Library Resources.

10 9 8 7 6 5 4 3 2

To the memory of my sister, Freddie Rothstein, who believed in the privacy and confidentiality of medical information

Contents

Foreword

Arthur C. Upton

Few developments are likely to affect human beings more profoundly in the long run than the discoveries resulting from advances in modern genetics. The increasingly powerful diagnostic, predictive, and life-enhancing tools generated by molecular genetics and biotechnology have already begun to revolutionize medicine, science, agriculture, animal husbandry, and a growing number of industries.[1]

Exemplifying the power of the new technologies are their uses to: (1) identify the specific strains and sources of microorganisms responsible for certain outbreaks of tuberculosis[2] and Legionnaire's disease;[3] (2) implicate the human papilloma virus in causing most cancers of the uterine cervix;[4] (3) elucidate many other aspects of carcinogenesis;[5] (4) clarify the causal mechanisms of certain allergic reactions;[6] and (5) give rise to increasing numbers of new and improved varieties of disease- and pest-resistant animals and plants.[7]

Although the developments in genetic technology promise to provide many additional benefits to humankind in coming years, their application to genetic screening poses ethical, social, and legal questions, many of which are rooted in issues of privacy and confidentiality. Still to be resolved, for example, is how much the highly personal information contained in one's genome differs in kind from other medical and legal information and, consequently, deserves greater protection against disclosure to one's employer, health insurer, family members, and others.[8]

Concerns about the disclosure of genetic information are prompted in large part by the fear that such knowledge could stigmatize the affected person and also, perhaps, members of his or her family, causing such persons to be barred from employment, denied insurance, or subjected to other discrimination.[9] Such concerns are heightened, moreover, by the fact that protection of the confidentiality of genetic information is being rendered increasingly difficult by the computerization and electronic transfer of medical records, coupled with the rapid growth of managed care and other sweeping changes in the organization of the health care delivery system.[10]

Also complicating the issue is the tension that exists under certain circumstances between the desire to respect the confidentiality of genetic information and the competing need or responsibility to share the information. For example: (1) a parent who possesses a disease-causing gene may be under the moral obligation to share the information with his or her child if the health of the child would otherwise be jeopardized;[11] (2) newborn infants in most states are required by law to undergo genetic screening for phenylketonuria;[12] (3) members of the military are required to contribute specimens of their DNA to a central armed forces repository in order to facilitate the identification of their bodies if they are killed in the line of duty;[13] (4) criminal offenders are required in many states to contribute DNA to databases maintained for forensic purposes by law enforcement agencies;[14] and (5) persons in all walks of life are increasingly being called upon to contribute to DNA data banks for research purposes.[15] Although most DNA banks and DNA databases are generally acknowledged to serve important and beneficial purposes, the adequacy of existing safeguards for protecting the confidentiality of the genetic information they contain is not without question.[16]

Also subject to question are the circumstances under which genetic information should, or should not, be disclosed to the affected individual.[17] For example, should a person who is found on genetic testing to carry a gene mutation that may predispose him or her to a disease of uncertain likelihood, for which no methods of treatment or prevention are known, be told of the condition, even if the disclosure under such circumstances might possibly do the person more harm than good? Also, by extension, if the same allele might pose a risk to other members of the person's family, who also happened to be carriers of the same mutation, should they too be notified?[18]

The ethical, practical, and legal ramifications of these and related questions—which are at the forefront of contemporary medicine and medical research—are explored in depth in the chapters that follow. The broad range of topics covered in these chapters includes: the privacy and confidentiality of genetic information, considered from an ethical standpoint and also in the framework of the patient-physician relationship, public health, the family, and society at large; the challenges to privacy and confidentiality that may be projected to result from the emerging genetic technologies and from the application of such technologies to exposure surveillance, population screening, and forensic problems; the role of informed consent in protecting the confidentiality of genetic information in the clinical setting, including the issues surrounding the right to know or not to know; the potential uses of genetic information by third parties, including employers, insurers, and schools; the implications of changes in the health care delivery system for privacy and confidentiality; relevant national and international developments in public policies, professional standards, and laws; recommendations for addressing problems in each of these subjects areas; and the identification of research needs. The chapters that follow address the privacy and confidentiality of genetic information of all types, considering the full range of their social, ethical, and legal ramifications.

NOTES

1. Philip Kitcher, *The Lives to Come: The Genetic Revolution and Human Possibilities* (New York: Simon and Schuster, 1996); U.S. Congress, Office of Technology Assessment, *New Developments in Biotechnology: Patenting Life—Special Report* (Washington, D.C.: U.S. Government Printing Office, 1989).

2. Agnes Genewein et al., "Molecular Approach to Identifying Route of Transmission of Tuberculosis in the Community," *Lancet* 342 (1993): 841–44.

3. W. Gary Hlady et al., "Outbreak of Legionnaire's Disease Linked to a Decorative Fountain by Molecular Epidemiology," *American Journal of Epidemiology* 138 (1993): 555–62.

4. Mark Schiffman et al., "Epidemiologic Evidence Showing That Human Papillomavirus Causes Most Cervical Intraepithelial Neoplasia," *Journal of the National Cancer Institute* 85 (1993): 958–64.

5. John Mendelsohn et al., eds., *The Molecular Basis of Cancer* (Philadelphia: W. B. Saunders, 1995); I. Bernard Weinstein, "The Contribution of Molecular Biology to Cancer Epidemiology," *Annals of the New York Academy of Sciences* 768 (1995): 30–40.

6. Delores Graham and Hillel Koren, "Biomarkers of Inflammation in Ozone-Exposed Humans," *American Review of Respiratory Disease* 142 (1990): 152–56.

7. Kitcher, *Lives to Come.*

8. Institute of Medicine, Committee on Assessing Genetic Risks, *Assessing Genetic Risks: Implications for Health and Social Policy,* Lori Andrews et al., eds. (Washington, D.C.: National Academy Press, 1994).

9. Arthur L. Frank, "Scientific and Ethical Aspects of Human Monitoring," *Environmental Health Perspectives* 104, suppl. 3 (1996): 659–62; Harry Ostrer et al., "Insurance and Genetic Testing: Where Are We Now?" *American Journal of Human Genetics* 52 (1993): 565–77; Walter C. Zimmerli, "Who Has the Right to Know the Genetic Constitution of a Particular Person?" in Ruth F. Chadwick and Gregory Bock, eds., *Human Genetic Information: Science, Law, and Ethics* (Chichester: John Wiley and Sons, 1990).

10. Committee on Regional Health Data Networks, Institute of Medicine, *Health Data in the Information Age: Use, Disclosure, and Privacy,* Molla Donaldson and Kathleen Lohr, eds. (Washington, D.C.: U.S. Government Printing Office, 1994); John K. Iglehart, "Physicians and the Growth of Managed Care," *New England Journal of Medicine* 331 (1994): 1167–68; Institute of Medicine, National Academy of Sciences, *Health Data in the Information Age* (Washington, D.C.: National Academy Press, 1994).

11. Sonia M. Suter, "Whose Genes Are These Anyway? Familial Conflicts over Access to Genetic Information," *Michigan Law Review* 91 (1993): 1854–908.

12. Jean McEwen and Philip R. Reilly, "Stored Guthrie Cards as DNA 'Banks,'" *American Journal of Human Genetics* 55 (1994): 196–200.

13. Jean E. McEwen, "DNA Data Banks," Chapter 13 in this volume.

14. Jean E. McEwen, "Forensic DNA Data Banking by State Crime Laboratories," *American Journal of Human Genetics* 56 (1995): 1487–92.

15. McEwen, "DNA Data Banks."

16. Barry Scheck, "DNA Data Banking: A Cautionary Tale," *American Journal of Human Genetics* 54 (1994): 931–33.

17. Committee on Assessing Genetic Risks, *Assessing Genetic Risks.*

18. Zimmerli, "Who Has the Right to Know?"

Preface

The United States Department of Energy sponsored a highly successful workshop on Medical Information and the Right to Privacy at the National Academy of Sciences in Washington, D.C., on June 9–10, 1994. The idea to produce a volume exploring the full range of issues related to genetic privacy arose from that meeting. I was pleased to accept the Department of Energy's invitation to organize, solicit, and edit the manuscripts contained in this volume. Any opinions, findings, conclusions, or recommendations expressed in the book are solely those of the authors and do not necessarily reflect the views of the Department of Energy.

Several individuals were instrumental in compiling this work. Dan Drell and John Peeters of the Department of Energy gave me their unqualified support as well as the independence to pursue my vision of the book's structure and content. I am indebted to my chapter authors, who permitted me to intrude into their busy lives to produce a work for me. They also were willing to revise their work several times to integrate the chapters more closely. Several authors also reviewed drafts of the concluding chapter and offered valuable criticism.

At the Health Law and Policy Institute at the University of Houston, I am indebted to Cathy Rupf, who coordinated the publisher's and authors' agreements, and to Diana Huezo, who processed all the manuscripts. Harriet Richman, faculty services librarian at the University of Houston Law Library, supplied essential reference support. Laura F. Rothstein not only wrote an excellent chapter on Genetics and Schools but supplied much-needed encouragement in marshaling the talents of twenty-nine colleagues.

Part One **Background**

Chapter 1 Genes, Genomes, and Society

Leroy Hood and Lee Rowen

The ability to decipher human heredity will allow us to glimpse into the innermost workings of our bodies. Two pioneering scientific endeavors laid the framework for this venture, perhaps the most far-reaching scientific exploration ever undertaken. In 1953, Jim Watson and Francis Crick elucidated the structure of DNA (deoxyribonucleic acid), the informational molecule of human heredity.[1] From this work came the fundamental insight that DNA employs a digital code similar to that used by computers, except that a four-letter language, G, C, A and T (guanine, cytosine, adenine, and thymine), is employed rather than the two-digit language of computers, 0 and 1. Thirty-seven years later, in 1990, the Human Genome Project was initiated, a 15-year program to decipher the human DNA digital code by mapping and sequencing the 23 pairs of human chromosomes that reside in the nucleus of every human cell (fig. 1.1). These chromosomes contain the DNA code that directs the marvelous process of human development wherein each of us goes from one cell (the fertilized egg) at conception to 10^{14} cells as an adult.

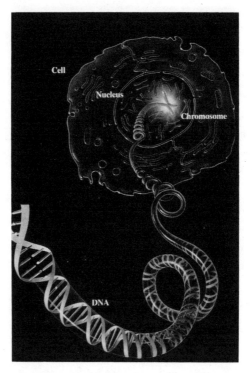

Figure 1.1 The cell, its nucleus, and the chromosomal strand extending from the nucleus (From Department of Health and Human Services, Public Health Service, National Institutes of Health, *The Human Genome Project: From Maps to Medicine,* NIH Publication no. 96-3897)

THREE TYPES OF BIOLOGICAL INFORMATION

There are three types of biological information that function in living organisms. The first type is the digital, or linear, information of the DNA backbone of our chromosomes (fig. 1.2). Its unit of information is the gene; it is estimated that human chromosomes contain perhaps 100,000 genes, or units of information. Genes are expressed in a differential manner; that is, in different cells (e.g., muscle and brain) different combinations of the genes are expressed and this leads to the different appearances and behaviors, or phenotypes, of these cells. The DNA molecules are composed of two strands oriented in opposite directions, in which G–C and A–T always pair, or exhibit molecular complementarity, across the strands (see fig. 1.2). If chromosomes are broken into small pieces and the two strands are separated, the correct partners can find one another through molecular complementarity and "zipper" back together, even

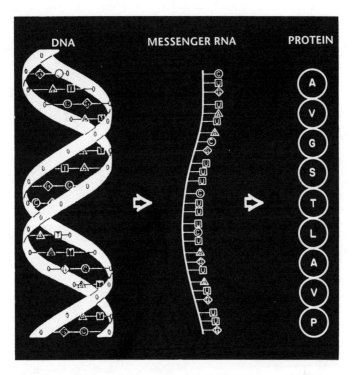

Figure 1.2 The flow of biological information from DNA to messenger RNA to protein

in a complex mixture of DNA fragments. This molecular complementarity is the basis for the DNA diagnostics that are discussed in later chapters. Each gene is expressed as messenger RNA, also exhibiting a four-letter language closely related to that of DNA. This mRNA molecule is processed by a specialized complex cellular machine, the ribosome, to generate the second type of biological information—the protein molecule—initially formed as a linear string of protein letters (see fig. 1.2). The genetic code dictionary connects the DNA and protein languages (e.g., three adjacent DNA letters encode one protein letter).

The molecular language of proteins is more complex than that of DNA, with 20 letters instead of four. The particular order of these letters in each protein string directs it to fold into a unique three-dimensional shape (fig. 1.3). Each protein is a three-dimensional molecular machine; these machines catalyze the chemistry of life and give the body shape and form. As we shall see, deciphering the DNA code may give us new insights into two of the most fundamental problems of proteins: (1) how does the order of the protein letters direct the three-dimensional folding into a precise shape (the protein folding problem)?

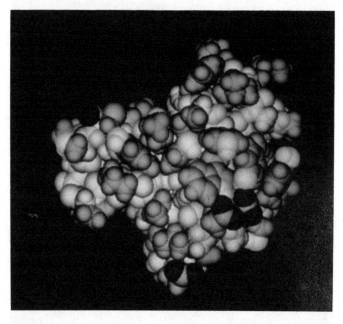

Figure 1.3 The three-dimensional structure of an enzyme, lysozyme, that cleaves sugar molecules

and (2) how does the three-dimensional structure of a protein permit it to execute its function (the structure-function problem)? Proteins and other biological macromolecules assemble together to create the functional units of living organisms, their cells (see fig. 1.1).

The third type of biological information resides in the complex systems and networks that arise from complex cellular interactions. For example, the human brain is composed of a $3 \times$ million million (10^{12}) nerve cells that form 10^{15} connections (synapses) to create an incredibly complex network (fig. 1.4). The interactions of these nerve cells lead to the so-called emergent properties of the brain (e.g., memory, consciousness, and the ability to learn). One could study one particular nerve cell for 20 years to learn everything it could do. Yet this study would provide no insights into these emergent properties because they arise as a consequence of the network interactions of many different cells. The information of complex systems and networks, or biological complexity, is, in a sense, four-dimensional—it changes in both time and space.

Studying complex systems and networks is difficult: (1) the components and their connections must be defined; (2) biological experiments must probe how

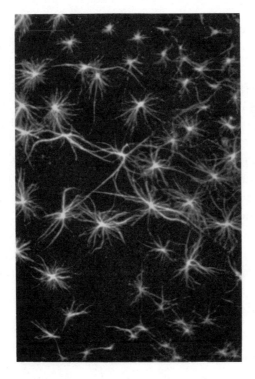

Figure 1.4 Stained nerve cells and their communicating extensions

emergent properties arise from the network; (3) mathematical modeling will be needed to thoroughly define complex systems; and (4) these models must ultimately be tested against biological reality by experimentation. Interestingly enough, many of the powerful new tools that scientists need to analyze biological complexity are emerging from technologies developed by the Human Genome Project.

DECIPHERING BIOLOGICAL INFORMATION

The Human Genome Project has catalyzed a quantum jump in our ability to decipher the one-dimensional biological information of DNA. However, the deciphering of biological information actually has two separate meanings for each of the three types of information. For DNA, it is one thing to determine the order of DNA letters across each of the chromosomes (e.g., the DNA sequence) and quite another to decipher the biological meaning that 3.7 billion years of evolution has inscribed in our DNA. For protein, it is one thing to identify a three-dimensional structure and quite another to understand how this structure carries out its function. For a network, it is one thing to define the components and their connections and something else to understand how the emergent properties arise from these biological networks. Applied mathematicians and computer scientists will play a critical role in deciphering each of these types of biological information because they will create the powerful tools needed for complex analyses of large data sets.

Deciphering the biological information of complex systems and networks will be the central challenge in biology and medicine as we move into the twenty-first century. Analyzing biological complexity will require breaking the systems down into more experimentally tractable subsystems whose properties still reflect those of the system as a whole. We will also have to identify key bottlenecks, or control points, in the complex systems, both to understand their biology and to manipulate the system for twenty-first-century medicine. The tools of the Human Genome Project, or genomics, are beginning to allow us to tackle biological complexity.

THE HUMAN GENOME PROJECT

The Human Genome Project is a worldwide research activity; in the United States it is funded largely by the National Institutes of Health and the Department of Energy. The goal of the enterprise is to map and sequence the 24 different human chromosomes (22 autosomes and the two sex chromosomes, X and Y). Humans have 46 chromosomes; half come from the mother, the other half from the father. Homologous chromosomes differ on average by one in 1,000 letters of the DNA sequence. These variations within the human population are called polymorphisms. Because humans have 3 billion (3×10^9) DNA letters in the maternal or paternal complement of chromosomes, typically 3 million (3×10^6) polymorphisms distinguish the maternal and paternal chromosome sets. The genes may occupy only 3–5% of the DNA, however, with the result that most of the polymorphisms will lie outside genes and therefore will have little effect on the functioning or appearance (phenotype) of the organism. A few polymorphisms, however, will predispose to human genetic diseases, such as cystic fibrosis or certain kinds of cancer, and are therefore medically important.[2]

The Human Genome Project is creating three types of maps for each chromosome (fig. 1.5). The genetic map has identified approximately 6,000 polymorphic markers spread evenly across all human chromosomes (except Y).[3] A

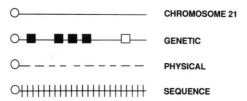

Figure 1.5 The three types of maps being determined by the Human Genome Project

polymorphic marker is, typically, a particular site on an individual chromosome where a single DNA letter or small group of letters varies among members of the human population (fig. 1.6). The genetic map can then be used to identify genes that predispose to disease. The perfect co-segregation, or passage of adjacent pairs of genetic markers, through families together with a disease

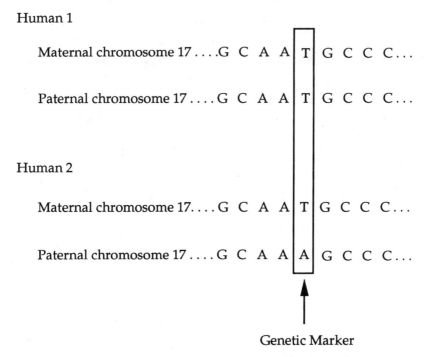

Genetic Marker

Figure 1.6 A hypothetical polymorphic site or genetic marker on a human chromosome. Similar portions of the same chromosome are given for the maternal and paternal chromosomes for two individuals. One of these four chromosomes has a single letter substitution, or polymorphism.

trait allows the localization of the disease-predisposing gene between the two polymorphic markers. Genetic markers further from the disease gene do not co-segregate in families because their association is lost by chromosomal recombination—that is, apparently random breakage and reunion between the paternal and maternal chromosomes that scrambles the associations between particular forms of genetic markers. (In other words, the further the markers are from the disease gene, the more likely it is that recombination will have unlinked an association.) Genes that predispose to disease are first crudely localized by analyzing them against approximately 400 genetic markers scattered across the genome. Once the general location is identified, more genetic markers in that region can be studied to narrow the location of the disease gene. This process is termed "genome-wide genetic mapping." It provides an approximate localization of disease-predisposing genes (to a region of perhaps 1 million DNA letters; the gene may only be 50,000 letters long). The actual gene must then be localized by other methods (e.g., DNA sequencing).

The physical map is made up of overlapping human DNA fragments that, taken together, span the length of the chromosomes (see fig. 1.5). These DNA fragments can be used to physically localize disease genes. These fragments are also the source of material for the final map, the sequence map.

The sequence map for each chromosome represents the order of the letters of the DNA language all the way along each chromosome—this is termed the "DNA sequence" of the chromosome. The average human chromosome contains 130 million DNA letters. Current DNA sequencing machines can read only about 500 letters in each DNA fragment at a time.[4] For this reason, the DNA sequence maps constitute by far the largest challenge the Human Genome Project faces. Indeed, the genetic and physical maps should be complete in a few years; another decade will be spent on the sequence maps. As the sequence maps are completed, computational approaches and biological experiments will allow the identification of the 100,000 human genes.

MODEL GENOMES

The Human Genome Project also proposes to map and sequence the genomes of five model organisms (table 1.1). Four are simple organisms with significantly smaller genomes than humans. The bacterium, yeast, simple roundworm (nematode), and fruit fly (*Drosophila*) all have genes that are similar to a subset of human genes. Hence, these simple model organisms can be used to gain insights into how the evolutionarily related genes in humans may function.

Table 1.1 Genome sizes of model organisms

Organism	Megabases (millions of bases)
E. coli	5
yeast	15
nematode (worm)	100
Drosophila (fruit fly)	180
mouse	3,000
human	3,000

The sequence of the yeast genome has been completed,[5] as have the sequences of three prokaryotic genomes.[6]

The fifth model organism, the mouse genome, is as complex as the human genome. Accordingly, the mouse can serve as a valid model organism to study the function of many genes that control complexities not found in the simple model organisms. The mouse can also serve as a model for studying disease genes—how they cause pathology—and as a vehicle to search for drugs to prevent the disease. Experiments can be done in the mouse that are impossible or impermissible in humans.

TECHNOLOGY DEVELOPMENT FOR GENOMICS: IMPLICATIONS FOR BIOLOGY AND MEDICINE

The study of genomes has, necessarily, led to the development of technologies that have the capacity to decipher large amounts of biological information from DNA. In the past, biologists tended to focus on the analysis of one gene or protein for extended periods of time. Today the tools of genomics permit the analysis of thousands to billions of units of information per day (table 1.2). For example, the Genome Center in the Department of Molecular Biotechnology at the University of Washington, Seattle, where we both work, has 10 DNA sequencers that provide the capacity to sequence 360,000 (10 × 36,000) DNA letters per day. Likewise, our four genetic mappers can analyze more than 4,000 genetic markers per day.

Our large-scale DNA arrayer can place 20,000 human DNA fragment clones in one hour on a filter about the size of this page. DNA fragments can be obtained from two sources. First, DNA from chromosomes can be fragmented

Table 1.2 Tools of genomics

Tools	Throughput
Large-scale DNA sequencer	36,000 DNA letters per day
Genome-wide genetic mapping	1,200 genetic markers per day
Large-scale DNA arrays	2,000 hybridizations per day
Computational (similarity analyses)	3×10^{12} DNA letters per day

and cloned into a recombinant DNA vector that can be grown in an appropriate host (e.g., bacteria). This is called a "genomic library." Second, mRNA can be copied into DNA to make copies of all the genes expressed in a tissue, cell type, or even tumor. This is called a "copy DNA (cDNA) library." The presence of an mRNA in a tissue indicates that the gene coding for that mRNA is expressed in that tissue—that is, is used to produce a protein. Hence, for example, to examine the differences between the genes expressed in normal and tumor cells, 20,000 cDNA clones from a normal prostate gland can be arrayed on a filter and used to analyze the cDNA information present in hundreds of prostate tumors by molecular complementarity or hybridization. Ten identical normal cDNA filters can easily be prepared in one day and compared against the cDNA libraries from 10 tumors, thus making 200,000 comparisons of informational units (20,000 × 10 hybridizations). A second approach to DNA arrays is the synthesis of 100,000-oligonucleotide (e.g., each oligonucleotide may be a string 20 DNA letters long) arrays on a glass or silicon chips the size of a thumbnail (fig. 1.7).[7] In time, the expression patterns of all 100,000 human genes can be studied with these DNA chips. From these studies, insights into which proteins play key roles in cellular development, both normal and cancerous, will be obtained on a scale not heretofore possible.

Powerful computational analyses can also be carried out on DNA sequences. For example, the 360,000 DNA letters per day coming from 10 DNA sequencers can be matched against the more than 600 million letters in the genome database to determine whether any of the new sequences match the preexisting sequences. The DNA sequence in the database comes mostly from very short stretches of experimental human genes or from the genomes of the model organisms. Only about 1% of the human genome has been sequenced to date.

The important point about these large-scale instruments is they can be used to study complex biological systems and networks. Indeed, the Human Ge-

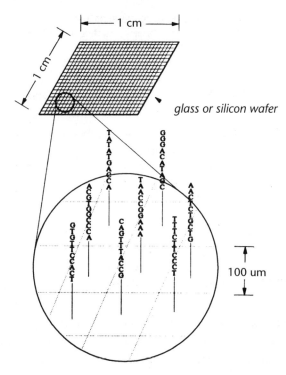

Figure 1.7 A DNA chip, or oligonucleotide array. Different short DNA sequences (of about 20 letters) can be synthesized on a glass or silicon chip and then used to detect messenger RNA (or their DNA copies) or DNA fragments that are complementary in sequence by hybridization.

nome Project is already beginning to revolutionize the practice of biology and medicine—and will have even more of an impact as we move toward completion of the human and model organism genomes early in the twenty-first century.

GENOMICS AND BIOLOGY

The major challenge genomics presents to biology is the identification of the functions of all 100,000 human genes (fig. 1.8). This is very hard. The functions of a few of these genes are understood to varying levels of sophistication. The functions of some others can be guessed at because they resemble genes whose functions are known. The functions of many genes are unknown. In the past, biologists would study a function, develop an assay (way of measuring) for it, through the assay purify the protein, and through the protein obtain the gene.[8]

**BIOLOGY WILL HAVE TO DEVELOP TOOLS AND
STRATEGIES TO DETERMINE PROTEIN FUNCTION
FROM GENE SEQUENCE**

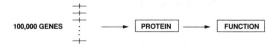

Figure 1.8 Challenge presented by the Human Genome Project through the identification of the 100,000 or so human genes, including the correlation of genes with their proteins, proteins with their structures, and protein structures with their functions

Thus, function was tied to gene identification. Genomics has inverted this pathway (fig. 1.8). There are three discrete challenges: (1) correlating genes with their proteins; (2) determining the three-dimensional structures of proteins; and (3) understanding how particular three-dimensional protein structures execute their functions. There may be shortcuts in correlating genes with presumptive functions. For example, computational methods can be used to determine whether the gene (or its protein translation via the genetic code dictionary) is similar to a gene (or protein) previously studied. If so, this may give a clue as to function. If not, one may use large-scale DNA arrays to identify the cells or tissues in which the gene is expressed.

The localization of the gene product to particular cells may give additional clues as to function. Then biological experiments must be performed to elucidate the function. For example, the gene can be rendered nonfunctional ("knocked out") in a mouse to determine whether it has any noticeable effect on the phenotype (appearance or behavior) of the mouse. Indeed, experiments are now under way to knock out each of the 6,000 yeast genes to determine their effect on yeast biology. Genes and their proteins can now be readily linked in yeast (because the entire genome has been sequenced). For example, two-dimensional protein separation gels, those which separate complex protein mixtures in one dimension by size and in a second dimension by charge, isolate relatively pure yeast protein spots (fig. 1.9). Individual proteins can be extracted from gels and cut with protein-cutting enzymes, the fragment sizes can be analyzed in a mass spectrometer, and, because the genome has been sequenced, the corresponding gene can be identified from computational comparisons of predicted and experimental protein fragment sizes. The behavior of particular proteins (levels of expression, chemical modifications that alter function) can be followed on two-dimensional gels over the time necessary for a cell or

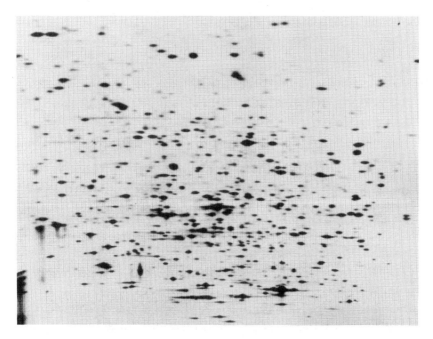

Figure 1.9 A two-dimensional protein gel. The proteins (dark spots) are separated in one dimension by size and in a second dimension by electrical charge.

organism to carry out a complex function in order to correlate protein behavior with particular functions. In this way the worlds of DNA and protein can be joined. It will be some time before we can use similar tools to analyze human genes (at least until most of the human genome is sequenced).

Several computational approaches may facilitate our understanding of gene-protein-function relations. The regulatory sequences (usually lying immediately to one side or even within the gene) determine when in development (time), where in the tissues (space), and how much of the gene is to be expressed (magnitude). As we develop systems analyses for the problems of gene regulation (studying, for example, the interactions of DNA regulatory sequences and the proteins that operate on these sequences to trigger the control decisions for gene expression of time, space, and magnitude), we will begin to decipher the regulatory code. Perhaps there will be a time when this code can be deciphered directly from the gene sequence to predict these three parameters of gene expression for every gene (fig. 1.10).

A second computational approach will be to attempt to identify the lexicon

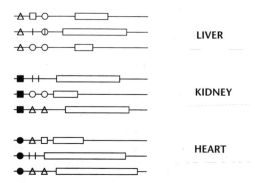

Figure 1.10 The DNA regulatory code that governs the expression of particular genes in different tissues. The long rectangles represent genes, and the squares, triangles, and circles represent various regulatory elements. (Adapted from Daniel J. Kevles and Leroy Hood, eds., *The Code of Codes, Scientific and Social Issues in the Human Genome Project* [Cambridge: Harvard University Press, 1992], fig. 19)

of motifs that are the fundamental building blocks of genes and proteins (fig. 1.11). A motif is a segment of protein sequence that causes a particular fold and/or facilitates a particular function. The train provides an analogy. The train is made up of many different cars that have discrete functions (caboose, engine, boxcar). In a similar fashion, a protein is often composed of several domains, each with a discrete function. Each car in the train has smaller

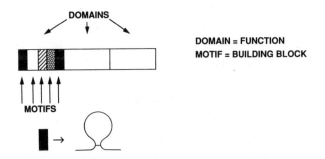

Figure 1.11 A schematic illustration of the domains and motifs of a hypothetical protein (Adapted from Daniel J. Kevles and Leroy Hood, eds., *The Code of Codes, Scientific and Social Issues in the Human Genome Project* [Cambridge: Harvard University Press, 1992], fig. 20)

Immunoglobulin Gene Superfamily

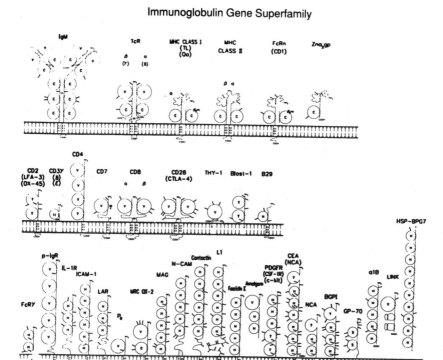

Figure 1.12 Members of a related set (the immunoglobulin super family) of very successful proteins that are encoded by genes and gene families scattered across the human genome (From Michael W. Hunkapiller and Leroy Hood, "Diversity of the Immunoglobulin Gene Superfamily," *Advances in Immunology* 44 [1981]: 9)

components that facilitate function (e.g., the windows, stove, chimney, doors, and walls of the caboose). So a protein domain has as its building block motifs that may vary in size from a few letters to 100 or more letters (see fig. 1.11). Perhaps a few hundred motifs out of a possible 10^3–10^4 have been identified (e.g., the zinc finger motif found in proteins that bind DNA).[9] These motifs correlate with defined structure and can sometimes facilitate a function. Motifs can be difficult to identify because many of them are highly degenerate; that is, out of 10–30 amino acid letters, perhaps only a few are conserved or partly conserved.

Two advances will facilitate the identification of the entire lexicon of motifs. The first is finishing the sequences of the genomes of the human and other model organisms. Cross-species comparisons can be useful in identifying motifs, as can identification and cross-comparison of all the individual members of gene families within a species. Gene families arise when one gene has been very successful. Often many copies of that gene are made at the same chromosomal site and the individual genes diverge to carry out distinct but related functions. This group of genes is termed a "gene family." Highly successful gene families can make copies of themselves that move to different chromosomal sites (fig. 1.12). Second, the determination of many more three-dimensional structures for proteins will permit cross-comparisons of one-dimensional patterns and three-dimensional structures to facilitate motif identification. This lexicon of protein motifs could play a key role in solving the protein-folding problem and in linking three-dimensional structures of proteins to their functions.

The tools of genomics, therefore, will let us approach in new and powerful ways the analysis of complex biological systems and networks. Such areas as immunity, development, and nervous system function can all be approached from the systems viewpoint using many of the powerful tools of genomics. Virtually every area of biology can be attacked with these new tools and approaches.

Last, it has been said that the history of much of our past evolution is buried in our genome. The complete genome sequence will let us identify all of the families of related genes and delineate the nature of their molecular archaeology (fig. 1.12). Comparisons with the genome sequences of the model organisms will enrich our understanding of molecular evolution enormously. As a product of evolution, the digital information of human chromosomes actually contains many different languages, some discrete and others overlapping. For example, the coding regions of genes represent one language; the regulatory code a second; the major features of genome evolution a third; and the chromosomal machinery necessary for rapid DNA replication from many sites a fourth. The initial efforts to decipher the multiplicity of languages present in human chromosomes have proved challenging. Look, for example, at figure 1.13, a schematic illustration of the 700,000 letters of the DNA alphabet spanning one important gene family of immune receptors. The vertical bars on the first line indicate the 94 gene elements found in this family. The lower colored bars all represent distinct types of digital information present in the longest contiguous stretch of human sequence analyzed to date.[10] Knowing all the members of this gene family gives us the ability to interrogate and manipulate the immune system with striking new strategies. This is moving us toward a preventive medicine of the twenty-first century.

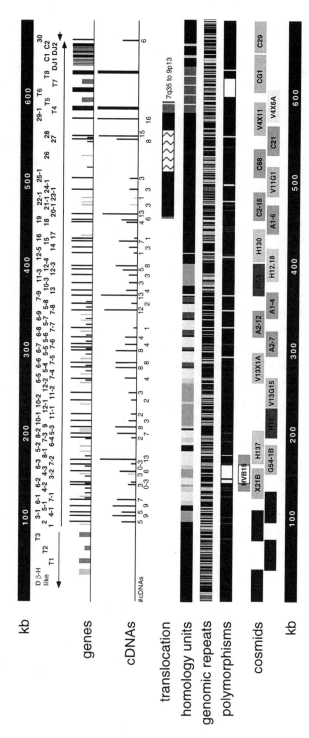

Figure 1.13 The human β T-cell receptor gene family. The vertical bars represent genes, the colored patterns various other types of biological information. (Adapted from Lee Rowen et al., "The Complete 685 Kilobase Sequence of the Human Beta T-Cell Receptor Locus," *Science 272* [1996]: 1755)

GENOMICS AND MEDICINE

The tools of genomics provide the large-scale capacity to study human poly-morphisms to determine which are irrelevant, which cause variations within the range of normal physiology (e.g., height and longevity variations), and which correlate with diseases or the predisposition to diseases. As we identify all 100,000 human genes, we will have the tools to study variation in large human populations (using large-scale DNA sequencing or even large-scale DNA ar-rays, or chips, to detect polymorphisms; see fig. 1.7). Indeed, with the use of DNA chips to study polymorphisms, it should be possible to increase the throughput of genetic marker analyses a hundredfold. Thus, genes that cause or predispose to disease could, given appropriate numbers of families with the disease, be identified rapidly.

Some sequence variations (polymorphisms) within genes invariably cause disease. For example, some defects in the structure of collagen, a protein required for building bones, have been traced to small deletions in the DNA coding for the protein.[11] A person who inherits this mutation from either parent will suffer from osteogenesis imperfecta, a bone disease. Such a situation of so-called autosomal dominance is rare. More commonly, a defective version of a gene inherited from one parent can be fully or partially compensated by the normal version of the gene inherited from the other parent. Thus, many diseases are caused only if a defective gene is inherited from both parents.

Alternatively, inheritance of a defective gene may result in a continuous gradient of phenotype ranging from no effect to explicit disease. For example, the severity of some diseases, such as Huntington disease and fragile X syn-drome, which causes mental retardation, has been correlated with an increase in the number of consecutive repeats found in a group of three DNA letters tied to a specific location within the gene.[12] Below a certain number of consecutive repeats, no disease symptoms are manifested. Above this, as the number of repeats increase, so does the severity of the disease.

Finally, some polymorphisms are associated with a *probability* of getting a disease. In these cases, terms such as *susceptibility* or *predisposition* may be used to describe the propensity to disease. For example, when the mutant (altered) form of the breast cancer 1 gene (BRCA1) is present in one defective copy, this gene predisposes that by age 60, a woman has a 70% chance of getting breast cancer.[13] The 70% probability figure may arise from one or both of two possibilities. First, women with the defective BRCA1 gene may require one or more environmental factors to trigger the disease process. Presumably, the overall probability that women with the defective gene will experience those factors is 70%. Second, perhaps other genes have the ability to modify the expression (or function) of the BRCA1 gene so as to enhance or limit its ability to cause cancer. By this alternative, the overall probability of having the requisite "bad" set of genes, without an offsetting collection of "good" genes, is 70%.

Complicating matters further, when larger numbers of families with a particular disease phenotype are studied by genetic analyses, it often turns out that multiple genes can predispose to the same apparent disease. For example, the BRCA1 and BRCA2 genes both can cause breast cancer,[14] and four genes have been identified as predisposing to Alzheimer's disease.[15] In essence, some diseases, such as cancers and dementias, appear to result from any number of defective genes, possibly in combination with environmental triggers. Along this same line, some diseases, such as multiple sclerosis, are likely to be multigenic in origin, requiring that two or more separate genes be defective, for the disease to occur.

Sequence variations in genes can thus lead to diseases that have an all-or-none symptamatology, a degree in the severity of symptoms, or a likelihood of causing symptoms if other genetic or environmental factors exacerbate or fail to ameliorate the effects of the defective genes.

If we look two to three decades into the future (or perhaps less), we can imagine a time when perhaps 100 (or more) polymorphic variations in genes will have been identified as predisposing to common diseases—cancer, cardiovascular diseases, autoimmune diseases, and so on. It will certainly be possible to identify these defective genes in individuals and deduce a future "probable health history" complete with numerical assignments to the probabilities. Many of these "probable health histories" can be quite complex and thus difficult to interpret. In the future, there will be therapeutic interventions or preventive measures that will circumvent the effects of many of these disease-predisposing genes.

Today, however, there exists a gap between the ability to diagnose the predisposition to diseases such as breast cancer and the ability to prevent the disease. The debate on whether to use DNA diagnostic tests to identify susceptible women is framed in terms of this gap between diagnostic capacities and the ability to intervene therapeutically. For complex diseases, this gap may span decades. The preventive measures will, in all likelihood, employ the manipulation of the three types of biological information (table 1.3). In this scenario, one of the major functions of medicine would be to keep people well (today medicine generally treats the sick). That is, preventive intervention would be

Table 1.3 Molecular therapies

---

1   Antisense
     Gene therapy
3   Protein engineering
     Applied molecular evolution
     Hormones
     Neurotransmitters
4   Stem cells
     Immunomanipulation

Note: 1, 3, and 4 indicate the three
types of biological information

given before the disease symptoms appear in persons whose genes conduce to a
high probability of causing a disease.

Genomics will thus provide powerful tools for correlating DNA polymorphisms with disease followed by subsequent manipulations of biologic information and environmental factors (such as diet) to prevent disease. This approach is not likely to change the natural life span. Rather, it will reduce the toll
of chronic illnesses that often strike in middle age. It will presumably let
individuals live well into their seventies and eighties mentally alert and physically healthy. Society will then, as it is now, be challenged to deal with an
expanding population of 70- and 80-year-old people capable of contributing to
society in a productive and creative manner.

ETHICAL AND SOCIAL IMPLICATIONS OF HUMAN VARIATION

The tools of genomics will provide powerful and large-scale means for deciphering human polymorphisms that predispose to disease. This biological
information must be acquired, stored, analyzed, and distributed from
computers. As we learn more about how human polymorphisms correlate with
disease, increasingly comprehensive knowledge can be gained about the predicted health history of each individual if appropriate DNA tests are carried
out. If preventive or therapeutic measures were available to circumvent the
deleterious effects of disease-predisposing genes (readily available to all), then
the question of privacy of genetic information would not be compelling. However, we do not now have preventive measures or therapies for most genetic
diseases, nor will we in the near future. DNA testing has begun and presumably

will continue. Databases are now accumulating DNA testing information. The issue of genetic privacy accordingly presents a compelling challenge. Because these and related issues are considered in detail in following chapters, we shall merely outline a few of the issues surrounding the deciphering and use of biological information after the following reflection on values.

VALUES AND POLICY MAKING

How does an individual or a society decide whether a particular action (to test or not? to abort or not? to inform or not?) is right? Typically, the rightness or wrongness of actions is evaluated in light of probable consequences. Will the action cause the most good and the least harm to self and others? Will the action cause immediate good but long-term harm, or vice versa? Will the action benefit many or only a privileged few? What might be the unintended consequences of a course of action? How are benefits and costs to be defined and assessed? What happens when different assumptions about what is best for individuals and society dictate conflicting courses of action? What is more important—the benefits to individuals or the benefits to society, if there is a conflict between the two? What benefits are most important to the long-term health of a society—fairness? optimal distribution of resources? protection of individual rights? prevention of harm to others? Judgments such as these are difficult to make for highly informed and reflective individuals. They are even harder for persons who lack the necessary background of information required to sensibly evaluate contrasting viewpoints or who lack the will or ability to think critically about ethical issues. Nonetheless, decisions regarding the uses of genetic information must and will be made, and many of these decisions will be embodied in public policy.

Policy decisions about genetic information are complicated by many factors: legal precedents, to which analogies will be made; current and future social, economic, and political realities that play into the content of various policies and into the processes by which consensus regarding the content of policies is achieved; and the inherent complexity of the issues posed by the future explosion of genetic data, techniques, and concepts.

The precedents in place surrounding such issues as testing and consent (e.g., testing newborns for phenylketonuria, a disease whose deleterious effects can be largely ameliorated by dietary modifications, or testing blood donations for hepatitis and HIV) may apply well to some genetic disease-causing polymorphisms but not others. Determining the validity of the analogical reasoning that ties precedents to new situations requires both an understanding of the ethical, political, and social issues at stake and an understanding of the scientific and technical nuances that pertain to a particular disease and its predisposing genes. Attaining the required depth and breadth of understanding is difficult, especially when such understanding is frequently not held or agreed upon even by the experts in the field. Because of an urgent need to make policy (so that such industries as insurance companies can be regulated and laws can be consistently applied to individual cases), decisions will be made in the absence of complete information and social reflection about the underlying values. As a result, new precedents may be set that turn out to be shortsighted or deleterious but that will be extremely difficult to overturn.

Factors inherent to social, economic, and political reality affect policy formation. For example, although American citizens may all be created equal in terms of possessing certain rights, we are not all created equal in terms of life circumstances, and our genes comprise an important and irreversible component of those life circumstances. In the arena of genetic information, many policy decisions will require a clarification of the application of the concept of a "right." Do citizens have a right to privacy of information about their genes even if the withholding of that information causes harm to others? Do citizens have a right to health care, even if that care is expensive? Who is obligated to pay for the care? Do fetuses have a right to life even if their life will be miserable due to some genetically caused disease? Does society have the right to say that certain fetuses must be aborted because the care of individuals with debilitating genetic diseases is too great a burden for its limited resources, resources that should instead be placed where they will do the most good? Addressing these questions and others will force an examination of our social values and commitments. Ideally, a consensus will emerge that optimizes benefits for both individuals and society over the long term. There will be costs, however, perhaps to individual liberty, perhaps to a conception of the sanctity of life, perhaps to our resources in the form of increased obligations toward those who, through no fault of their own, bear the burden of genetic diseases.

Last, the data and concepts emerging from the Human Genome Project will challenge many of our beliefs about human nature. We will discover the ways in which we humans are special, gifted with abilities not possessed by other species. We will also discover how very similar we are to other species inhabiting our planet. We believe that two fascinating issues will dominate social policy discussions in the twenty-first century. One is our capacity to shape our evolution as a species. Decisions may be made about who should live to adulthood and who should die, either through permissible or mandatory abortion or through the withholding of therapeutic intervention for life-threatening genetic diseases in the interest of rationing the precious resources of health care. Policies may be considered regarding the regulation of who should be allowed to bear children. And it may become possible to develop and implement techniques aimed at altering the DNA in the chromosomes passed on through inheritance, thus potentially eliminating some disease-causing genes from the gene pool, at least for several generations.

The second issue concerns the age-old free-will versus determinism and nature versus nurture debates. A vastly increased understanding of the relations between genes and behavior will bring these debates to the fore, with social implications for education, therapeutic intervention, and legal adjudications. Distinctions between normal and deviant behavior might be drawn, in part, along the lines of genetic polymorphisms. Just as with genetic diseases, some polymorphisms may promote an all-or-none phenotype with regard to a particular behavioral trait, and some may affect degrees of expression of a behavioral trait. Decisions may be made that certain behaviors are intolerable for society and, thus, that therapeutic intervention modifying the behavior will be mandatory. It will take purpose, resourcefulness, and soul-searching on the part of society's policy makers to find an ethical path through the thorny issues created by the notion that there might be identifiable genetic predispositions to certain behaviors.

We turn now to a brief listing of specific issues arising from the deciphering and use of biological information.

Screening. Who should get genetic tests? When is it advisable to screen the members of a family with genetic disease? When is it appropriate to use genetic screening for prenatal diagnostics? When is it appropriate to carry out population-wide genetic screening?

Privacy. Who should or will have access to genetic information beyond the patient and his or her physician? An insurance company or employer? A family or a future spouse? These are complex questions. It appears obvious at first glance that only an individual and his or her physician should know about one's genetic information. Yet this approach creates complications. For example, if the entire population knew who had good and bad genes but the insurance companies did not, would it not be possible for those with more bad genes to carry far more insurance than those with few bad genes, thus placing insurance companies at a disadvantage? Alternatively, suppose an individual knowingly chooses to work for a company with an environment unhealthy for him or her because of a defective gene. If the individual becomes sick, is the company responsible if it had no right to deny employment based on defective genes? This relates to the complex question of how responsible an individual is for his or her choices. Several bills addressing the issue of genetic privacy are now before Congress.

Counseling. How does one explain genetics and the probability of acquiring genetically transmitted diseases to the lay public? Where will the trained experts come from to handle the volume of potential future patients?

Physicians. How can one effectively train physicians about the complexities of human genetic disease and biological information? Physicians' education will have to change dramatically as we move to the preventive medicine of the twenty-first century; education will need to become more analytic and conceptual; physicians' ability to use computers will become critical; and training in how to educate and communicate with patients will become more important.

Abortion. As the 100,000 human genes are identified, it will be possible to screen in utero for increasing numbers of human genetic diseases. How can the boundary conditions for permissible therapeutic abortions be determined? Will wrongful life suits be permissible if a fetus with a genetic defect is not aborted? In some cases, most reasonable individuals could agree that abortion is not appropriate (e.g., to obtain the desired sex). In other cases, most reasonable individuals, apart from those with religious convictions against abortion, would agree that abortion is appropriate when a severe, untreatable disease is involved (e.g., Tay-Sachs disease is a rapidly progressive neurological disease that generally kills infants within their first few years of life). How can society set the boundary conditions between these extremes (assuming that abortion remains legal)?

Genetic engineering. Genetic engineering or gene therapy involves the replacement of defective genes by good ones. There are two types of genetic engineering: gene replacement in the cells of the body (somatic cell engineering) and gene replacement in the sex (sperm and egg) cells (germ cell engineering). Somatic cell engineering is in one sense simply an extension of contemporary medical therapies. Changes made in genes die with the individual. Limited somatic cell engineering has been carried out, but many technical problems remain to be solved.

Germ cell engineering modifies the human gene pool. These changes can alter human heredity. Germ cell genetic engineering is unlikely to be practiced (in humans) for a long while, if ever. First, enormous technical difficulties must be solved before it is safe in just the technical sense. Second, most interesting human traits (e.g., intelligence, emotional stability, and physical attractiveness) are complex multigenic traits that will probably not be completely understood in our lifetimes. Hence, they could not be engineered. There may come a time, however, when society could engineer human heredity to modify fundamentally human traits. Society will then have to determine whether this is appropriate and, if so, establish reasonable rules and guidelines for such changes.

Genes and behavior. Genes do appear to influence behavior. For example, genes appear to contribute to homosexuality[16] and thrill-seeking.[17] In 1995 a scientist at Johns Hopkins University created a strain of mice in which the gene that synthesized an important neural transmitter (the signal molecules brain cells use to communicate with one another) was destroyed.[18] Mutant male mice killed normal males they were caged with and brutally attacked females. The loss of this neural transmitter apparently caused the mice to become extremely violent. A similar observation has been made for humans. In 1993, a Dutch geneticist reported on a large family with eight males predisposed to extremely violent behavior (e.g., armed robberies, brutal assaults, rapes).[19] The violent males all had defects in a gene that breaks down a particular neural transmitter. None of the normal (nonviolent) family members tested had this defect. Accordingly, it does appear likely that genes may influence some aspects of human behavior. This poses an interesting challenge for our society and judicial system. Because our system of law is based on the ideas of free will and individual responsibility, could criminals in future plead extenuating circumstances because their genes made them commit criminal acts?

Forbidden science. Are some types of biological research considered so dangerous (e.g., connections between genes and behavior) or so socially inappropriate (such as, to some, the use of fetuses for investigation) that research into these areas should be banned? We would argue that the fundamental knowledge of how our genes and human development work is so important to dealing with some of humanity's most deadly and devastating diseases that few, if any, restrictions should be placed on fundamental research. Society should control how this knowledge is applied, not its acquisition.

SCIENTISTS AND SOCIETY

Never have the research opportunities been greater in the biological and medical sciences. And yet scientists face a skeptical general public. Surrounded by pollution, disease (cancer and AIDS), and poorly understood new technologies that appear to have a touch of science fiction to them (think of *Jurassic Park*), they may wonder whether science has really brought tangible benefits. People are vaguely aware of the ethical issues emerging from human genetics but often lack sufficient knowledge of this science to think rationally about them. We believe the fundamental contract between scientists and society has changed markedly, even in the past five to ten years. Scientists must reach out to society and educate the public about the opportunities (wonders) and benefits of science, as well as the ethical challenges.

When we founded the Department of Molecular Biotechnology at the University of Washington, one of us (Hood) had two objectives: (1) to create an interdisciplinary environment for developing and applying tools to study systems complexity in biology and medicine; and (2) to create an environment to encourage scientists to spend 5–10% of their time bringing science to society. The most effective way we have found to do this is to catalyze system change in K–12 schools in Seattle. One example is our elementary school program, funded by a $4.25-million grant from the National Science Foundation to bring hands-on, inquiry-based science through 100 hours of instruction to each of the 1,400 elementary teachers in the Seattle Public School District over the next five years. This educational program is a collaborative effort of the school district, Boeing Corporation, the Fred Hutchinson Cancer Research Center, and our department, together with nine other departments at the university. In addition, we are also teaching high school students and teachers how to sequence the human genome. Twenty schools are participating in an endeavor to sequence an unknown gene that causes deafness in a large Costa Rican family. Another exercise is to group students in fours and ask them to imagine that they are a family with Huntington disease. The students learn how to analyze the situation ethically and then have to decide whether they want to know if they (hypothetically) have the defective gene. The experience is a challenging and educational adventure. We hope that these students will realize that science is not about answers but rather about asking questions. We hope that they will be excited by challenges, curious about the world, and aware that learning is a lifelong commitment. As these children become adult citizens, they will be able to face the complexities of their changing world.

We would argue that scientists (and other academicians) should make a commitment to bring science (and the benefits of education) to the public. It is perhaps the only way we can make our case to society about the fundamental importance of science to our shared future. We can, at the same time, prepare tomorrow's citizens to appreciate and deal with the opportunities and challenges arising from the recent and exponentially increasing explosion in deciphering biological information.

NOTES

1. James D. Watson and Francis C. Crick, "Molecular Structure of Nucleic Acids: A Structure for Deoxyribose Nucleic Acids," *Nature* 171 (1953): 737–38.
2. John R. Riordan et al., "Identification of the Cystic Fibrosis Gene: Cloning and Characterization of Complementary DNA," *Science* 245 (1989): 1066–73.
3. Colette Dib et al., "A Comprehensive Genetic Map of the Human Genome Based on 5,264 Microsatellites," *Nature* 380 (1996): 152–54.
4. Tim W. Hunkapiller et al., "Large-Scale and Automated DNA Sequence Determination," *Science* 254 (1991): 59–67.
5. Nigel William, "Yeast Genome Sequence Ferments New Research" [News], *Science* 272 (1996): 481.
6. Robert D. Fleischmann et al., "Whole-Genome Random Sequencing and Assembly of Haemophilus Influenzae Rd," *Science* 269 (1995): 496–512; Claire M. Fraser et al., "The Mycoplasma Genitalium Genome Sequence Reveals a Minimal Gene Complement," *Science* 270 (1995): 397–403; Carol Bult et al., "Insights into the Origins of Cellular Life from the Complete Genome Sequence of the Methanogenic Archeon. *Methanoccoccus jannaschii*" (in press).
7. Stephen P. Fodor et al., "Light-Directed, Spatially Addressable Parallel Chemical Synthesis," *Science* 251 (1991): 767–73.
8. Michael W. Hunkapiller et al., "A Microchemical Facility for the Analysis and Synthesis of Genes and Proteins," *Nature* 310 (1984): 105–11.
9. Frank Eisenhaber, Bengt Persson, and Patrick Argos, "Protein Structure Prediction: Recognition of Primary, Secondary, and Tertiary Structural Features from Amino Acid Sequence," *Critical Reviews in Biochemistry and Molecular Biology* 30 (1995): 1–94.
10. Lee Rowen, B. F. Koop, and Leroy Hood, "The Complete 685 kilobase DNA Sequence of the Human Beta T-Cell Receptor Locus," *Science* 272 (1996): 1750–62.
11. Darwin J. Prockop and Kari I. Kivirikko, "Heritable Diseases of Collagen," *New England Journal of Medicine* 311 (1984): 376–86.
12. Neal G. Ranen et al., "Anticipation and Instability of IT-15 (CAG)n Repeats in Parent-Offspring Pairs with Huntington Disease," *American Journal of Human Genetics* 57 (1995): 593–602; E. Pintado et al., "Instability of the CGG Repeat at the FRAXA Locus and Variable Phenotype Expression in a Large Fragile X Pedigree," *Journal of Medical Genetics* 32 (1995): 907–8.
13. Mary-Claire King, Sarah Rowell, and Susan M. Love, "Inherited Breast and Ovarian Cancer: What Are the Risks? What Are the Choices?" *Journal of the American Medical Association* 269 (1993): 1975–80.
14. Oshio Miki et al., "A Strong Candidate for the Breast and Ovarian Cancer Susceptibility Gene BRCA1," *Science* 266 (1994): 66–71; S. V. Tavtigian et al., "The Complete BRCA2

Gene and Mutations in Chromosome 13q-Linked Kindreds," *Nature Genetics* 12 (1996): 333–37.

15. Marcia Barinaga, "Missing Alzheimer's Gene Found" [News], *Science* 269 (1995): 917–18.

16. Dean H. Hamer et al., "A Linkage Between DNA Markers on the X Chromosome and Male Sexual Orientation," *Science* 261 (1993): 321–27; Stella Hu et al., "Linkage Between Sexual Orientation and Chromosome Xq28 in Males But Not in Females," *Nature Genetics* 11 (1995): 248–56.

17. Richard P. Ebstein et al., "Dopamine D4 Receptor (D4DR) Exon III Polymorphism Associated with the Human Personality Trait of Novelty Seeking," *Nature Genetics* 12 (1996): 78–80; Jonathan Benjamin et al., "Population and Familial Association Between the D4 Dopamine Receptor Gene and Measure of Novelty Seeking," *Nature Genetics* 12 (1996): 81–84.

18. Olivier Cases et al., "Aggressive Behavior and Altered Amounts of Brain Serotonin and Norepinephrine in Mice Lacking MAOA," *Science* 268 (1995): 1763–66; Randy Nelson et al., "Behavioural Abnormalities in Male Mice Lacking Neuronal Nitric Oxide Synthase," *Nature* 378 (1995): 383–86.

19. H. G. Brunner et al., "X-Linked Borderline Mental Retardation with Prominent Behavioral Disturbance: Phenotype, Genetic Localization, and Evidence for Disturbed Monoamine Metabolism," *American Journal of Human Genetics* 52 (1993): 1032–39.

Chapter 2 Genetic Privacy: Emerging Concepts and Values

Anita L. Allen

The age of science and computers has given rise to the concept of genetic privacy. The term *genetic privacy* appears pervasively in discussions of the paramount ethical, legal, and social implications of genetics research and technology.[1] For example, a bioethicist has urged recognition of a moral right to "genetic privacy."[2] George Annas, Leonard H. Glantz, and Patricia A. Roche have drafted a "Genetic Privacy Act."[3] Members of the U.S. Senate and House of Representatives have introduced various "genetic privacy" bills into Congress. Health professionals have debated ethical guidelines for safeguarding "genetic privacy" in research, medicine, and counseling.[4] The popular press has also employed the term.[5]

Exactly what is genetic privacy? Why is it thought to be so important? Across the varied contexts in which it is found, "genetic privacy" carries no single meaning. It holds multiple meanings. The goal of this chapter is to identify and illuminate those meanings. First, I identify the most common emergent understandings of "genetic privacy." Toward this end, I distinguish the informational, decisional, physical, and proprietary dimensions of privacy evident in recent academic scholarship and public policy relating to genetics. Second, to illuminate the broad significance of genetic privacy, I identify ethical and legal values cited on behalf of genetic privacy protection.

Genetic science has already produced reliable techniques of prenatal diagnosis, paternity testing, and forensic identification. The highest hope for gene science is that its practical applications will someday dramatically improve the ability to prevent, predict, treat, and cure serious disease and disorders.[6] In some communities, the risk of harm from violent crime exceeds the risk of serious genetic illness. For this reason, a second paramount hope for gene science is that sophisticated forensic applications will deter crime, or bring about its just punishment, by making accurate identification of criminal offenders routine.[7]

Science inspires hope, but also fear.[8] Developments in gene science have prompted predictions that human beings increasingly will "play God," interfering with nature by genetically reengineering the natural world.[9] Although few people object to the goal of reducing the risk of early onset debilitating diseases, many object to genetic manipulation seemingly aimed at cleansing the human race of medically and socially imperfect people.[10] Gene science has led to fears that the future will be marked by eugenic intolerance.[11] Gene science has also led to fears that unsubstantiated claims for the genetic determination of human traits will lead to social attitudes and policies that discriminate against poor people and racial minorities.[12]

Another major fear prompted by human genetics is the fear of lost privacy.[13] Genetic science indeed augurs diminished privacy. In the wake of privacy losses come the potential for social stigma,[14] discrimination in employment,[15] barriers to health insurance,[16] and other problems. Novel applications of gene science could become pervasive before appropriate ethical and legal safeguards are in place to protect valued forms of privacy. Moreover, the splendid benefits of science could blind society to some of its social costs, lowering expectations of privacy below levels philosophers describe as just and ethical. The fate of privacy in our age of science is mainly, but not solely, a worry of elite ethicists, health care providers, and lawyers. Public awareness of genetic policy problems is limited, but opinion polls suggest that the general public views threats to privacy as significant issues.[17] Because of what Dorothy Nelkin calls the "social power" of information, personal privacy merits protection from employers, insurers, researchers, health care providers, schools, businesses, and government.[18] Just how much of what kinds of privacy merit protection and by whom are complex questions with controversial answers. Modern clinical medicine and research require that patients and human subjects yield personal information and a degree of control over their bodies and lives.[19] Nevertheless, consensual professional relationships merit safeguards against breaches of confidentiality and other privacy intrusions of the sort described below.[20]

THE FOUR DIMENSIONS OF GENETIC PRIVACY

The word *privacy* has a wide range of meanings.[21] It is used ambiguously in law and morals to describe and prescribe, denote and connote, praise and blame. "Genetic privacy" is no less rich with ambiguity than "privacy." Although the expression "genetic privacy" is a product of recent developments in science, it does not stand for a wholly new concept. "Genetic privacy" signifies applications of the familiar concept of privacy to genetic-related phenomena.

When used to label issues that arise in contemporary bioethics and public policy, "privacy" generally refers to one of four categories of concern. They are: (1) informational privacy concerns about access to personal information; (2) physical privacy concerns about access to persons and personal spaces; (3) decisional privacy concerns about governmental and other third-party interference with personal choices; and (4) proprietary privacy concerns about the appropriation and ownership of interests in human personality. "Genetic privacy" typically refers to one of these same four general categories.

"Genetic privacy" often denotes informational privacy, including the confidentiality, anonymity, or secrecy of the data that result from genetic testing and screening.[22] Substantial limits on third-party access to confidential, anonymous, or secret genetic information are requirements of respect for informational privacy. However, family members may possess moral rights to undisclosed genetic data that patients and the professionals who serve them legitimately withhold from other third parties.[23]

George Annas had informational privacy in mind when he warned that "control of and access to the information contained in an individual's genome gives others potential power over the personal life of the individual by providing a basis not only for counseling, but also for stigmatizing and discrimination."[24] Likewise, Alan Westin was thinking of informational privacy when he defined "genetic privacy" by reference to what he called the "core concept of privacy"—namely, "the claim of an individual to determine what information about himself or herself should be known by others."[25] Westin's definition captures well much of the informational dimension of genetic privacy and its connection to ideals of self-determination. Although it is adequate for purposes of a discussion of informational privacy, Westin's definition leaves important physical, decisional, and proprietary dimensions of genetic privacy in the shadows.

The genetic privacy concerns heard today range far beyond informational privacy to concerns about physical, decisional, and proprietary privacy. Briefly, issues of physical privacy underlie concerns about genetic testing, screening, or treatment without voluntary and informed consent. In the absence of consent, these practices constitute unwanted physical contact, compromising interests in bodily integrity and security. Decisional privacy concerns are heard in calls for autonomous decision making by individuals, couples, or families who use genetic services. A degree of choice with regard to genetic counseling, testing, and abortion are requirements of respect for decisional privacy. The fourth category of privacy concern, proprietary privacy, encompasses issues relating to the appropriation of individuals' possessory and economic interests in their genes and other putative bodily repositories of personality.[26]

Closer accounts of each of these four dimensions of genetic privacy—informational, decisional, physical, and proprietary—will follow an overview of the privacy values at play in American law and morals. The human genome contains many mysteries that await scientific discovery. The air of mystery that shrouds gene science often shrouds discourse about genetic privacy, too. Yet genetic privacy is only an expansive concept, not an unfathomable one.

PRIVACY IN LAW AND MORALS

Morality and Privacy

Privacy has emerged in bioethics and policy assessment as a yardstick against which to measure the adequacy of rules and practices. This is particularly true in domains related to health and medicine. Genetic privacy functions as a yardstick too. Privacy concerns figure prominently in public debates over whether and how we ought to collect, store, use, and share genetic information.

In spite of the pervasiveness of privacy concerns, bioethicists, lawyers, and policy makers continue to advance competing definitions of the meaning of privacy.[27] They also continue to advance competing theories of the moral and legal value of the many things they consider to be individual, group, and organizational privacy. The scholarly literature prescribing ideal definitions of privacy is extensive and inconclusive.[28] Proposed definitions of privacy range from "anything that offends decency" and "being let alone" to "control over information" and "restricted access to persons and personal information."[29]

Some definitions are more defensible than others.[30] Yet the time has probably come to recognize that the quest for an ideal, all-purpose philosophical or legal definition of privacy is futile. Rather than devoting attention to whether particular values and states should be labeled "privacy," we ought to shift resources fully to the task of deciding whether the values and states that are in fact labeled "privacy" warrant ethical or legal protection.

The prevailing viewpoint is that many forms of privacy indeed merit protection. Numerous theorists have undertaken to explain the value of the one or more forms of privacy that they believe warrant protection.[31] A few theorists depict privacy as denoting a basic human good whose value is intrinsic.[32] However, most theorists describe privacy as denoting conditions of life that are valued as a good or evil depending on whether they satisfy the extrinsic demands of, for example, moral respect for persons[33] or economic utility.[34] The idea that moral respect for persons demands broad protection for privacy appears in many of the most influential accounts of the value of privacy.[35] These accounts maintain that opportunities for physical, informational, decisional, and proprietary privacy promote two things. They promote, first, ideals of personhood, consisting of rational, self-determining, morally autonomous individuals.[36] Second, they promote ideals of human relationships, consisting of intimate association, complementing appropriately confidential and anonymous ties.[37]

Theories that base the value of privacy on the importance of promoting individual personhood and relationships presuppose highly individualistic understandings of human flourishing. Yet communitarian and care-based understandings of human flourishing also entail privacy protection.[38] Men and women are embedded in social worlds replete with responsibilities for self and others. Without privacy for purposes of rest, reflection, experimentation, and independent action, individuals would be less fit for meeting their responsibilities as citizens and caretakers. A degree of privacy may be needed to facilitate the flourishing of self-determining, autonomous individuals; but a degree of privacy also seems necessary to facilitate the flourishing of responsible members of families and wider communities.[39] Legal rules of privacy can be viewed as shared understandings of the privacy needed to create and preserve social civility.[40]

Normative accounts of decisional privacy—less so informational, physical, and proprietary privacy—commonly stress political values. Some political accounts of the value of decisional privacy emphasize the importance within a liberal democracy of self-determination and individual autonomy respecting reproduction, sex, and health care. Others stress the importance of a limited and neutral government. Collective toleration of a wide range of popular and unpopular choices empowers individuals, thereby keeping in check potentially totalitarian government and tyrannical majorities.[41]

General theories and theoretical debates about the value of privacy can seem far removed from concrete concerns about genetic privacy. The privacy of genetic information has a tangible relation to affordable health care and jobs. In a society in which men and women are insecure in the conditions of health and self-respect, neither individualistic nor communitarian grand conceptions of human flourishing are immediately meaningful. A just government and fair-minded business, research, and health care entities would ideally cooperate to minimize the number of lives marked by dependency,[42] discrimination,[43] and stigma.[44]

The normative assessment of privacy has not always proceeded on the assumption that individuals' genetic privacy claims are equally coherent or legitimate. As to their coherence, decisional and proprietary privacy claims pose serious conceptual and jurisprudential challenges.[45] As to their legitimacy, it has been argued that absolute claims to genetic privacy are not defensible in light of the interests in public health, family disclosure, and rational insurance.[46] Leading feminists have voiced ambivalence about privacy as a regulative ideal in constitutional law.[47] Catharine MacKinnon and other feminist legal theorists argue that decisional privacy doctrines reinforce an ideal of lives free from government intervention, thereby legitimating community neglect of women, children, and the poor.[48] Still, bioethicists specializing in women's issues, including Alta Charo, Ruth Faden, Dorothy Roberts, and Karen Rothenberg, have tended to favor policies that treat women's decision making about abortion and prenatal testing as deeply and beneficially private.[49]

LEGAL PRINCIPLES AND VALUES

Privacy is not a merely local value.[50] The law of nearly every nation provides for a degree of physical, informational, and decisional privacy by limiting government access to homes, possessions, and persons.[51] Limiting government by limiting government access to people and personal information is a major function of the Constitution of the United States. Physical, proprietary, and informational privacy themes figure importantly in the Bill of Rights. Decisional privacy themes are the heart and soul of the Fourteenth Amendment privacy doctrines. Genetic privacy losses suffered at the hands of state and federal government potentially run afoul of constitutional norms.

Privacy protection has a long and complex history in the United States.[52] The original Constitution fostered privacy values but without mentioning the word *privacy*. The First Amendment provides that "Congress shall make no law . . . abridging the freedom of speech . . . or the right of the people peaceably to assemble." The Supreme Court has held that this provision guarantees a right of free association for individuals and a right of privacy for groups. Individuals may form exclusive political, social, or civic groups whose meeting places and membership lists are beyond the reach of state and federal government. The "inviolability of privacy in group association may in many circumstances be indispensable to the preservation of freedom of association."[53] Restricted access to meeting places is the demand of physical privacy; restricted access to membership lists, the demand of informational privacy.

According to the eighteenth-century thinker James Otis: "A man's house is his castle; and while he is quiet, he is as well guarded as a prince in his castle."[54] This conception of the physical privacy of the home is reflected in the Third Amendment's strictures on access to private houses: "No Soldier shall, in time of peace be quartered in any house, without the consent of the Owner, nor in time of war, but in a manner to be prescribed by law." The Third Amendment appears in the Constitution as a direct result of England's refusal in the eighteenth-century to treat American colonists' homes as unbreachable safe-havens, for in 1774, Parliament enacted the Quartering Act, authorizing the housing of British soldiers anywhere in the American colonies, including private dwellings. The Third Amendment therefore "carved out a sharp distinction between public and private . . . [and] symbolized an emergent sense of privacy among the Revolutionary generation."[55]

The privacy norms that motivated the Third Amendment are highly consonant with the privacy norms behind the Fourth Amendment. Also carving out a sphere of physical household privacy, the Fourth Amendment asserts that "the right of the people to be secure in their persons, houses, papers, and effects, against unreasonable searches and seizures, shall not be violated, and no Warrants shall issue, but upon probable cause, supported by Oath or affirmation, and particularly describing the place to be searched, and the persons or things to be seized." Fourth Amendment cases have ascribed to individuals a right to a "reasonable expectation of privacy."[56] To fall under the protection of the Fourth Amendment's limit on search and seizure, "a person must . . . exhibit . . . an actual (subjective) expectation of privacy and . . . the expectation

[must] be one that society is prepared to recognize as 'reasonable.'"[57] Traditionally private areas, such as homes and public restrooms, are not the only places with respect to which a person has a reasonable expectation of privacy. Activity in public places or publicly accessible places may be protected by the Fourth Amendment's strictures on search and seizure if a person has justifiably relied on his or her sense of privacy.

The Fifth Amendment restricts access to personal information by limiting the government's power to compel persons to provide evidence against themselves that would lead to their prosecution in a criminal proceeding: "nor shall any person . . . be compelled in any criminal case to be a witness against himself." The Fifth Amendment privilege "respects a private inner sanctum of individual feeling and thought and proscribes state intrusion to extract self-condemnation."[58] Speaking the truth is not inherently demeaning. However, human personality arguably is compromised by compulsory self-disclosure: "personal dignity and integrity, both intimately tied to the ability to keep information about ourselves from others, are demeaned when the state is permitted to use tactics that make the unwilling incriminate themselves."[59] Also compromised are the nontotalitarian ambitions of liberal democratic society. The amendment "enables the citizen to create a zone of privacy which government may not force him to surrender to his detriment."[60]

Surveillance technologies developed in the early twentieth century empowered police and federal authorities to detect criminal wrongdoing with greater ease. At the same time, wiretapping and sensory-enhancing technologies created a new level of constitutional concern about government invasion of physical and informational privacy. In a 1928 wiretapping case, Supreme Court Justice Louis Brandeis declared in dissent that "discovery and invention have made it possible for the Government, by means far more effective than the rack, to obtain disclosure in court of what is whispered in the closet."[61]

It was not until 1965 that the Supreme Court expressly recognized a constitutional right of privacy. In the landmark decision Griswold v. Connecticut, the Supreme Court ruled that the Bill of Rights entails a broad right to privacy that prohibited states from criminalizing an individual's decision to use contraception.[62] Citing the Fourteenth Amendment, Roe v. Wade held in 1973 that the right to privacy prohibits blanket criminalization of abortion.[63] An important 1977 case, Whalen v. Roe, upheld a New York law requiring that pharmacists report to the state the names of persons purchasing certain prescription drugs.[64] Recognizing the distinct informational, physical, and decisional dimensions of privacy, the Court distinguished the "interest in avoiding disclosure of personal matters" from the "interest in independence in making certain kinds of important decisions."[65] The Court affirmed that both interests are protected by the Constitution but concluded that the state's confidentiality safeguards rendered New York's data-collection requirements constitutional.

Decades before the Supreme Court explicitly recognized an express constitutional right to privacy, state courts recognized a common law privacy right. In addition, the earliest state privacy-protection statutes preceded congressional privacy-protection legislation by more than 50 years.

The word *privacy* scarcely existed in the law before 1890, when new technologies contributed to an explosion of interest in privacy among intellectuals and lawyers.[66] Genetic technologies are not the first technologies to spark concerns about the demise of personal privacy. Nineteenth-century printing and photographic innovations generated passionate concern that privacy would be lost in a world of unchecked curiosity, gossip, and publicity.

In 1890, magazine editor E. L. Godkin decried mass printing and photographic techniques employed by "a particular class of newspapers."[67] He wrote that "personal dignity is the fine flower of civilization, and the more of it there is in a community the better off the community is."[68] Godkin characterized informational and physical privacy as a moral right:

> The right to decide how much knowledge of [a man's] personal thought and feeling, and how much knowledge, therefore, of his tastes, and habits, of his own private doings and affairs, and those of his family living under his roof, the public at large shall have, is as much one of his natural rights as his right to decide how he shall eat and drink, what he shall wear, and in what manner he shall pass his leisure hours.[69]

Also in 1890, lawyers Samuel Warren and Louis Brandeis published an influential law review article arguing for the creation of a new legal right "to be let alone," the right of privacy.[70] Warren and Brandeis warned of the coarsening effects of "recent inventions and business methods" on "inviolate personality." Humankind's spiritual nature was at stake,[71] since:

> The intensity and complexity of life, attendant upon advancing civilization, have rendered necessary some retreat from the world, and man, under the refining influence of culture, has become more sensitive to publicity, so that solitude and privacy have become more essential to the individual; but modern enterprise and invention have, through invasions upon his privacy, subjected him to mental pain and distress, far greater than could be inflicted by mere bodily injury.[72]

In 1903, the New York legislature enacted a proprietary privacy statute, creating, for the first time, civil liability for commercial appropriation of a person's name, portrait, or picture.[73] In 1905, the Supreme Court of Georgia became the first state court to recognize a common law right to privacy.[74] Within a few decades after the publication of Warren and Brandeis's article, "privacy" and "the right to privacy" had become solid fixtures of the legal lexicon.

By 1960, the legacy of Warren and Brandeis included the scholarly and judicial recognition of four common law privacy torts, collectively referred to as "the right to privacy." In 1960, William Prosser asserted in an article that state courts were imposing civil liability for: (1) intrusion upon the plaintiff's seclusion or solitude, or into his or her private affairs; (2) public disclosure of embarrassing private facts about the plaintiff; (3) publicity that places the plaintiff in a false light in the public eye; and (4) appropriation, for the defendant's advantage, of the plaintiff's name or likeness.[75] Virtually all state courts currently recognize some or all of these invasion of privacy torts.[76] In theory, the privacy torts offer legal protection for interests in good reputation, as well as in physical, informational, and proprietary privacy.

Further developments in surveillance technologies, together with computer information technologies, spawned a fresh round of privacy concerns in the 1960s and 1970s. Milton Konvitz and Alan Westin offered early assessments of privacy as a philosophical concept with a place in the law. Citing the Bible, Konvitz identified privacy with the concealment of the true, transcendent self.[77] Writing on a more practical than spiritual plane, Westin analyzed how the privacy of individuals and entities functions to control information.[78]

Since the 1970s, a number of states have amended their constitutions to include right of privacy provisions. Moreover, state legislatures have enacted hundreds of privacy-related statutes.[79] Every state has statutes governing the confidentiality of medical records. A few have specific confidentiality laws governing access to information about HIV and AIDS. Generally, state statutes limit disclosure of information contained in school, adoption, tax, library, video rental, bank, and criminal records. Many states have statutes governing employer polygraph testing and government wiretapping. Although informational privacy is the object of most privacy-protection statutes, such statutes as Virginia's Natural Death Act protect interests in decisional privacy.[80]

The federal law includes both congressional statutes and agency regulations that govern privacy. Incidental privacy-protection provisions can be found in federal communications laws and in the tax code. Major federal legislation regulates physical and informational privacy. Examples include Title III of the Omnibus Crime Control and Safe Streets Act,[81] the Privacy Act,[82] the Freedom of Information Act,[83] the Family Educational Rights and Privacy Act,[84] the Right to Financial Privacy Act,[85] and the Electronic Communications Privacy Act.[86] Bills to create a comprehensive genetic privacy code have thus far failed. Americans still live without national medical privacy legislation, under which aspects of individuals' genetic privacy would presumably receive protection.

Most of the statutes denominated "privacy" statutes restrict access to people and personal information. A few restrict government interference with decision making. Some legislation denominated "privacy" legislation establishes qualitative standards for the collection, use, transfer, and storage of information.[87] Policy makers call these standards "fair information practices." Where privacy is conceived as a set of fair information practices, showing respect for privacy entails adhering to policies that grant the individual a degree of control over the quality and dissemination of acquirable personal information.

The federal Code of Fair Information Practices of 1973 exhorted data collectors to: (1) disclose the existence of record-keeping systems containing personal data about individuals; (2) grant the individuals about whom data are collected access to those records; (3) limit the nonconsensual use of data to the purposes for which they have been collected; (4) protect personal information from public exposure, unauthorized transfers, and abuse; and (5) take reasonable steps to verify and update information.[88] The federal Fair Credit Reporting Act of 1970 requires that credit agencies comply with some of these fair information practices.[89] Moreover, a number of fair information practices are statutorily mandated by the Privacy Act. The Privacy Act governs the accessibility of information contained in systems of federal government records.

INFORMATIONAL GENETIC PRIVACY

"Genetic privacy" can mean informational privacy. Genetic information includes facts discovered in the context of genetic testing, screening, sampling, and research. Genetic data are often considered "personal" because of what they may reveal about a person's health and family.

Genetic science and its applications challenge expectations of the confidentiality, secrecy, and anonymity of genetic information about individuals. They also challenge traditionally individualistic conceptions of fair information practices, the "right to know," and the "right not to know."[90] In the context of genetics, fairness and nonmaleficence to family members may require genetic self-education to determine personal or familial health risks. It also may require the patients or their health care providers to disclose information to third parties.[91]

Privacy and confidentiality are treated sometimes as distinct concepts and sometimes as synonyms. The same is true of both privacy and secrecy, and privacy and anonymity. Here I discuss the confidentiality, secrecy, and anonymity of genetic information under a general rubric of informational privacy. That each is a mechanism for limiting access to personal information might be thought to justify a common privacy rubric.[92]

CONFIDENTIALITY

The efficient delivery of adequate health services depends on the free exchange of information.[93] For this reason, one should presume that restrictions on ready access to genetic information have a cost. It is a special policy-making challenge to efficiently transfer vital information collected by researchers and clinicians to third parties who need it without utterly sacrificing personal interests in nondisclosure. It is also a special policy-making challenge to decide whose claims to need for genetic information should be respected. Should insurers' claims be respected if they plan to exclude from coverage persons or families at serious risk for costly genetic diseases? Should employers' if they plan to eliminate adequate insurance or employment opportunities? Should distant relatives' if medical science offers them no prevention or treatment options?

It is widely agreed as a general proposition that genetic information acquired in a medical or research context should be kept confidential.[94] To maintain "confidentiality" is to limit access to information to a community of authorized knowers, often a specific group of two or more persons in a professional or intimate relationship. Genetic information in which family members may have an urgent health interest poses special concerns. Comprehensive ethical guidelines for genetic medicine and services developed by Dorothy C. Wertz, John C. Fletcher, and Kare Berg recommend that the confidentiality of genetic information be maintained except when there is a high probability of serious harm to family members at genetic risk and the information could be used to avert this exact harm.[95]

Applying this principle would permit a provider to disclose information about early onset genetic breast disease to the adult children of a carrier, though not to a health insurer that might use the information to increase premiums or reduce or eliminate coverage. Some in the health law field maintain that insurers should not be permitted to ask individuals about their genetic traits, even under conditions of informed consent.[96]

Physicians and other health care providers generally maintain individual, written medical records concerning their patients. As a matter of both professional practice and state law, access to these records is usually limited. As genetic testing and screening become more commonplace, confidential patient records kept by physicians and hospitals are increasingly likely to contain sensitive genetic information. Proposed privacy and confidentiality guidelines for clinical genetics services include the guidelines that patient information and records should be maintained in secured, lockable locations and that computerized data be accessible only to authorized personnel.[97] Genetic privacy, and indeed all medical privacy, can be easily compromised by the transmittal of medical records by telephone, fax, and e-mail.[98] The use of postcards and return addresses can inadvertently reveal the occurrence of otherwise confidential genetic testing.[99]

SECRECY

An undiscovered scientific truth is a kind of secret.[100] One can thus refer to the "secrets" of the human genome that the Human Genome Project is expected to uncover.[101] But the secrecy of greatest ethical concern is the intentional concealment brought about by human agents. The intentional concealment of genetic facts is a way of protecting self-esteem and important relationships. Deliberate concealment is also a way of gaining advantage over others to their serious detriment. Although insurers and health care workers have access to a great deal of personal medical information, individuals are able to limit access to what they learn about themselves in the course of seeking professional medical services. Secrecy of this sort enables us to go about into the world with our reputations and dignity intact. But secrecy has moral limits. This is particularly true when it comes to intrafamilial secrecy.[102]

To illustrate the moral limits of secrecy, one commentator has described cases of selfish disregard for others and calculated maleficence, including a "hypothetical case of a man with a mild form of adrenoleukodystrophy [a disease inherited on the X chromosome that can lead to deteriorating brain function and childhood death] who wants the fact kept secret. . . . Years after he is diagnosed, his two nieces both have children with severe forms of the disorder, leading to bitter resentment. In [a] . . . real example, . . . someone withheld details of their genetic disorder out of malice."[103] Genetic maleficence could also be cited by Richard Posner as an illustration of the major premise of his argument that personal privacy does not merit special protection because individuals use privacy to conceal adverse information about themselves and to gain advantages over others.[104]

Posner argues that people generally use privacy to conceal "bad" facts about themselves. The concealment of "bad" facts—including "bad" genes—gives a person potentially undesirable "market" advantages over those with whom he or she deals. In a related vein, Judith Andre's critique of privacy emphasizes the belief that accurate mutual knowledge is imperative for social relations. Andre concluded that "there is no right to privacy nor to control over it" since "a society without mutual knowledge would be impossible."[105] The point she made about society could perhaps be made about the family—that there is no right to privacy within a family because a family without mutual knowledge would be impossible.[106] Malicious secrecy poisons family and other social ties. Yet some privacy between fellow citizens and family members is surely called for. Patterns of selective intimate disclosure and nondisclosure are not obviously per se inimical to families or societies.

ANONYMITY

Anonymity joins confidentiality and secrecy as yet another kind of informational privacy. Anonymity is privacy in the well-recognized sense of restricted access to identifying information, such as a person's name or Social Security number. Wertz, Fletcher, and Berg maintain that anonymous testing or screening of genetic material for epidemiological purposes should not require informed consent.[107] The assumption behind this argument is that anonymity perfectly protects individuals' interests in informational privacy and freedom from discrimination and stigma.

Anonymity is not an ethical panacea, however. Anonymous testing and screening would raise physical and decisional privacy concerns were persons compelled to submit to needle pricks or cheek scrapings stored and used anonymously. In addition, ethical concerns are raised by research that uses anonymous genetic materials for unauthorized purposes. Ellen Wright Clayton has forcefully argued that limits on the use of anonymous genetic samples are called for by respect for the autonomy and values of human subjects.[108] One concern Clayton raises is whether techniques of eliminating identifiers are likely to result in true anonymity. A larger issue she raises has to do with the potentially exploitative character of unauthorized uses of persons' samples.

Individuals ought to know, in advance, about the uses to which their samples will be put. Advance knowledge affords them an opportunity to decline to provide samples for uses of which they strongly disapprove. Indeed, an African-American woman might strongly object to the use of her genetic samples in research about the alleged genetic bases of intelligence.[109]

FAIR INFORMATION PRACTICES

The terms *data protection*[110] and *fair information practices*[111] are used in a variety of contexts to refer to institutional practices designed to maintain the confidentiality, security, and accuracy of information collected and held for business, commercial, or governmental purposes. Proposed ethical guidelines require that individuals be given information regarding the length of time their biological samples are likely to be stored and future access to information derived from banked biological material.[112] Because the maintaining of accurate information is a fair information practice, policies may call for making what amounts to "hearsay" pedigree information accessible to third parties.[113]

Fair information practices protect interests in knowing and not knowing information held about individuals. These interests are sometimes referred to as "the right to know"[114] and "the right not to know."[115] A woman contemplating childbirth may have a right to know from her family members of serious genetically carried disorders from which her offspring might die in childhood. Persons with late-onset heritable health risks for which there is no real treatment or cure may have a "right not to know" their genotype and susceptibility. Knowledge of adverse genetic facts about oneself can lead to self-stigma and problematic self-identity.[116] Still, some ethicists advocate that "all clinically relevant information that may affect the health of an individual should be disclosed."[117] The argument for disclosure to patients can be frankly paternalistic: it enables the patient to engage in better-informed decision making.

Some ethicists conclude that only test results with a "direct relevance to health" need be disclosed. Although they advocate disclosure of all "clinically relevant" information, Wertz, Fletcher, and Berg assert that a genetic test that provides information regarding "nonpaternity, [and] fetal sex (in the absence of X-linked disorders) may be withheld if this appears necessary to protect a vulnerable party."[118] The involvement of vulnerable minors raises special issues of decisional and informational privacy. It seems ethically troubling, though, to withhold genetic information from adults on general grounds of "vulnerability." Suppose a woman with externally normal female sex characteristics experiences infertility and undergoes genetic testing that reveals the presence of the male chromosome. One might argue that in such cases the truth of her disorder could be concealed with justification in the interests of potential risks to emotional health. Yet it is arguable that she should be told about her condition simply because it is a clinical fact about herself and because she is an adult voluntarily using professional services to understand the causes of her inability to bear children.

PHYSICAL GENETIC PRIVACY

The human body, like information, is an object of privacy. Physical senses of privacy are among the paradigmatic ones.[119] The term *privacy* commonly denotes conditions of physical separation, bodily integrity, seclusion, solitude, intimacy, isolation, or confinement.[120] *Genetic privacy* frequently means informational genetic privacy—confidentiality, secrecy, anonymity, and fair information practices. In this section, I point to instances in which the genetic privacy at issue is a physical form of privacy.

Physical contact with others should be consensual. This is a principle of both morality and law. American law cloaks the human body in a protective shield, by ascribing rights and remedies that recognize the profound personal interest in bodily integrity and collateral peace of mind. The general rule within legal doctrine is that, in the absence of consent, intentionally harmful or offensive physical contact with another is tortious battery; uninvited entry onto another's property is trespass; and intrusion into anothers' seclusion, especially by searching, prying, or remote surveillance, is an invasion of privacy.

Much of the current concern about genetic privacy relates to the provision of health services. Health care presupposes close physical contact between patient and provider. In order for medical contacts to pass legal muster, informed consent is required.[121] Our bodily integrity and security are compromised when an unwanted procedure is thrust upon us. Procedures that sustain our lives against our wills, test us for substance abuse, or screen us for a disease may be defensible health care strategies, and yet they amount to unethical means to an end.

In the context of genetics, physical privacy is plainly at issue in relation to population screening or the testing of adults without informed consent. Physically assaultive care should be strenuously avoided. These principles are behind the general ethical guideline proposed by Wertz, Fletcher, and Berg that "all genetics services, including screening, counseling, and testing, should be voluntary, with the exception of screening newborns for conditions for which early and available treatment would benefit the newborn."[122]

In the literature on genetic privacy, moral and legal concerns about physical privacy take a back seat to concerns about informational and decisional privacy. The reason for this is simple. Genetic testing and screening can be painlessly performed on blood or other cell samples acquired for other consensual purposes or, failing that, by means of virtually painless clinical procedures, such as needle pricks and cheek scrapes. Rather than focusing on the bare fact that persons subjected to mandatory testing or screening are compelled to present themselves for a medical procedure on their bodies, commentators tend to focus on the social and economic consequences of testing and screening. How will the patient view himself or herself after testing? Who will have access to the genetic information, profiles, and samples obtained? What consequences will ensue if the patient's employers and health insurers have access to genetic information? Who will participate in the important decisions that he or she might make as a result of testing?

In sum, the key difficulty ethicists have had with mass population screening is not the physical invasions but, rather, the harms that may flow from invasions. Ethicists weigh the potential harm to the health and economic interests of third parties in light of the potential for stigma and discrimination that obtains in the wake of lost physical privacy.

DECISIONAL GENETIC PRIVACY

The proliferation of genetics services has entailed the proliferation of genetic choices. Many choices must be made related to genetics services. Choices about "counseling, screening, testing, contraception, assisted procreation, and abortion following prenatal diagnosis" are among those that must be made and that many argue should be "available on a voluntary basis and should be respected."[123] The freedom to make decisions about health, reproduction, and family life autonomously, free of unwanted governmental or other third-party interference, is often referred to as privacy. This decisional brand of privacy is a major component of what some authors have meant by genetic privacy.

The expression *privacy* is used in current constitutional law to refer to the autonomous or nongovernmental decision making protected by the Fourteenth Amendment's guarantee of liberty. This kind of privacy has been recognized in cases relating to abortion and the "right to die."[124] Some philosophers object to the decisional usage of privacy, preferring to reserve the term for its paradigmatic informational and physical uses. In this vein, Ruth Gavison's restricted access definition of privacy invasions includes "such 'typical' invasions of privacy as the collection, storage, and computerization of information; the dissemination of information about individuals; peeping, following, watching, and photographing individuals; intruding or entering 'private' places; eavesdropping, wiretapping, reading of letters, drawing attention to individuals, required testing of individuals; and forced disclosure of information."[125] Her definition intentionally excludes such "decisional" privacy invasions as "prohibitions on conduct such as abortions, use of contraceptives and unnatural sexual intercourse . . . [and] regulation of the way family obligations should be discharged."[126]

Gavison maintains that a lack of rigor and clarity is the inevitable consequence of using "privacy" as a shorthand for the concept of liberty or freedom from outside interference with private choice. She doubts that it would be possible to give a philosophic account of the concept that distinguishes privacy from the concepts of liberty, freedom, and autonomy, if privacy were allowed a decisional rendering. In spite of criticisms like Gavison's, the idea of decisional privacy has taken hold in ordinary language, bioethics, constitutional theory, and law.

Decisional privacy concerns relating to autonomous decision making and limited government loom large in connection with mandatory genetic testing and screening. Mandatory testing and screening also raise concerns of physical privacy. Handing over our bodies or samples taken from our bodies compromises the desire for physical seclusion and bodily integrity. But mandatory genetic testing and screening also violate conceptions of decisional privacy. These place the decision to test or screen in the hands of government or other third-party decision makers, even though the impact of the decisions is most felt by individuals and their families. Some have argued that screening programs are just only when voluntary testing cannot adequately prevent serious harm to vulnerable people.

American constitutional law defines the decision whether to procreate as legally private. The right to the decisional privacy of abortion has been entrusted to women, nearly absolutely in the early stages of pregnancy.[127] The rationale is both to respect women's physical privacy and bodily integrity for their own sake and to recognize the reality that women are the first and primary caretakers of children. Arguably, decisional privacy with respect to the decision to abort a fetus with serious disabilities or risk of disorders appropriately belongs to individual pregnant women because women in our society have a special position as caregivers for children with disabilities.[128]

In spite of women's special interest in control over the fate of potential offspring, there are serious arguments against enabling pregnant women to select medical procedures for sex selection.[129] Yet the notion of a positive right to subsidized choice, never endorsed by the Supreme Court, is advanced as necessary to make genetic privacy meaningful.[130] Choice, some argue, is more than the absence of coercion. It includes the positive right to affordable genetic services, safe abortions, and medically indicated care for children with disabilities.[131]

PROPRIETARY GENETIC PRIVACY

According to legal doctrine, to appropriate a person's name or likeness is a way of invading his or her privacy.[132] Privacy, it appears, has something to do with controlling one's identity. Leading nineteenth-century defenses of moral and legal rights of privacy equated the protection of privacy with protecting "inviolate personality" and humankind's supposed "spiritual" nature.[133] These understandings forged links between privacy norms and the human essence that have yet to be entirely severed.

The question whether our genes comprise our identities is a difficult one.[134] Proprietary genetic privacy is suggested by the idea that the human DNA is a repository of valuable human personality.[135] Proprietary genetic privacy is further suggested by the related notion that human DNA is owned by the persons from whom it is taken, as a species of private property.[136]

If DNA is the human essence—that is, the thing that makes individuals special and perhaps unique—it arguably ought to belong to the individual from whom it was ultimately derived. If DNA "belongs" to individual sources, it might belong to them exclusively and inalienably. Or DNA could qualify as alienable property that others can acquire both lawfully through voluntary private transactions and wrongfully through nonconsensual appropriation. Linking human essence with DNA invests DNA with importance. But there are dangers. If human essence is equated with genotype, low self-esteem and self-stigma might easily result from an individual's learning of his or her imperfect, mutated genes.

Notwithstanding its apparent dangers, the idea that genetic materials are valuable repositories of human personality has enjoyed wide appeal as both literal and metaphorical truth. George Annas trades on the "repository of personality" idea when he likens our DNA molecules to future diaries.[137] The intentionally oxymoronic "future diary" metaphor has the potential for confusion. As Caroline Whitbeck has observed, the metaphor perpetuates confusion of genotype with phenotype.[138] People do not record their phenotypes in their diaries; they record their socially mediated experiences. I would add that keeping a diary is a voluntary, even artistic social practice. A process of creative selection decides what goes in and what does not. We control what goes into our diaries and may choose not to include narratives of our health and illness. By contrast, we do not control—write—what goes into our genetic makeups. A person's future medical history is not a self-selected, self-initiated narrative. For these reasons our genes are inaptly likened to coded passages of a future diary.

Proprietary privacy issues are frequently raised in discussions of rights respecting stored tissue samples and information gleaned from families with genetic disorders. The proposed Genetic Privacy and Nondiscrimination Act of 1995 would have created rights of confidentiality, but without assigning ownership of genetic information or DNA samples to anyone. The proposed Genetic Privacy Act expressly places ownership of DNA in the person from whom samples are derived. Principles established by the American Society of Human Genetics' Ad Hoc Committee on DNA Technology assign ownership and "property" of DNA deposited in a data bank to the depositor or donor. The proprietary interest in deposited DNA is protected under ASHG principles by traditional rules of medical confidentiality.[139]

There are at least two reasons to invest ownership in DNA to the sample source. One is to protect expectations. It has been argued that "a reasonably prudent person positioned as a potential supplier of a tissue sample for a study involving DNA banking would tend to think, in our judgment, that at least to some degree he or she would continue to 'own' the blood sample or other tissue sample being solicited by a genetics investigator, even after the tissue was stored in the investigator's laboratory."[140] A second reason is to indicate that there are limits on exploitative appropriation.

Yet "it could be argued that the human genome is our common heritage and collective property; genetic information is, therefore, in the public domain."[141] Placing genetic information in the public domain may avoid the need to confront limits on the sale of cells, cell lines, tissues, and fetuses. If genetic materials are owned privately, one might also think that they can be bought and sold. And if genetic materials may be sold, it might seem to follow that cells and cell lines can be sold; if cells and cell lines can be sold, what of aborted fetuses and undiseased organs?

CONCLUSION

Genetic privacy is a new concept of broad application. Its roots extend deeply into law and morals. Just what is genetic privacy? The answer I have offered is descriptive. Indeed, my central aim has been to describe current patterns of linguistic usage rather than to dictate definitions and values.

Mirroring the semantic dimensions of "privacy," "genetic privacy" has emergent informational, physical, decisional, and proprietary dimensions. The confidentiality, secrecy, and anonymity of genetic information are major privacy concerns addressed in pending legislation, policy guidelines, and codes of professional ethics. The physical, decisional, and proprietary aspects of genetic privacy receive less attention than its informational aspects. But judging by wide-ranging topics addressed in the scholarly and professional literature, the regulation of all four modes of privacy is of special interest.

Genetic science and technology have spawned ethical, legal, and social concerns that penetrate every corner of the present-day conceptual domain of privacy. Language is malleable; language changes. In time, "genetic privacy" may take on a broader, narrower, or different set of meanings than the emergent ones gathered here.

NOTES

1. The concept of genetic privacy is at play in many ethical discussions in which the words *genetic privacy* do not appear. See, e.g., Task Force on Genetic Testing, NIH-DOE Working Group on the Ethical, Legal, and Social Implications of Human Genome Research, "Interim Principles," 1996, 33, available at http://www.med.jhu.tfgtelsi.

2. Walther C. Zimmerli, "Who Has the Right to Know the Genetic Constitution of a Particular Person?" in Ruth F. Chadwick and Gregory Bock, eds., *Human Genetic Information: Science, Law, and Ethics* (Chichester: John Wiley and Sons, 1990), 93–102.

3. George J. Annas, Leonard H. Glantz, and Patricia A. Roche, *The Genetic Privacy Act and Commentary* (Boston: Boston University School of Public Health, 1995). See also George J. Annas, Leonard H. Glantz, and Patricia A. Roche, "Drafting the Genetic Privacy Act: Science, Policy and Practical Considerations," *Journal of Law, Medicine, and Ethics* 23 (1995): 360–66. Cf. Neil A. Holtzman, "The Attempt to Pass the Genetic Privacy Act in Maryland," *Journal of Law, Medicine, and Ethics* 23 (1995): 367–70.

4. Cf. Dorothy C. Wertz et al., "Guidelines on Ethical Issues," in Dorothy C. Wertz, John C. Fletcher, and Kare Berg, *Guidelines on Ethical Issues in Medical Genetics and the Provision of Genetics Services* (Geneva: World Health Organization, 1995); Kare Berg,

"Medical Genetics: Practice of Medical Genetics," in Warren T. Reich, ed., *Encyclopedia of Bioethics,* rev. ed., 5 vols. (New York: Macmillan, 1995), 3:1646–52.

5. See, e.g., Stephen E. Bajardi, "Why We Need Genetic Privacy," *New York Times,* Oct. 16, 1992, A30, col. 4; David Brown, "Individual Genetic 'Privacy' Seen as Threatened," *Washington Post,* Oct. 20, 1991, A6.

6. Carol A. Tauer, "The Human Significance of the Genome Project," *Midwest Medical Ethics* 8, no. 1 (1992): 3–12.

7. Paul R. Billings, ed., *DNA on Trial: Genetic Identification and Criminal Justice* (Plainview, N.Y.: Cold Spring Harbor Laboratory, 1992); Dan L. Burk, "DNA ID Testing: Assessing the Threat to Privacy," *Toledo Law Review* 24 (1992): 87–102; JoAnn Marie Longobardi, "DNA Fingerprinting and the Need for a National Data Base," *Fordham Urban Law Journal* 17 (1989): 323–57.

8. Sandra Byrd Petersen, "Your Life as an Open Book: Has Technology Rendered Personal Privacy Obsolete?" *Federal Communications Law Journal* 48 (1995): 164.

9. Theodore Friedmann, "Opinion: The Human Genome Project—Some Implications of Extensive 'Reverse Genetic' Medicine," *American Journal of Human Genetics* 46 (1990): 407–14.

10. See, e.g., Dorothy C. Wertz and John C. Fletcher, "Fatal Knowledge? Prenatal Diagnosis and Sex Selection," *Hastings Center Report* 19 (May–June 1989): 21–27.

11. See George J. Annas, "Genetic Prophecy and Genetic Privacy: Can We Prevent the Dream from Becoming a Nightmare?" *American Journal of Public Health* 85 (1995): 1196–97; Neil A. Holtzman and Mark A. Rothstein, "Eugenics and Genetic Discrimination," *American Journal of Human Genetics* 50 (1992): 457–59; Curt S. Rush, "Genetic Screening, Eugenic Abortion, and Roe v. Wade: How Viable Is Roe's Viability Standard?" *Brooklyn Law Review* 50 (1983): 113.

12. NIH-DOE Joint Working Group on the Ethical, Legal, and Social Implications of Human Genome Research, "Statement on *The Bell Curve*" (unpublished MS, 1995).

13. Lori B. Andrews et al., eds., *Assessing Genetic Risks: Implications for Health and Social Policy* (Washington, D.C.: National Academy Press, 1994), 146–84, 247–89; George J. Annas, "Genetic Prophecy and Genetic Privacy," *Trial* (January 1996): 18–24; Thomas H. Murray, "Ethical Issues in Employment and Insurance," in Mark A. Rothstein, ed., *Legal and Ethical Issues Raised by the Human Genome Project* (Houston: Health Law and Policy Institute, 1991), 398–412; Thomas H. Murray, "The Human Genome Project and Genetic Testing: Ethical Implications," in *The Genome, Ethics, and the Law* (Washington, D.C.: American Association for the Advancement of Science, 1992), 49–78.

14. See Regina H. Kenen and Robert M. Schmidt, "Stigmatization of Carrier Status: Social Implications of Heterozygote Genetic Screening Programs," *American Journal of Public Health* 68 (1978): 1116–20.

15. See Joseph Kupfer, "The Ethics of Genetic Screening in the Workplace," *Business Ethics Quarterly* 3 (1993): 17–25; Marc Lappé, "Ethical Issues in Testing for Differential Sensitivity to Occupational Hazards," *Journal of Occupational Medicine* 25 (1983): 797–808; Gilbert Omenn, "Genetic Testing and Screening: Predictive and Workplace Testing," in *Encyclopedia of Bioethics,* 2:995–1000; David Orentlicher, "Genetic Screening by Employers," *Journal of the American Medical Association* 263 (1990): 1005; Mark A. Rothstein,

"Genetic Screening in Employment: Some Legal, Ethical, and Societal Issues," *International Journal of Bioethics* 1 (1990): 244.

16. Nancy E. Kass, "Insurance for the Insurers: The Use of Genetic Tests," *Hastings Center Report* 22 (November–December 1992): 6–11; Jennifer Landes, "Genetic Testing Thorny for Insurers: Privacy Issues vs. Value of New Information," *National Underwriter—Life and Health Insurance Edition,* Nov. 26, 1990, 3: J. A. Lowden, "Genetic Discrimination and Insurance Underwriting," *American Journal of Human Genetics* 51 (1992): 901–3; Harry Ostrer, "Insurance and Genetic Testing: Where Are We Now?" *American Journal of Human Genetics* 52 (1993): 565–77.

17. Alan F. Westin, "A Privacy Analysis," in Jack Ballantyne, George Sensabaugh, and Jan Witkowski, eds., *DNA Technology and Forensic Science* (Plainview, N.Y.: Cold Spring Harbor Laboratory Press, 1989), 25–36; Alan F. Westin, "Privacy and Genetic Information," in Mark S. Frankel and Albert H. Teich, eds., *The Genetic Frontier: Ethics, Law, and Policy* (Washington, D.C.: American Association for the Advancement of Science, 1994), 53–76.

18. Dorothy Nelkin, "The Social Power of Genetic Information," in Daniel J. Kevles and Leroy Hood, eds., *The Code of Codes: Scientific and Social Issues in the Human Genome Project* (Cambridge: Harvard University Press, 1992), 177–90.

19. Anita L. Allen, "Privacy in Health Care," in *Encyclopedia of Bioethics,* 4:2064–73.

20. Dorothy C. Wertz, "Medical Genetics: Ethical and Social Issues," in ibid., 3:1652–56.

21. See generally Anita L. Allen, "Defining Privacy," in Anita L. Allen, *Uneasy Access: Privacy for Women in a Free Society* (Totowa, N.J.: Rowman and Littlefield, 1988).

22. See David B. Resnik, "Genetic Privacy in Employment," *Public Affairs Quarterly* 7 (1993): 47–56; Task Force on Genetic Testing, *Interim Principles,* 33.

23. Task Force on Genetic Testing, *Interim Principles,* 34; Mary Pelias, "Duty to Disclose in Medical Genetics: A Legal Perspective," *American Journal of Medical Genetics* 39 (1991): 347–54; Mary Pelias, "The Duty to Disclose to Relatives in Medical Genetics: Response to Dr. Hecht," ibid. 42 (1992): 759–60.

24. George J. Annas, "Privacy Rules for DNA Databanks: Protecting Coded Future Diaries," *Journal of the American Medical Association* 270 (1993): 2346–50.

25. Westin, "Privacy and Genetic Information," 54.

26. See Lori B. Andrews, "My Body, My Property," *Hastings Center Report* 16 (1986): 728; Catherine Valerio Barrad, "Genetic Information and Property Theory," *Northwestern University Law Review* 87 (1993): 1037–86. Cf. Rebecca S. Eisenberg, "Patenting the Human Genome," *Emory Law Journal* 39 (1990): 721.

27. Allen, *Uneasy Access;* Allen, "Privacy in Health Care."

28. See numerous sources cited in Allen, "Privacy in Health Care," and Allen, *Uneasy Access,* chaps. 1, 2.

29. These characterizations of privacy derive from, respectively, James Fitzjames Stephen, *Liberty, Equality and Fraternity* (Cambridge: Harvard University Press, 1967 [orig. publ. 1873]), 18, 32, 60; Samuel Warren and Louis Brandeis, "The Right to Privacy," *Harvard Law Review* 4 (1890): 193–220; Alan F. Westin, *Privacy and Freedom* (New York: Atheneum, 1967), 18, 37, 39, 61, 68; and Ruth Gavison, "Privacy and the Limits of Law," *Yale Law Journal* 89 (1980): 421, 428, 438–39. A striking list of 16 varied proposed

definitions of privacy is included in Richard C. Turkington, George B. Trubow, and Anita L. Allen, *Privacy: Cases and Materials* (Houston: John Marshall, 1992), 60–62.

30. I attempt to defend a general purpose "restricted access" privacy definition in Allen, *Uneasy Access*, 11–30.

31. For varied accounts of values relating to the concept of privacy in some of its several dimensions, see Joel Feinberg, "Autonomy, Sovereignty and Privacy: Moral Ideals in the Constitution," *Notre Dame Law Review* 58 (1983): 445–90; Charles Fried, *An Anatomy of Values* (London: Oxford University Press, 1970); James Rachels, "Why Privacy Is Important," *Philosophy and Public Affairs* 4 (1975): 323–33; Julie Inness, *Privacy, Intimacy, and Isolation* (New York: Oxford University Press, 1992); Howard B. Radest, "The Public and Private: An American Fairy Tale," *Ethics* 89 (1979): 280–88; and Judith Thomson, "The Right to Privacy," *Philosophy and Public Affairs* 4 (1995): 295–314.

32. See Allen, *Uneasy Access*, 37–41, for a discussion of theories of this type and the concept of intrinsic value. Cf. Robert Post, "The Social Foundations of Privacy: Community and Self in the Common Law of Tort," *California Law Review* 77 (1989): 957.

33. Stanley I. Benn, *A Theory of Freedom* (Cambridge: Cambridge University Press, 1988), 292–93.

34. See Richard Posner, *The Economics of Justice* (Cambridge: Harvard University Press, 1981), 231–347.

35. See J. Roland Pennock and John W. Chapman, eds., *Privacy: Nomos XIII* (New York: Atherton Press, 1971); Ferdinand Schoeman, *Philosophical Dimensions of Privacy: An Anthology* (Cambridge: Cambridge University Press, 1984); and John Young, ed., *Privacy* (Chichester: John Wiley and Sons, 1978).

36. Edward J. Bloustein, "Privacy as an Aspect of Human Dignity: An Answer to Dean Prosser," *New York University Law Review* 39 (1967): 34. See also Bernd R. Beier, "Genetic Testing and the Right of Self-Determination: The Experience in the Federal Republic of Germany," *Hofstra Law Review* 16 (1988): 601.

37. Irwin Altman, "Privacy—A Conceptual Analysis," *Environment and Behavior* 8 (1976): 7, 8; C. Keith Boone, "Privacy and Community," *Social Theory and Practice* 9 (1983): 1, 6–24; Michael Sandel, *Democracy's Discontent* (Cambridge: Harvard University Press, 1996), 91–119.

38. Dorothy C. Wertz and John C. Fletcher, "Privacy and Disclosure in Medical Genetics Examined in an Ethics of Care," *Bioethics* 5 (1991): 212–32; Boone, "Privacy and Community."

39. See Allen, *Uneasy Access*, 47–52; cf. Boone, "Privacy and Community."

40. Post, "Social Foundations of Privacy."

41. See David A. J. Richards, *Toleration and the Constitution* (New York: Oxford University Press, 1986); Jed Rubenfeld, "The Right to Privacy," *Harvard Law Review* 102 (1989): 737–807.

42. Karen Lebacqz, "Genetic Privacy: No Deal for the Poor," *Dialog: A Journal of Theology* 33 (1994): 39–48.

43. See Paul R. Billings, "Genetics and Insurance Discrimination," in R. Steven Brown and Karen Marshall, eds., *Advances in Genetic Information: A Guide for State Policymakers* (Lexington, Ky.: Council of State Governments, 1992), 43–64; and Paul R. Billings et al.,

"Discrimination as a Consequence of Genetic Testing," *American Journal of Human Genetics* 50 (1992): 476–82. Also see Mark A. Rothstein, "Genetic Discrimination in Employment and the Americans with Disabilities Act," *Houston Law Review* 29 (1992): 23–84; Mark A. Rothstein, "Discrimination Based on Genetic Information," *Jurimetrics* 33 (1992): 13; and Mark A. Rothstein, "Genetics, Insurance, and the Ethics of Genetic Counseling," *Molecular Genetic Medicine* 3 (1993): 159–77. And see Lawrence O. Gostin, "Genetic Discrimination: The Use of Genetically Based Diagnostic and Prognostic Tests by Employers," *American Journal of Law and Medicine* 17 (1991): 109; and Lawrence O. Gostin et al., "Privacy and Security of Personal Information in a New Health Care System," *Journal of the American Medical Association* 270 (1993): 2487–93.

44. See Kenen and Schmidt, "Stigmatization of Carrier Status."

45. See Judith DeCew, "Defending the 'Private' in Constitutional Privacy," *Journal of Value Inquiry* 21 (1987): 171–84; Robert Dixon, "The Griswold Penumbra: Constitutional Charter for an Expanded Law of Privacy," *Michigan Law Review* 64 (1965): 197–231; John Hart Ely, "The Wages of Crying Wolf: A Comment on Roe v. Wade," *Yale Law Journal* 89 (1973): 920; and Louis Henkin, "Privacy and Autonomy," *Columbia Law Review* 74 (1974): 1410.

46. Lawrence O. Gostin, "Health Information Privacy," *Cornell Law Review* 80 (1995): 451; Wertz, Fletcher, and Berg, *Guidelines on Ethical Issues.*

47. See Elizabeth M. Schneider, "The Violence of Privacy," *Connecticut Law Review* 23 (1991): 973–98.

48. Catharine A. MacKinnon, *Feminism Unmodified: Discourses on Life and Law* (Cambridge: Harvard University Press, 1987), 96–102; Ruth Colker, "Feminism, Theology, and Abortion: Toward Love, Compassion and Wisdom," *California Law Review* 77 (1989): 1017–75; Ruth Colker, *Abortion and Dialogue* (Bloomington: Indiana University Press, 1992); Francis Olsen, "Unraveling Compromise," *Harvard Law Review* 103 (1989): 105–35.

49. Ruth R. Faden, Gail Geller, and Madison Powers, "AIDS, Women and the Next Generation," in Faden, Geller, and Powers, *Aids, Women, and the Next Generation: Towards a Morally Acceptable Public Policy for HIV Testing of Pregnant Women and Newborns* (New York: Oxford University Press, 1991); Sherrill Cohen and Nadine Taub, *Reproductive Law for the 1990s* (Clifton, N.J.: Humana, 1989).

50. Cross-cultural anthropological perspectives are advanced in Barrington Moore, *Privacy: Studies in Social and Cultural History* (New York: M. E. Sharpe, 1984). See discussions of international privacy policy norms in Dennis Campbell and Joy Fisher, *Data Transmission and Privacy* (Boston: M. Nijhoff, 1994).

51. Albert P. Blaustein and Gisbert H. Flanz, *Constitutions of the Countries of the World* (Dobbs Ferry, N.Y.: Oceana, 1994).

52. David H. Flaherty, *Privacy in Colonial New England* (Charlottesville: University Press of Virginia, 1972).

53. These are the words of Justice Harlan, writing for the majority in NAACP v. Alabama, 357 U.S. 449, 462 (1958).

54. Cited in L. Kinvin Wroth and Hiller B. Zobel, eds., *Legal Papers of John Adams*, vol. 2 (Cambridge: Belknap Press of Harvard University Press, 1965), 142.

55. Robert A. Gross, "Public and Private in the Third Amendment," *Valparaiso University Law Review* 26 (1991): 215, 220.
56. Katz v. United States, 389 U.S. 347, 351 (1967).
57. Ibid.
58. Couch v. United States, 409 U.S. 322, 327 (1973).
59. Mark Berger, "The Unprivileged Status of the Fifth Amendment Privilege," *American Criminal Law Review* 15 (1978): 191, 213.
60. Griswold v. Connecticut, 381 U.S. 479, 484 (1965).
61. Olmstead v. United States, 277 U.S. 438 (1928).
62. 381 U.S. 479, 484 (1965).
63. 410 U.S. 113 (1973).
64. 429 U.S. 589 (1977).
65. Ibid., 589–90.
66. But see Thomas M. Cooley, *A Treatise on the Law of Torts, or the Wrongs Which Arise Independent of Contract* (Chicago: Callaghan, 1880), 29.
67. E. L. Godkin, "The Rights of the Citizen, IV.—To His Own Reputation," *Scribner's Magazine* 8 (July 1890): 58, 65–66.
68. Ibid.
69. Ibid.
70. Warren and Brandeis, "Right to Privacy."
71. Ibid., 195, 211.
72. Ibid., 196.
73. N.Y. Civ. Rights Law, §§ 50–51 (McKinney 1992 and Supp. 1996).
74. Pavesich v. New England Life Ins. Co., 50 S.E. 68 (Ga. 1905).
75. William L. Prosser, "Privacy," *California Law Review* 48 (1960): 383, 422.
76. See *Restatement (Second) of Torts,* §§ 652B, C, D, E (St. Paul, Minn.: American Law Institute, 1977) (recognizing "intrusion upon seclusion," "appropriation of name or likeness," "publicity given to private life," and "publicity placing person in false light" as invasions of privacy).
77. Milton R. Konvitz, "Privacy and the Law: A Philosophical Prelude," *Law and Contemporary Problems* 31 (1966): 272.
78. Westin, *Privacy and Freedom.*
79. Robert E. Smith, *Compilation of State and Federal Privacy Laws* (Washington, D.C.: Privacy Journal, 1988).
80. Va. Code Ann. §§ 54.1–2981–91 (Michie 1995).
81. 18 U.S.C. §§ 2510–21 (1994).
82. 5 U.S.C. § 552a (1994).
83. 5 U.S.C. § 552 (1994).
84. 20 U.S.C. § 123g (1994); 34 C.F.R. Part 99 (1996).
85. 12 U.S.C. §§ 3401–22 (1994).
86. 18 U.S.C. § 2510(12) (1994).
87. C. Bennett, *Regulating Privacy: Data Protection and Public Policy in Europe and the United States* (Ithaca, N.Y.: Cornell University Press, 1992).
88. Government sources cited in G. Grossman, "Transborder Data Flow: Separating the

Privacy Interests of Individuals and Corporations," *Journal of International Business* 4 (1992): 1, 11.

89. 15 U.S.C. §§ 1681–81t (1994).

90. See Norman Fost, "Ethical Issues in Genetics," *Medical Genetics* 39 (1992): 79–89.

91. Robert Wachbroit and David Wasserman, "Patient Autonomy and Value-Neutrality in Nondirective Genetic Counseling," *Stanford Law and Policy Review* 6 (1995): 103; Leroy Walters, "Ethical Obligations of Genetic Counselors," in Diane M. Bartels, Bonnie S. LeRoy, and Arthur L. Caplan, eds., *Prescribing Our Future: Ethical Challenges in Genetic Counseling* (New York: de Gruyter, 1993), 131–47; Jon R. Walz and Carol R. Thigpen, "Genetic Screening and Counseling: The Legal and Ethical Issues," *Northwestern University Law Review* 68 (1973): 696; David D. Weaver et al., "Minimum Guidelines for the Delivery of Clinical Genetics Services," *American Journal of Human Genetics* 53 (1993): 287–89; Jeffrey M. Weinberg, "Breaking Bonds: Discrimination in the Genetics Revolution," *Journal of the American Medical Association* 268 (1992): 1767.

92. I argue as much in *Uneasy Access*, 18–25.

93. Cf. Gostin, "Health Information Privacy," 451.

94. See, e.g., Lori B. Andrews, *Medical Genetics: A Legal Frontier* (Chicago: American Bar Foundation, 1987), 187–220; George J. Annas, "Problems of Informed Consent and Confidentiality in Genetic Counseling," in Aubrey Milunsky and George J. Annas, eds., *Genetics and the Law* (New York: Plenum, 1976); Alexander M. Capron, "Autonomy, Confidentiality, and Quality Care in Genetic Counseling," in Alexander M. Capron and Marc Lappé, eds., *Genetic Counseling: Facts, Values and Norms* (New York: Alan R. Liss, 1979); P. Michael Conneally, "The Genome Project and Confidentiality in the Clinical Setting," in Rothstein, ed., *Legal and Ethical Issues,* 184–96; and Bartha M. Knoppers, "Confidentiality," *American Journal of Human Genetics* 49 (1991): 8.

95. Wertz, Fletcher, and Berg, *Guidelines on Ethical Issues,* 79.

96. Kathy L. Hudson et al., "Genetic Discrimination and Health Insurance: An Urgent Need for Reform," *Science* 270 (1995): 391–93.

97. Weaver et al., "Minimum Guidelines for Delivery of Clinical Genetics Services."

98. Wertz, Fletcher, and Berg, *Guidelines on Ethical Issues,* 46.

99. Ibid., 46.

100. For a general account of secrecy, defined as "intentional concealment," see Sissela Bok, *Secrets: On the Ethics of Concealment and Revelation* (New York: Random House, 1982).

101. See Gerry M. Doot, "The Secrets of the Genome Revealed: Threats to Genetic Privacy," *Wayne Law Review* 37 (1991): 1615–45; Elaine Draper, "Genetic Secrets: Social Issues of Medical Screening in a Genetic Age," *Hastings Center Report* 22 (July–August 1992): S15–18.

102. Segolene Ayme et al., "Diffusion of Information About Genetic Risk Within Families," *Neuromuscular Disorders* 3 (1993): 571–74.

103. Jeremy Webb, "Genetics Is a Family Affair," *New Scientist* 11 December 1993, 9.

104. Posner, *Economics of Justice.*

105. Judith Andre, "Privacy as a Value and as a Right," *Journal of Value Inquiry* 20 (1986): 309–17.

106. Cf. Lori B. Andrews, "Gen-Etiquette: Genetic Information, Family Relationships, and Adoption," Chapter 14 in this volume.

107. Wertz, Fletcher, and Berg, *Guidelines on Ethical Issues,* 75.

108. Ellen Wright Clayton, "Panel Comment: Why the Use of Anonymous Samples for Research Matters," *Journal of Law, Medicine and Ethics* 23 (1995): 375–381.

109. Clayton uses a similar example to illustrate her point.

110. Bennett, *Regulating Privacy,* 13.

111. Grossman, "Transborder Data Flow," 11.

112. R. F. Weir and J. R. Horton, "Genetic Research, Adolescents, and Informed Consent," *Theoretical Medicine* 16 (1995): 347–73; J. R. Yates, S. Malcolm, and A. P. Read, "Guidelines for DNA Banking: Report of the Clinical Genetics Society Working Party on DNA Banking," *Journal of Medical Genetics* 26 (1989): 245–50.

113. Wilson, "The Problem of Extended Information in Genetic Counseling," in Dennis A. Robbins and Allen R. Dyer, eds., *Ethical Dimensions of Clinical Medicine* (Springfield, Ill.: C. C. Thomas, 1981), 82–92.

114. Zimmerli, "Who Has the Right to Know?"

115. Rita Kielston and Hans-Martin Sass, "Right Not to Know or Duty to Know?" *Journal of Medicine and Philosophy* 17 (1992): 395–405.

116. See Jeffrey M. Weinberg, "Breaking Bonds in the Genetic Revolution," *Journal of the American Medical Association* 268 (1992): 1767; and Sonia M. Suter, "Whose Genes Are These Anyway? Familial Conflicts over Access to Genetic Information," *Michigan Law Review* 91 (1993): 1854–1908.

117. Wertz, Fletcher, and Berg, *Guidelines on Ethical Issues,* 79.

118. Ibid., 78.

119. Allen, *Uneasy Access,* chap. 1.

120. Ibid.

121. Mary Anne Bobinski, "Genetics and Reproductive Decision Making," in Thomas H. Murray, Mark A. Rothstein, and Robert F. Murray, Jr., eds., *The Human Genome Project and the Future of Health Care* (Indianapolis: Indiana University Press, 1996); Ellen Wright Clayton, "Informed Consent and Genetic Research," Chapter 7 in this volume; Madison Powers, "Privacy and the Control of Genetic Information," in Mark A. Frankel and Albert H. Teich, eds., *The Genetic Frontier: Ethics, Law, and Policy* (Washington, D.C.: American Association for the Advancement of Science, 1994), 77–100.

122. Wertz, Fletcher, and Berg, *Guidelines on Ethical Issues,* 35, 79.

123. Ibid., 79.

124. Cruzan v. Missouri Dep't of Health, 497 U.S. 261 (1990) (right to die); Roe v. Wade, 410 U.S. 113 (1973) (abortion).

125. Ruth Gavison, "Privacy and the Limits of Law," *Yale Law Journal* 89 (1980): 421, 428, 438–39.

126. Ibid., 438–39.

127. Planned Parenthood v. Casey, 505 U.S. 833 (1992); Roe v. Wade, 410 U.S. 113 (1973).

128. See R. Alta Charo and Karen H. Rothenberg, "The Good Mother: The Limits of Reproductive Accountability and Genetic Choice," in Karen H. Rothenberg and Eliz-

abeth M. Thomson, eds., *Women and Prenatal Testing: Facing the Challenge of Genetic Technology* (Columbus: Ohio State University Press, 1994), 105–30; and Patricia A. King, "Ethics and Reproductive Genetic Testing: The Need to Understand the Parent-Child Relationship," in ibid., 98–104.

129. See the discussion of sex selection in an international context in Wertz, Fletcher, and Berg, *Guidelines on Ethical Issues,* 57–60.

130. Rust v. Sullivan, 500 U.S. 173 (1991); Webster v. Reproductive Health Services, 492 U.S. 490 (1989); Harris v. McRae, 448 U.S. 297 (1980); Maher v. Roe, 432 U.S. 464 (1977).

131. See Wertz, Fletcher, and Berg, *Guidelines on Ethical Issues,* 79.

132. See *Restatement (Second) Torts,* §§ 652 B, C, D, and E. Section 652 B states that "one who appropriates to his own use or benefit the name or likeness of another is subject for liability for invasion of his privacy."

133. Warren and Brandeis, "Right to Privacy."

134. Dan W. Brock, "The Human Genome Project and Human Identity," *Houston Law Review* 29 (1992): 7–16; Howard L. Kaye, "Are We the Sum of Our Genes?" *Wilson Quarterly* 16 (1992): 77–84.

135. Suter, "Whose Genes Are These Anyway?"

136. See generally Robert F. Weir and Susan C. Lawrence, eds., *Genes and Human Self-Knowledge* (Iowa City: University of Iowa Press, 1994).

137. George J. Annas, "Privacy Rules for DNA Databanks: Protecting Coded Future Diaries," *Journal of the American Medical Association* 270 (1993): 2346–50.

138. Caroline Whitbeck, "Genetics, Scientism, and Self-Understanding" (unpublished paper on file with author).

139. Ad Hoc Committee on DNA Technology, American Society of Human Genetics, "DNA Banking and DNA Analysis: Points to Consider," *American Journal of Human Genetics* 42 (1988): 781–83.

140. Robert F. Weir and Jay R. Horton, "DNA Banking and Informed Consent" (unpublished paper on file with author).

141. Ibid.

Chapter 3 Genetic Exceptionalism and "Future Diaries": Is Genetic Information Different from Other Medical Information?

Thomas H. Murray

A few years ago, at a meeting to discuss the larger implications of the Human Genome Project, the head of the Federal Bureau of Investigation's laboratories leaned over to me and related this story. The FBI lab had conducted analyses of samples connected to the bombing of the World Trade Center in Manhattan. They had an envelope in which an incriminating document had been sent. With a technology known as PCR, polymerase chain reaction, they were able to amplify enough DNA from the back of the stamp to link it with one of the chief suspects through a genetic fingerprint. They also learned that someone else had licked the envelope itself.

In other words, if someone cares enough to go to the trouble, it is possible to get substantial information about a person's genetic makeup from the tiny bits of genetic material we scatter around us without much thought. The cells mixed in with our saliva and the bulbs at the base of the hairs we continuously shed are two widely distributed sources of raw material for creating genetic information about each of us.

Of course, at least some other medically relevant information about us is just as readily available. We may be pallid and cachectic, morbidly obese, rosy-cheeked, or missing limbs. We may be depressed or manic, delusional or paranoid, sharp as a tack or forgetful and confused. So the mere fact that people can learn things about us that are medically relevant would not seem to distinguish genetic data from other kinds of health-related information.

What, if anything, makes genetic information different from other health-related information? Can it, in concept and in practice, be singled out? Regardless of whether it really is different from medical information, are there characteristics of genetic information or of the society into which it will flow that should lead us to act *as if* it were different?

I was chair of the Task Force on Genetic Information and Insurance of the NIH-DOE Joint Working Group on the Ethical, Legal, and Social Implications of the Human Genome Project. The task force used the term *genetic exceptionalism* to mean roughly the claim that genetic information is sufficiently different from other kinds of health-related information that it deserves special protection or other exceptional measures. After many attempts to make the case for genetic exceptionalism, the task force abandoned the effort. At least for the purpose of deciding who should receive health care coverage, we concluded that genetic information did not differ substantially from other kinds of health-related information.[1] For many reasons, we were reluctant to reach this conclusion. Our expertise lay in genetics, our mandate came from the Human Genome Project, and the problem of genetics and health insurance, as big as it was, was nevertheless tiny compared to the prospect of trying to comprehend—much less change—the entire American health care system. I will explain why we abandoned genetic exceptionalism shortly. But first I want to explore why it is that so many thoughtful and knowledgeable commentators think it is important to treat genetic information as special.

In an article on genetic privacy, Lawrence Gostin predicts a move to longitudinal, electronic clinical records for each individual that would "contain all data relevant to the individual's health collected over a lifetime . . . continually expanded from prebirth to death, and accessible to a wide range of individuals and institutions."[2] George Annas, Leonard Glantz, and Patricia Roche, authors of a model Genetic Privacy Act, conclude a rousing defense of genetic exceptionalism with this claim: "To the extent that we accord special status to our genes and what they reveal, genetic information is uniquely powerful and uniquely personal, and thus merits unique privacy protection."[3] The model Genetic Privacy Act, like other legislation intended to protect against genetic discrimination, insists both that genetic information *can* be distinguished from other medical information and that it *ought* to be so distinguished. Just why is genetic information, in these authors' words, "uniquely powerful and uniquely personal"? Annas, Glantz, and Roche offer three reasons.

First, they liken a person's genetic profile to a "future diary" and claim that genetic information "can predict an individual's likely medical future for a variety of conditions." They go on to argue that we should think of DNA as a "coded probabilistic future diary because it describes an important part of a person's unique future and, as such, can affect and undermine an individual's view of his/her life's possibilities. Unlike ordinary diaries that are created by the writer, the information contained in one's DNA, which is stable and can be stored for long periods of time, is in code and is largely unknown to the person. Most of the code cannot now be broken, but parts are being deciphered almost daily."[4] Let us call this, borrowing a phrase from Nancy Wexler, the concern about genetic prophecy.

The second reason Annas, Glantz, and Roche cite for regarding genetic information as unique is that "it divulges personal information about one's parents, siblings, and children."[5] The biology of the claim is straightforward enough: we get half of our genes from each biological parent, and we pass half of ours on to each of our biological children. Genetic information about each of us, then, is also to some extent information about our ancestors, descendants, and other such biological relations as sisters and brothers. Call this the concern for kin.

As their third reason, the authors cite a history of genetics being used to stigmatize and victimize people. Whether they have in mind eugenics programs, ill-conceived genetic screening, or the use of genetic information by employers, insurers, or others, they do not say. Call this the concern about genetic discrimination.

Other authors have offered their own lists of reasons supporting genetic exceptionalism. Gostin, for example, offers these "compelling justifications" for protecting the privacy of genetic information: "the sheer breadth of information discoverable; the potential to unlock secrets that are currently unknown about the person; the unique quality of the information enabling certain identification of the individual; the stability of DNA rendering distant future applications possible; and the generalizability of the data to families, genetically related communities, and ethnic and racial populations."[6] The first two factors—breadth and the potential to unlock secrets—seem to be expansions of the concern about genetic prophecy. The last concern mentioned, the generalizability of the data, is an interesting expansion of the concern for kin. In

Gostin's view, the concern does not stop at the family's door but extends to those larger groupings of people who share a certain genetic heritage. I agree. A focus on genetics emphasizes racial and ethnic differences, a very sensitive matter both now and possibly in the future. Stressing the genetics of race has the potential to intensify those divisions, while reinforcing the view that perceived differences are not mere accidents of culture and circumstance but are grounded in biology, which is itself seen as somehow fundamental and unalterable. Looking toward the future, people might be concerned that genetic information about race and ethnicity could fall into the hands of groups or governments with hostile or totalitarian ambitions. The recent experience of ethnic conflict in Eastern Europe and Africa, as well as enduring racism in the United States, reinforces that concern.

Gostin's third and fourth factors—the "unique quality" that permits identification of the individual and the possible future uses of stable DNA—require some explanation. The "unique quality" is what enabled the FBI in the World Trade Center bombing case to confirm who licked the stamp and who licked the envelope. Gostin notes an interesting feature of genomic *sequence* information. Genetic fingerprinting operates by detecting differences in the DNA sequences of individuals in a number of regions of the genome known to be highly variable. If a database contained sufficient information about the sequence, even if the person's name were not attached to the file, it might be possible to identify the individual whose sequence it is, in a manner similar to the method of genetic fingerprinting. So, although the practice of removing identifying information is usually thought to confer anonymity by making the records impossible to trace to an individual, that may not be the case with records containing significant chunks of DNA sequence data. (Of course, this problem is not limited in principle to genomic information. It is not hard to conceive of databases that, while containing no names, still contain enough information—e.g., community, neighborhood, age, marital status, number and ages of children, occupation, make, model and year of cars—to allow individuals to be identified.)

It is also useful to distinguish between two types of genetic collections. One form is databases of genetic information that either exist in electronic form or are readily translatable into a computer-searchable database. Such databases might, in the future, include DNA sequence information about identifiable individuals; they are unlikely to do so now. Researchers and others are less interested in raw sequence than in variants of important genes—mutations and benign polymorphisms—or in short stretches of DNA that are useful for genetic fingerprinting. The other type is collections of tissue samples containing DNA. Each sample could yield, in principle, an entire sequence for each individual. Gostin asserts correctly that such tissue samples contain sufficient information to study any and all genes, as well as the DNA needed to do a genetic fingerprint, which could then be linked to the individual *if* his or her matching genetic fingerprint were on file. But it is crucial to understand that the information in such collections of genetic materials is opaque. Considerable work and expense are needed to get any of the latent information from a sample.[7] Gostin's worry about the durability of DNA is correct on the bare facts. In the World Trade Center bombing case, the FBI, after all, was able to take microscopic bits of DNA and identify two individuals. But without the motivation and resources required to analyze the DNA, we do not have genetic information per se, merely the raw materials from which genetic information could be derived. (But, then, we would not need a fancy tissue bank either. One of the most massive collections would be in the hands of the Publisher's Clearinghouse—all those stamps and envelopes, with return addresses yet!)

Are the arguments in favor of genetic exceptionalism persuasive? The strong form of genetic exceptionalism claims that genetic information is unique— "uniquely powerful and uniquely personal," as Annas, Glantz, and Roche have written. We could admit to hyperbole in that statement and look for a weaker form of genetic exceptionalism, one that claims that genetic information is sufficiently distinctive from other information that it ought to receive greater privacy protection. The policy question, after all, is the one we are most concerned with. Genetic information does not have to be unique in order to warrant special protection, but it does have to be distinctive and especially sensitive. In evaluating the arguments, we should consider the case that could be made if only the weaker form of genetic exceptionalism is supported.

The argument from genetic prophecy is not compelling. Genetic information is neither unique nor distinctive in its ability to offer probabilistic peeks into our future health. Many other things afford equally interesting predictions. Some of them would be impossible to conceal and so fall outside the concern of privacy—some people, for example, are avid skydivers or parasailers. Other types of information would be hidden, just like most genetic information; examples include asymptomatic hepatitis B infection, early HIV infection, and even one's cholesterol level. These have implications for future health that are every bit as cogent and sensitive as genetic predispositions.

Perhaps genetic risks ought to be treated differently because there are potentially so many of them, and such a massive prospective difference in quantity effectively makes a qualitative difference. Or perhaps what is most worrisome is that our genetic risks are occult, hidden; attributes that others could know even as we remain ignorant about them. Here lurks an image of genetic information as a mysterious, powerful, and inexorable force that will dominate and control our futures. Keep this image in mind. We will return to it.

The second argument for genetic exceptionalism is concern about kin—not merely our immediate family but perhaps also the larger ethnic community. Again, it is difficult to claim uniqueness, or even special importance and sensitivity, for genetic information. That one member of a family has tuberculosis is certainly relevant to the rest of the household, all of whom are in danger of infection, along with everyone who works with or goes to school with the infected individual. Likewise, if one partner in a marriage has a sexually transmitted disease, that information is important for the other partner. Or suppose the main wage earner in the household showed early signs of heart disease that could bring disability and death. Wouldn't the other family members have a profoundly important stake in knowing this? They might make very different career training or employment choices if they knew the breadwinner was likely to be struck down soon.

Although the concern for kin could amplify the sensitivity of genetic information, it does not render that information unique. It can be very important, to be sure, but whether genetic information is important and sensitive enough to distinguish it from other sorts of information is not yet clear.

The fear of discrimination is the third of the candidates for the unique character of genetic information. Here again, genetics is not alone. Institutions and individuals can and have used all sorts of information, both visible and occult, as the basis for discrimination. In underwriting for health insurance, for example, insurers use evidence of current disease or future disease risk— whether it is genetic or nongenetic doesn't matter—to decide who gets a policy, what that policy covers, and how much it costs. Whether this discrimination should be regarded as fair or unfair is debated. But it is difficult to make the argument that it is fair to discriminate on nongenetic factors but unfair to discriminate on genetic ones.

Some nongenetic factors, to be sure, can be thought of as a matter of choice, in contrast with one's genes. Such risky behaviors as smoking, thrill-seeking, and the like do seem different from being struck by Huntington disease, over which we have no control. But there are plenty of nongenetic risks that no more reflect genuine individual choice than genetic risks. If the air we breathe and the water we drink are polluted, if our parents or co-workers are heavy smokers, if we are reasonably prudent but injured in an accident nonetheless, it is hard to say that we bear any significant measure of responsibility for the resulting illnesses. Likewise, most links between genes and disease are likely to be very different from the link in Huntington disease. Most will be probabilistic associations rather than straightforward causal connections. And many may be modifiable by the individual's actions. No simple equation exists between genetic factors and inexorable fate, or nongenetic factors and being open to individual choice and action. If we are less inclined to worry about discrimination on the basis of health risk factors that are open to modification and individual choice, then let us recognize *that* as the relevant difference, and not confuse it with the distinction between genetic and nongenetic factors.

The concern for genetic information and discrimination may help explain some of the interest in genetic privacy because it broadens and sharpens important perceptions. First, it broadens the pool of possible factors that might be used to discriminate against an individual, and it likewise expands the pool of individuals who might become the subjects of discrimination. Second, it sharpens the widely held moral intuition that we should not be punished for things beyond our control. (This does not contradict the warning just stated about oversimplifying the connection between genes and illness. Health insurers, for example, work on probabilities. It might be enough that a woman has a mutated form of the breast cancer 1 gene [BRCA1], hence an approximately 85% lifetime risk of breast cancer, for an insurer to deny her coverage. Whose "fault" it might be is irrelevant.)

Perhaps what really frightens and galls us about discrimination on the basis of genetic information is its reliance on information about us over which we have no control and may not even know ourselves. Here again is the hidden and mysterious nature of genetic information, joined with its aura of power and ubiquity, lurking close beneath the surface of our discomfort. George Annas's metaphor of our genes as our future diary captures the power and ambiguity of the personal significance of genetic information.

Recall the description of an individual's genome as his or her "coded probabilistic future diary because it describes an important part of a person's unique future and, as such, can affect and undermine an individual's view of his/her life's possibilities. Unlike ordinary diaries that are created by the writer, the information contained in one's DNA . . . is in code and is largely unknown to the person."[8] The metaphor is ingenious, powerful, and provocative. What features of genetic information does it capture? What is the source of its power? Does it mislead in any way?

Diaries are intimate, private places where we confide what is most important about who we are, who and what we love, and what we do. Those same confidences are also just those things we may be most reluctant to broadcast. There may come a time when we choose to share what we have recorded in our diary, but we want to be able to say when and with whom we share it.

The future diary metaphor captures several sources of our uneasiness about genetic privacy. Our "genetic diary" was written not by us but by an agency completely outside our control. It can be read not only by others but without our permission or even knowledge. Last, it is possible for strangers, whose purposes are not ours, to use those genetic "secrets" to harm us. Little wonder that we want to protect whatever is written in that "diary."

But the metaphor also misleads. It implies that the contents of that future diary reflect what is most intimate, central, and important about us—that it reveals, in some fundamental way, our social and personal identity, our loves and interests, and our actions. In fact, our genomes have little or nothing to say about any of these crucial matters. The metaphor also promotes genetic determinism. In complex disorders with many contributing factors, such as many cancers and heart disease, genetic information may indicate only a rough range of probabilities, something that falls far short of a "probabilistic future."

So much for the case in favor of genetic exceptionalism. What about the case against it? When the Task Force on Genetic Information and Insurance rejected genetic exceptionalism, it did so with reluctance. At least for the purpose of deciding who should have access to health care coverage, the task force could find no sound way to distinguish genetic from nongenetic diseases and risks. Genetic exceptionalism depends on what we have come to call the "two-bucket theory" of disease. According to this model, there are two buckets—one labeled "genetic," the other labeled "nongenetic"—and we should be able to toss every disease and risk factor into one of the two.[9] So, Huntington disease goes into the "genetic" bucket and getting run over by a truck goes into the "non-genetic" one. But many diseases and risks don't fit neatly into either bucket. Take breast cancer. Some cases of breast cancer have strong genetic roots, but others have no clear genetic connection. For that matter, not every woman with a mutated BRCA1 gene will develop breast cancer. And some apparent risk factors have little or no link to genetics. Similar complexity exists for heart disease: cholesterol is a risk factor, and one's cholesterol level can be modified by diet, exercise, and other factors; but our genes have as much or more to do with the level of cholesterol circulating in our blood as our environment or behavior. Into which bucket, then, should we toss breast cancer? Heart disease? Cholesterol level?

On conceptual grounds, the task force agreed that the argument for distinguishing genetic from nongenetic information was dubious. Certainly, there were cases of relatively unambiguous and pure genetic or nongenetic diseases and risk factors. But in many more cases, including many of the most interesting and important ones, the two-bucket theory was hopelessly inadequate.

Efforts to legislate genetic privacy have confronted the two-bucket problem by confining themselves more or less to whatever fit neatly into the genetic bucket. Karen Rothenberg notes this in her study of state laws, which typically limit the definition of genetic information to the results of DNA testing.[10] The draft Genetic Privacy Act itself began with a conceptually rich, inclusive definition but moved to a much narrower one. This is how the act's authors describe the decision they faced: "either create a definition for genetic information that is consistent from the viewpoint of theory and principle, but not of much practical value, or design provisions that are capable of practical application that would have the effect of protecting the most private and potentially stigmatizing genetic information." Their definition reads: "The term *private genetic information* means any information about an identifiable individual that is derived from the presence, absence, alteration, or mutation of a gene or genes, or the presence or absence of a specific DNA marker or markers, and that has been obtained: (1) from an analysis of the individual's DNA; or (2) from an analysis of the DNA of a person to whom the individual is related."[11] They acknowledge that this definition leaves out biochemical tests for genes—potentially a massive gap, because what we will often be interested in clinically are the products of the genes, not the genes themselves. But they observe ruefully that amending the definition of private genetic information to include testing for gene products "makes the distinction between genetic information and medical information generally more difficult to justify."[12]

This conceptual problem has fed another difficulty with genetic exceptionalism: how to identify and keep separate genetic from nongenetic information in the medical record. If it could not be determined whether some piece of information belonged in one category or the other, it seemed practically infeasible to divide medical records into those portions that were genetic (hence off-limits), from those portions that were nongenetic (therefore available to prospective insurers). More recently, Lawrence Gostin argued that laws offering special protection to genetic information may be problematic because "different standards would apply to data held by the same entity" depending on whether it met the definition of genetic information; because "other health conditions raise similar sensitivity issues" such as HIV and mental illness; and because it could create enormous practical problems in record keeping and information flow.[13]

The task force had another reason for abandoning genetic exceptionalism: we concluded that there was no good moral justification for treating genetic information, genetic diseases, or genetic risk factors as categorically different from other medical information, diseases, or risk factors.[14] If someone genuinely needed health care, it did not matter whether one could find a genetic root for the disease or whether it was the product of nongenetic bad luck or accident. Some people regard so-called self-inflicted or lifestyle-related maladies as exceptions. The argument here turns on both moral and policy premises—roughly, that to the extent that people are responsible for their own misfortune, there is no moral obligation to share the cost of their care, and that the point of access to health insurance is the proper place to extract that cost or to inflict punishment. Whether everyone finds this position persuasive is, however, not the crucial point. Our need for health care in most cases will be the product of a complex mix of factors, genetic and nongenetic, both within the scope of our responsibility and outside of that scope. The distinction between genetic and nongenetic factors is not the crucial one. We are inclined to regard it as crucial only when we fall for the overselling of genetics—when we fall prey, that is, to genetic reductionism and genetic determinism.

Resounding statements about the significance of genetic information are not hard to find. Lawrence Gostin, for example, claims that "the features of a person revealed by genetic information are fixed—unchanging and unchangeable."[15] George Annas, Leonard Glantz, and Patricia Roche write: "To the extent that we accord special status to our genes and what they reveal, genetic information is uniquely powerful and uniquely personal, and thus merits unique privacy protection."[16]

Some scholars worry that the significance of genetics has been oversold. In their book *The DNA Mystique: The Gene as a Cultural Icon,* Dorothy Nelkin and Susan Lindee bemoan what they see as genetic hype:

As the science of genetics has moved from the laboratory to mass culture, from professional journals to the television screen, the gene has been transformed. Instead of a piece of hereditary information, it has become the key to human relationships and the basis of family cohesion. Instead of a string of purines and pyramidines, it has become the essence of identity and the source of social difference. Instead of an important molecule, it has become the secular equivalent of the human soul.[17]

Other scholars have voiced similar concerns. In a study of factors contributing to the social power of genetics, Eric Juengst identifies genetic determinism and genetic reductionism, along with their familial implications, as the sources of the anxiety caused by genetics. He notes that the link of genetics to disease in the public mind is defined by examples such as Huntington disease, in which having the mutated gene effectively determines the outcome: if one lives long enough, one will get the disease. "This history still affects the way many people think about genetic risk information, by leading them to assume that genetic diagnostics of any kind have more predictive power than other kinds of health risk assessments."[18] Juengst notes that images of crystal balls and "future diaries" bolster this deterministic image of genetic information. He also remarks that such images invite fatalism and social stigmatization. Because genetic risks encourage an explanation of disease in biological terms, they are open to reductionistic accounts of both diseases and persons. That is, genetic risks may come to be seen as *the* explanation for complex multifactorial diseases. They may also be seen as fundamental, defining characteristics of the persons who have such risks, essentially reducing those persons to their genetic propensities.

Carl F. Cranor considers the concept of causation in genetics and looks critically at both those who underemphasize and those who overemphasize the causal role of genes. He acknowledges the concerns of those worried about possible social misuses of genetic explanations but worries that those critics place too much importance on minimizing the *causal* significance of genes, when they should be criticizing the misuses they fear. Cranor urges us to "recognize that genes, for at least some single-gene diseases (even if rare), appear to make discernible causal contributions to some diseases, but to deny that this settles all questions concerning scientific understanding, recommendations about research agendas, and the important normative and practical issues as to how such diseases should be treated or 'engineered,' if at all."[19] That is, we do not have to pretend that genes are unimportant to avoid determinism or reductionism. We should give genes their due, but no more than that.

Evelyn Fox Keller points out the simplistic premises of genetic determinism: "The idea of 'a gene for X' already presupposes the existence of an organism capable of identifying, translating, interpreting, and making productive use of a particular gene." As she goes on to explain, "All biological functions are composite functions, involving the correct 'reading' of many genes. The more complex the function, the more genes are likely to be involved. What genetics can and often does enable us to do is to identify aberrations in some component part that lead to failure of the composite function—always, however, relative to the other components of that function and almost always relative to particular environmental conditions." Keller warns of the consequences of a too-hasty acceptance of genetic reductionism: "a far more radical depersonalization of medicine than that initiated by the earlier and more general march of medicine from art to science." This step would invite the effacement of not only the patient's environment and history but also the patient him or herself.[20]

The paths I have explored lead to one destination. Genetic information is special because we are inclined to treat it as mysterious, as having exceptional potency or significance, not because it differs in some fundamental way from all other sorts of information about us. Portions of that mystery and power come from the opaqueness of genetic information, the possibility that others will know things about the individual that he or she does not know, and how genetic information connects individuals to immediate family and more distant kin. The more genetic information is treated as special, the more special treatment will be necessary. Yet none of these factors is unique to genetic information.

I propose that genetic exceptionalism—the plea to treat genetic information as different from other health-related information—is an overly dramatic view of the significance of genetic information in our lives. It is a reflection of genetic determinism and genetic reductionism at least as much as the product of genuinely distinctive features of genetic information. There is a disturbing corollary to this thesis: there is a vicious circularity in insisting that genetic information is different and must be given special treatment. The more we repeat that genetic information is fundamentally unlike other kinds of medical information, the more support we implicitly provide for genetic determinism, for the notion that genetics exerts special power over our lives.

I therefore suggest a revision of the "future diary" metaphor for genetic information. Why not regard our genes as a list of the obstacles we are likely to encounter and perhaps as a somewhat better prediction of how long we will have to do what matters to us, to be with the people we love, and to accomplish the tasks we have set for ourselves? Our genes no more dictate what is significant about our lives than the covers and pages of a blank diary dictate the content of what is written within. Our genes might be regarded metaphorically as the physical, but blank, volume in which we will create our diary. Some volumes have fewer pages in which to write, some more. Certain pages, often toward the back of the volume, may be more difficult to write on. And some leaves may require great skill and effort to open at all. But the physical volume is not the content of the diary. The content we must write ourselves.

NOTES

1. *Task Force Report: Genetic Information and Insurance* (Bethesda, Md.: Genetic Information and Health Insurance, National Institutes of Health, National Center for Human Genome Research, 1993).

2. Lawrence O. Gostin, "Genetic Privacy," *Journal of Law, Medicine and Ethics* 23 (1995): 320, 321.

3. George J. Annas, Leonard H. Glantz, and Patricia A. Roche, "Drafting the Genetic Privacy Act: Science, Policy, and Practical Considerations," *Journal of Law, Medicine and Ethics* 23 (1995): 360, 365.

4. George J. Annas, "Privacy Rules for DNA Databanks: Protecting Coded 'Future Diaries,'" *Journal of the American Medical Association* 270 (1993): 2346–50; Annas, Glantz, and Roche, "Drafting the Genetic Privacy Act," quotation on p. 360.

5. Annas, Glantz, and Roche, "Drafting the Genetic Privacy Act."

6. Gostin, "Genetic Privacy," 326.

7. Thomas H. Murray and Norman T. Mendel, "Introduction: The Genome Imperative," *Journal of Law, Medicine and Ethics* 23 (1995): 309–11.

8. Annas, Glantz, and Roche, "Drafting the Genetic Privacy Act," 360.

9. Thomas H. Murray, "Assessing Genetic Technologies: Two Ethical Issues," *International Journal of Technology Assessment in Health Care* 10 (1994): 573–82.

10. Karen H. Rothenberg, "Genetic Information and Health Insurance: State Legislative Approaches," *Journal of Law, Medicine and Ethics* 23 (1995): 312–19.

11. Robert J. Pokorski, "The Potential Role of Genetic Testing in Risk Classification," Report of the Genetic Testing Committee to the Medical Section of the American Council of Life Insurance, Hilton Head, S.C., June 10, 1989.

12. Annas, Glantz, and Roche, "Drafting the Genetic Privacy Act," 326.

13. Gostin, "Genetic Privacy," 324.

14. Thomas H. Murray, "Genetics and the Moral Mission of Health Insurance," *Hastings Center Report* 22, no. 6 (1992): 12–17.

15. Gostin, "Genetic Privacy," 324.

16. Annas, Glantz, and Roche, "Drafting the Genetic Privacy Act," 365.

17. Dorothy Nelkin and M. Susan Lindee, *The DNA Mystique: The Gene as a Cultural Icon* (New York: W. H. Freeman, 1995), 198.

18. Eric T. Juengst, "The Ethics of Prediction: Genetic Risk and the Physician-Patient Relationship," *Genome Science and Technology* 1, no. 1 (1995): 21, 30.

19. Carl F. Cranor, "Genetic Causation," in *Are Genes Us?: The Social Consequences of the New Genetics,* Carl F. Cranor, ed. (New Brunswick, N.J.: Rutgers University Press, 1994).

20. Evelyn Fox Keller, "Masters Molecules," in ibid., quotations on pp. 90, 91, 97.

Part Two **The Health Care Setting**

Chapter 4 Genetic Privacy in the Patient-Physician Relationship

David Orentlicher

What I may see or hear in the course of the treatment or even outside of the treatment in regard to the life of men, which on no account one must spread abroad, I will keep to myself holding such things shameful to be spoken about.
Hippocratic oath, fifth century B.C.E.

A physician should respect confidences and protect the patient's secrets. In protecting a patient's secrets, he must be more insistent than the patient himself.
Haly Abbas (Ahwazi), advice to a physician, tenth century C.E.

I will respect the secrets which are confided in me, *even after the patient has died.*
Geneva Declaration, World Medical Association, 1940

A physician shall respect the rights of patients, of colleagues, and of other health professionals, and shall safeguard patient confidences within the constraints of the law.
Principles of Medical Ethics, American Medical Association, 1980

The medical profession has traditionally exhibited great concern for patient privacy. Throughout history, codes of medical ethics have identified patient confidentiality as an essential element of the patient-physician relationship. Because medical information is often highly intimate and potentially embarrassing, physicians are required to maintain the secrecy of medical information that they learn from or about their patients. In the absence of express or implied patient consent or of a law requiring disclosure, physicians may not disclose information about their patients to other persons, and physicians must take measures to prevent the inadvertent disclosure of patient information. Discussions among a patient's health care providers must not occur in the presence of potential eavesdroppers, patient charts must be kept in a secure place, and information sent to insurers must be limited to the information necessary to process the patient's claim.

In addition to the duty of confidentiality, physicians assume other responsibilities to protect a patient's privacy rights in medical information. Patients may not only insist that information shared with a physician remain with the physician, they may also decide not to share certain medical information about themselves with their physician. Patients may simply not want to disclose the information to anyone, they may fear inadvertent breaches of confidentiality if they do disclose information to their physician, or they may fear that physicians will view them disfavorably once certain information is disclosed. For example, someone who is gay may fear that physicians will refuse care if they know of his or her sexual orientation. Patients may also refuse medical testing in order to maintain the secrecy of their medical information from themselves. In particular, patients may prefer not to know whether they are at risk for a disease for which no treatment is available, especially if disclosure of that information would result in invidious discrimination.

Because genetic information is unusually sensitive and subject to misuse, patient privacy is especially important for genetic information. Yet, as advances in genetics are increasing the ability of physicians to discover genetic information about their patients, threats to the privacy of that information are increasing from two sources—developments in information technologies and changes in health care reimbursement. In this chapter, I will discuss the fundamental importance of privacy in the patient-physician relationship and the concerns raised for the privacy of genetic information.

PRIVACY IN THE PATIENT-PHYSICIAN RELATIONSHIP

Privacy in the patient-physician relationship promotes three important values: patient control, patient property interests, and patient health.

Patient control. Privacy permits patients to retain control over the amount of intimate information they divulge about themselves and to whom they divulge it. Society demonstrates its respect for people when it gives them control over important aspects of their lives, including decisions about career, marriage, reproduction, and medical treatment. Control over personal information is of fundamental importance to individuals. It assures people that they can avoid the shame of having embarrassing intimate information disclosed publicly.[1] It also assures individuals that they can pursue deeply held beliefs that are politically unpopular or engage in behavior that is unconventional without risk of opprobrium or retaliation.[2] Privacy in personal information allows people the freedom of self-exploration as they shape their identity without the risk that, at some later date, they will be penalized for experiments with behavior or lifestyles that they later rejected.[3] Informational privacy is not only about shielding facts that might be viewed negatively by others, it is also about shielding facts that are generally viewed positively by others. For many people, for example, charity is noblest when given anonymously.[4] Most fundamentally, informational privacy is valuable regardless of whether the information it shields is viewed positively or negatively by others. Informational privacy allows people to pursue their education, careers, friendships, romances, and medical care without the oversight, interference, or other unwelcome involvement of others.[5] By controlling personal information, individuals can control the extent to which other people can participate in their lives.

The confidentiality of medical information is of special importance. A person's medical condition can involve the most intimate of personal information. Diagnosis of a venereal disease, for example, may reveal marital infidelity or suggest involvement with multiple sex partners. Disclosure of medical information may also lead to stigmatization and discrimination. People with HIV infection may be shunned by family, friends, and others, evicted from housing, fired from employment, and denied insurance. Even when reactions are less extreme, people frequently are treated differently once their friends and acquaintances discover that they have an illness. In many cases, the discovery leads to a welcomed response of sympathy and comfort, but it often leads to unwelcomed responses of avoidance or excessive solicitousness. In any case, for many people, any change in their relationships will be unwelcome, and they will choose not to disclose their illness to others.

Concerns about privacy in medical information are particularly present with genetic information. Genetic makeup is at the heart of personality. Genetics not only has a profound influence on such physical characteristics as height, weight,[6] skin color, and eye color, but it almost certainly affects less tangible traits, such as shyness,[7] altruism, sociableness, artistry, and intellectual skills.[8] Indeed, a chief argument against the cloning of embryos has been the concern that the creation of genetically identical sibling embryos deprives those individuals who develop from the embryos of their unique identity.[9] Individuals may not want to know whether they are at risk for a genetic disease, like Huntington disease, for which nothing can be done by way of prevention or treatment in advance. Such persons may conclude that they will be better off psychologically not knowing,[10] and they may therefore decline medical testing to discover genetic information about themselves.

Disclosure of genetic information to others is also of particular concern. One's genetic makeup may one day provide a detailed blueprint of the person, thereby enabling others to alter their relationship with the person on account of that genetic information. Employers may decide to fire or not hire persons with undesirable traits, and landlords may refuse to rent housing to them. Disclosures of genetic information also may lead to self-fulfilling categorizations or stigmatizations. People who are expected to develop certain traits will be perceived as having those traits and will be encouraged by others to develop those traits. For example, children for whom adults have low expectations and who are therefore not challenged educationally or otherwise will not do as well as if adults had high expectations for them.[11] Moreover, because genetic information can indicate tendencies for medical problems years or even decades in the future, disclosure of genetic risks for disease can elicit the stigmatization and discrimination that ordinarily result from actual illness far before the development of any illness or even in cases when a person at elevated risk for disease would not actually develop the disease.[12]

Genetic information also carries a high risk for discrimination because nonspecialists often misunderstand the significance of genetic information. For example, there have been cases in which individuals carried a single autosomal (a chromosome other than a sex chromosome) recessive gene and therefore were not affected by genetic disease but were still treated by potential employers as if they had two copies of the recessive gene and therefore as if they were affected by the genetic disease.[13] Similarly, people with asymptomatic expressions of a genetic disease have been treated by employers and insurers as if they had significant symptoms.[14]

Finally, a person's genetic makeup can implicate reproductive decisions and the response of others to those decisions. Although many people are willing to have a child even if it means passing on a genetic abnormality like Down syndrome or cystic fibrosis, others believe that it is wrong for couples to procreate under such conditions. Privacy about genetic status is critical to protect couples or women from harassment because they choose to procreate even when they risk having a child with a genetic disease.[15]

Privacy is especially important with genetic information also because an individual's genetic makeup reveals information not only about the individual but also about family members.[16] If a person carries the gene mutation for Huntington disease, it follows that one of the person's parents also carries the mutation, that each of the person's children has a 50% chance of carrying the mutation, and that each of the person's siblings also has a 50% chance of carrying the mutation. Violations of a patient's privacy with respect to genetic information may also mean that the privacy of many other persons has been violated.

Patient property interests. It is often assumed that patient privacy is protected as long as information about a patient is disseminated in a way that protects patient anonymity. If data about patients are aggregated, or if data about a patient are stripped of any identifying characteristics,[17] then there is arguably no violation of the patient's interests.

However, people have not only privacy interests in their personal medical information, they also have property interests. Because personal medical information, particularly genetic information, is closely linked to one's identity, it is important that individuals be able to control the uses to which their personal medical information is put.[18] When patients divulge information to their physicians, they do so for the purpose of enhancing their health. In effect, they sacrifice some of their property interests to facilitate physicians' efforts on their behalf. Physicians are entitled to use the information so long as they use it in diagnosing and treating the patient. When physicians start using the information to benefit persons other than the patient, they will often be misappropriating the patient's property interests in personal information.[19]

Patients might be particularly troubled when personal information, even nonidentifiable information, is sold by physicians to pharmaceutical companies to be used for marketing purposes. For example, companies might use the information to target their promotional activities at physicians who treat patients likely to be candidates for the companies' drugs. In such cases, both the physicians and the companies realize a profit from the patient's information, and patients might feel that they have been unfairly exploited. In addition, patients may feel that the information is being put to uses that are harmful to themselves or other patients. Pharmaceutical marketing efforts may result in treatment decisions that are not optimal in terms of medical effectiveness or cost.[20]

Patient health. Confidentiality is also critical to the patient-physician relationship because of its role in promoting patient well-being. Without assurances of confidentiality, many individuals would delay seeking, or avoid entirely, medical attention for their illnesses, especially when they have or suspect that they have diseases that carry stigma and to which others react negatively. Individuals with psychological problems may avoid counseling; individuals at risk for HIV-infection may refrain from being tested;[21] and such delay or avoidance often will compromise the patient's health or the health of third parties. Promises of confidentiality are therefore essential to assure patients that they can obtain necessary health care without risking serious harm to themselves.

Whether people will sacrifice their health even if they are not assured of confidentiality is, of course, a question.[22] There are several responses to this point. First, for many people, ostracization may be worse than sickness. Having better health may be small consolation when one is shunned by society and denied opportunities to pursue personal and professional goals. Just as people dying with cancer may choose a better quality of life over a longer life, so may other people accept diminished health to preserve their privacy. Second, the health benefits of medical attention may be relatively small for the individual with a disease but substantial for other persons who would benefit from the individual's seeking medical attention. For example, in the early days of the HIV epidemic, when little in the way of treatment was available, HIV testing and counseling provided much greater benefits for the uninfected public than the infected patient. In such circumstances, even assuming that people would not seriously compromise their health over a lack of confidentiality, people might well trade off a marginal benefit in health to maintain their privacy. Accordingly, confidentiality is important to ensure that individuals will seek health care when doing so is important to protect the public's health.

There is another important point about medical interventions that provide little benefit to the patient and that would be forgone in the absence of assurances of confidentiality. The tendency to forgo medical attention will likely persist for some time even after treatments have improved. Because there is always a lag between the availability of treatment and the awareness of affected individuals about that availability, many people will underestimate the benefits to themselves of seeking care when weighing those benefits against the costs of compromising their privacy. Confidentiality, then, ensures that people will come forward for medical care even when they mistakenly underestimate the benefits of obtaining care.

Last, although there is little empirical evidence on the effects of confidentiality policies, important evidence does indicate that confidentiality is important for the health of both the individual seeking care and society generally. When Maryland changed its law regarding confidentiality of treatment for past sexual abuse of children, the number of individuals seeking treatment declined dramatically. Before the change, therapists could maintain the confidentiality of a patient's disclosures that he or she had committed child sexual abuse before seeking treatment, and about seven persons a year sought counseling at the Johns Hopkins Sexual Disorders Clinic because they had engaged in child sexual abuse in the past. In contrast, during the first year that therapists were mandated to report patients who disclosed their sexual abuse of children before seeking treatment, no one sought treatment at Hopkins for past child sexual abuse.[23] As this case suggests, breaches of confidentiality to protect the public health may in fact be more likely to compromise the public health. If affected persons are discouraged from seeking care, then society is worse off by having them at large without any treatment than by having them under treatment with their confidentiality protected.[24] In the absence of mandatory reporting requirements, patients generally can trust that physicians will respect their privacy and preserve their confidentiality. Yet when the government requires the breach of confidentiality, patients may conclude that it is more prudent to withhold the reportable information from their physicians.

Confidentiality to protect patient and public health is important in genetics as in other areas of medicine. Because genetic information implicates highly personal information and may lead to discrimination in employment and access to insurance, an absence of confidentiality will likely discourage people from seeking genetic testing. If individuals are discouraged from undergoing genetic testing, then they are missing potentially important health care not only for themselves but also for their children and other relatives. Identification of genetic risks allows people to consider those risks in their reproductive decisions and to notify family members that they may carry the same or similar risks.

Trust in the patient-physician relationship. Confidentiality is important not only to protect patient privacy and patient property interests and to enhance the health of both the individual patient and the public. In addition, confidentiality is critical in assuring patients that they may safely place their trust in their physicians.

Physicians have long assumed a fiduciary role on behalf of patients in which the physician is expected to act primarily as an advocate for the interests of patients.[25] This fiduciary role derives naturally from the patient's condition and the physician's role. Patients are especially needy when they are sick; their health, indeed their life, often hangs in the balance. They are especially dependent on their physicians at such times. Physicians have the information needed to make the patient well. Although patients can often master the medical knowledge necessary to understand their illness, diminished physical capacity, mental capacity, or time constraints may leave them unable to undertake the necessary study. Moreover, even patients who have a sufficient understanding of their illness are profoundly dependent on physicians. Physicians possess a virtual monopoly not only on the expertise to treat illness but also on the use of medical therapies. Patients generally have no choice but to turn to physicians for treatment. Finally, patients' dependence rests on their inability to monitor their physicians' behavior. Because patients generally lack medical expertise and because it is generally difficult even for experts to assess whether physicians are providing quality care,[26] patients have little ability to check on their physicians' provision of care over time.

With so much at stake for the patient's welfare and so much power in the hands of physicians, patients will not be willing to rely on their physicians' judgment unless they can trust that physicians will use their power and authority on behalf of their patients, placing their patients' interests above competing interests. Accordingly, a wide range of professional responsibilities have been designed, in part, to assure patients that physicians will not compromise their interests in the pursuit of other goals. For example, physicians are prohibited from referring patients to laboratories or imaging facilities in which they have an investment interest,[27] from accepting cash gifts from drug companies,[28] or from engaging in sexual relationships with their patients.[29]

Confidentiality in the patient-physician relationship likewise plays a fundamental role in ensuring patients' trust in their physicians. The betrayal of a confidence is a signal to the patient that the physician is serving as an agent of interests that may conflict with the patient's interests. Reporting drug use to law enforcement authorities makes the physician an agent of the state, selling patient data to pharmaceutical companies makes the physician an agent of the drug industry, and disclosing genetic status to siblings or cousins makes the physician an agent of family members. When physicians become dual agents, they can no longer provide assurances to patients that it is safe to place their trust in their physicians.

Some breaches of confidentiality are of course necessary. Physicians may need to report patient information for the protection of the public health.[30] Nevertheless, it will be very difficult, if at all possible, to justify overriding the confidentiality of genetic information in the patient-physician relationship. First, the benefits of disclosure would probably be small. It is unlikely, for example, that withholding genetic information of individual patients will compromise public health. Moreover, the harm from disclosure would probably be high. Because of the intensely intimate nature of genetic information, any betrayal of confidentiality in that information will have substantial consequences for the willingness of patients to undergo other testing that would divulge genetic information about themselves. Betrayal of confidentiality will also have substantial consequences because patients's neediness and dependence force them to trust deeply in their physicians. The deeper the need for trust, the greater the need for assurances of physician loyalty. As a corollary, it is difficult to limit the impact of breaches of confidentiality. Patients can accept that their physicians have strengths in some areas of practice and weaknesses in other areas and rely on their physicians only in areas of strength; but perceptions of trust are global. People are generally viewed as either trustworthy or not trustworthy rather than as trustworthy on some matters but not on others. Accordingly, it is not critical whether genetic information is more or less private than other kinds of medical information. If trust is compromised in one area of concern for patients—like genetics—it will be compromised for other areas of concern (and vice versa).

THREATS TO CONFIDENTIALITY IN THE PATIENT-PHYSICIAN RELATIONSHIP

Although concerns about protecting confidentiality are always present, the public faces two major threats to confidentiality of genetic information: new information technologies and the greater intrusiveness of cost containment in the patient-physician relationship.

New information technologies. Key threats to confidentiality of patient information are posed by the computerization of health records and the development of health databases. Individuals stand to gain much in the way of improved health care through these developments. The benefits, however, will be accompanied by greater risks to privacy.

The computerization of medical records means that physicians can more readily access those records, helping them provide appropriate care. For example, if someone is brought unconscious to an emergency room after collapsing suddenly, the emergency room physicians need to know whether the person has been taking medication, whether he or she has a history of heart disease, diabetes, or other illnesses, and whether he or she has any allergies.[31] Quick access to medical records is especially important for patients who travel frequently or who have multiple residences.

Health databases offer an even wider array of benefits for the public. Databases about patients' demographic characteristics, medical histories and problems, treatments and outcomes can provide answers to many important questions. Likewise, people choosing a health plan or a physician can consider data regarding the plan's or physician's standing on a number of measures of quality. Public health specialists can more quickly recognize when an outbreak of infectious disease is developing in a community. A health care insurer can compare outcomes of different treatments for certain medical problems in deciding the treatments for which it will provide coverage. Planners at a state department of health can better assess the state's health care needs during the next five to ten years and allocate their development budget accordingly.[32]

Although the ready availability of patient data offers important benefits to patients, it also increases the risk of intrusions on patient privacy. The more ways that patient data can be used to improve patient care, the more people will be authorized to use the data. Indeed, more than a decade ago, one investigator found that, even within the limited setting of hospital care for a single patient, more than 75 persons had legitimate grounds for access to the patient's record.[33] In addition, persons without authorization have much easier access to medical records entered into computerized databases than those stored in a file cabinet.[34]

The concerns about new information technologies are not unique to genetic information, but they are more acute. The personal intimacy of genetic information makes confidentiality of that information particularly important. In addition, some data banks include blood or other tissue samples, which may or may not have been taken for purposes of genetic analysis and which can be reanalyzed at later dates as advances in genetics increase our ability to discover information about the person from whom the sample was taken.[35] A tissue database, in other words, has the capacity for dramatic self-expansion; people will have supplied the samples with no idea of the extent to which the samples may reveal personal information.[36]

Although the advent of new information technologies greatly increases the risks to informational privacy, safeguards can be adopted to limit the risks and draw an appropriate balance between the benefits and costs of ready access to medical information.[37]

Health care cost containment. A more serious threat to patient privacy comes from the increasing emphasis on health care cost containment, characterized by the shift in health care coverage to managed care from traditional indemnity insurance,[38] and the intrusiveness of cost containment techniques into the patient-physician relationship.

Under managed care, patients accept greater constraints on their autonomy in exchange for lower premiums, and physicians accept greater constraints on their autonomy in exchange for managed care plans that authorize reimbursement of their services to plan subscribers. Thus, unlike traditional indemnity insurance in which patients enjoy virtually unlimited freedom in choosing physicians and hospitals, in many health maintenance organizations (HMOs), patients are limited to seeing only those physicians employed by the plan and are required to obtain a referral from their primary care physician before seeing a specialist. For physicians, there is no longer reimbursement based primarily on the basis of what the physician decides to provide. Rather, there may be restrictions on the drugs that may be prescribed, the X-rays and other scans that may be ordered, and the number of days that may be allowed for hospitalization. Hospitalizations and surgeries may require advance authorization from utilization overseers.

These changes in health care and health insurance are critical for patient privacy and confidentiality because the more intensive the efforts to contain costs become, the more health care insurers intrude into the patient-physician relationship. As indicated, as a result of health care cost containment, insurers are no longer relying on physicians to allocate health care dollars. Instead, they are assuming more of the allocative responsibility by deciding which drugs can be used, when a patient can undergo surgery or be hospitalized, and how long a patient can remain in the hospital. Some of these decisions can be made on the basis of general rules, but many decisions need to be individualized. A patient's need for care often turns on his or her particular circumstances, and general rules for all patients will leave many patients underserved and other patients overserved. Accordingly, if insurers are to make fair decisions about reimbursement, they must receive detailed accounts of their subscribers' health care problems. Instead of deciding simply on the basis of the physician's diagnosis, the health care plan will need to look at summaries of the patient's medical history and physical examination, reports of laboratory tests and radiologic images, and descriptions of the patient's response to treatment in the past. Patients under chronic care will have an ongoing need for reevaluation.

The intrusiveness of managed care can compromise important privacy interests as well as patients' well-being. Physicians are being asked to disclose intimate information about their patients to health care reviewers. In one case, a psychoanalyst was asked to describe a patient's history of being sexually abused.[39] These reviewers will be similarly interested in knowing detailed information when patients undergo psychological counseling after learning about a serious genetic risk or when patients seek abortion services because of a genetic condition passed on to the fetus. Such disclosures can aggravate a patient's psychological distress and may discourage patients from initiating or continuing treatment.

Health care costs can be limited not only by using health care dollars wisely but also by excluding potentially high-cost subscribers from coverage. Pressures to contain health care costs will encourage insurers to increase their efforts to identify applicants who are at risk for disease. As genetic testing becomes more available in identifying risks of heart disease, cancer, and other illnesses, insurers will incorporate genetic information into the underwriting process. Insurers will review the medical records of applicants for genetic testing results and may insist on genetic testing as a condition of coverage. Individuals will be forced to choose between maintaining their genetic privacy and maintaining their health care coverage.

The genetic privacy of patients can be protected by effective enforcement of professional ethical standards. As the American Medical Association's Council on Ethical and Judicial Affairs has recognized, the ethical obligation of physicians to preserve patient confidentiality imposes an obligation to ensure that patient privacy is not lost for genetic information. Although insurers and employers may want genetic information, physicians need not and should not participate in efforts by insurers or employers to obtain genetic information from subscribers, employees, or applicants. Accordingly, under the AMA's Code of Medical Ethics, such participation is unethical for physicians.[40] With greater dissemination and enforcement of the AMA's guidelines by professional societies as well as by medical licensing boards, both of which have authority to discipline physicians for failing to meet their ethical obligations, insurers and employers may find that they are able to obtain little in the way of genetic information. The medical profession can do much to preserve the genetic privacy of patients; it merely needs to use its existing powers effectively.

NOTES

Note to epigraphs: The first three are from Warren T. Reich et al., eds., *Encyclopedia of Bioethics,* vol. 4 (New York: Free Press, 1978), 1731, 1735, and 1749 (emphasis in original); the last is from American Medical Association, Council on Ethical and Judicial Affairs, *Code of Medical Ethics: Current Opinions with Annotations,* vol. 14 (1994).

1. "Developments in the Law—Privileged Communications, Parts 1 and 2," *Harvard Law Review* 98 (1985): 1450, 1481.
2. Charles Fried, "Privacy," *Yale Law Journal* 77 (1968): 475, 483–84.
3. Alan F. Westin, *Privacy and Freedom* (London: Bodley Head, 1970), 34.
4. Fried, "Privacy," 483.
5. Westin, *Privacy and Freedom,* 33.
6. William Ira Bennett, "Beyond Overeating," *New England Journal of Medicine* (hereafter *NEJM*) 332 (1995): 673; Albert J. Stunkdard et al., "The Body-Mass Index of Twins Who Have Been Reared Apart," ibid. 322 (1990): 1483 (finding that as much as 70% of the variation among different persons in body weight can be attributed to genetic factors).
7. Researchers have identified a gene variant that is linked to impulsive, exploratory, fickle, excitable, quick-tempered, and extravagant behavior, described as the Novelty Seeking trait. Richard P. Ebstein et al., "Dopamine D4 receptor (D4DR) Exon III Polymorphism Associated with the Human Personality Trait of Novelty Seeking," *Nature Genetics* 12 (1996): 78; Jonathan Benjamin et al., "Population and Familial Association Between the D4 Dopamine Receptor Gene and Measures of Novelty Seeking," ibid., 81; Natalie Angier, "Variant Gene Tied to a Love of New Thrills," *New York Times,* Jan. 2, 1996, A1.
8. A number of genetic diseases, including Down syndrome and fragile X syndrome, are characterized by mental retardation. James J. Nora and F. Clarke Fraser, *Medical Genetics: Principles and Practice,* 4th ed. (Philadelphia: Lea and Febinger, 1994), 43, 130.
9. Daniel Callahan, "Perspective on Cloning; A Threat to Individual Uniqueness; An Attempt to Aid Childless Couples by Engineering Conception Could Transform the Idea of Human Identity," *Los Angeles Times,* Nov. 12, 1993, B7.
10. This belief may be mistaken. Some evidence suggests that resolution of uncertainty about risk may have positive effects even when the resolution indicates that the person will develop the disease for which the person is at risk. Sandi Wiggins et al., "The Psychological Consequences of Predictive Testing for Huntington's Disease," *NEJM* 327 (1993): 1401.
11. Linda C. Mayes et al., "The Problem of Prenatal Cocaine Exposure: A Rush to Judgment," *Journal of the American Medical Association* (hereafter *JAMA*) 267 (1993): 406, 407. A study of persons with visual impairment suggests that the extent to which a visually impaired person's activities are compromised may depend less on the person's actual degree of visual impairment than on the fact that the attitudes of others toward visual impairment socialize the person into the role of a blind person. Robert A. Scott, *The Making of Blind Men: A Study of Adult Socialization* (New York: Russell Sage Foundation, 1969), 71–89, 105–21.

12. Because of incomplete penetrance, genetic abnormalities do not always result in genetic disease. Moreover, even among those who develop genetic disease, there can be great variation in the extent of illness, from minimal to severe. David Orentlicher, "Genetic Screening by Employers," *JAMA* 263 (1990): 1005.

13. Paul R. Billings et al., "Discrimination as a Consequence of Genetic Testing," *American Journal of Human Genetics* 50 (1992): 476, 478. American Medical Association, Council on Ethical and Judicial Affairs, "Use of Genetic Testing by Employers," *JAMA* 266 (1991): 1827.

14. Billings et al., "Discrimination," 479.

15. American Medical Association, Council on Ethical and Judicial Affairs, "Prenatal Genetic Screening," in *Code of Medical Ethics: Reports,* vol. 4 (1993), 81, 87. Neil A. Holtzman and Mark A. Rothstein, "Invited Editorial: Eugenics and Genetic Discrimination," *American Journal of Human Genetics* 50 (1992): 457.

16. Anita L. Allen, "Privacy in Health Care," in Warren T. Reich, ed., *Encyclopedia of Bioethics,* rev. ed., 5 vols. (New York: Macmillan, 1995), 4:2064–73.

17. E.g., a physician might submit a case report of a patient and describe only the patient's age, sex, race, and medical problems.

18. Sissela Bok, *Secrets: On the Ethics of Concealment and Revelation* (New York: Pantheon Books, 1982), 24.

19. In some cases, society's interest in research may outweigh the individual's property interest. In most cases where others will benefit from patient information, people will waive their property rights, either out of altruism or because they have been properly compensated (as when the information is put to a commercial use).

20. Jerry Avorn, Milton Chen, and Robert Hartley, "Scientific Versus Commercial Sources of Influence on the Prescribing Behavior of Physicians," *American Journal of Medicine* 73 (1982): 4.

21. Neil A. Holtzman, *Proceed with Caution: Predicting Genetic Risks in the Recombinant DNA Era* (Baltimore: Johns Hopkins University Press, 1989), 186.

22. "Developments in the Law," 1543–44.

23. Fred S. Berlin, H. Martin Malin, and Sharon Dean, "Effects of Statutes Requiring Psychiatrists to Report Suspected Sexual Abuse of Children," *American Journal of Psychiatry* 148 (1991): 449, 451–54. Similarly, although about 17 patients a year in treatment disclosed relapses into child sexual abuse when such relapses were not reportable, no patients disclosed relapses in the two years after a statute was passed requiring that the disclosures be reported. Ibid., 451. Without the disclosures, the patients' therapists were unable to intervene clinically with hospitalization, drug treatment or removal of the patient from home to minimize the risk of additional abuse.

24. Tarasoff v. Regents of the Univ. of Cal., 551 P.2d 334, 359–60 (Cal. 1976) (Clark, J., dissenting).

25. Robert M. Veatch, "Physicians and Cost Containment: The Ethical Conflict," *Jurimetrics* 30 (1990): 461, 469–70.

26. Timothy Stoltzfus Jost, "Health System Reform: Forward or Backward with Quality Oversight?" *JAMA* 271 (1994): 1508, 1509.

27. American Medical Association, Council on Ethical and Judicial Affairs, "Conflict of Interest: Physician Ownership of Medical Facilities," *JAMA* 267 (1992): 2366, 2368.

28. American Medical Association, Council on Ethical and Judicial Affairs, "Guidelines on Gifts to Physicians from Industry: An Update," *Food and Drug Journal* 47 (1992): 445, 451.

29. American Medical Association, Council on Ethical and Judicial Affairs, "Sexual Misconduct in the Practice of Medicine," *JAMA* 266 (1991): 2741, 2745.

30. For example, states typically require reporting of certain infectious diseases and violent injuries.

31. Institute of Medicine, Committee on Regional Health Data Networks, *Health Data in the Information Age: Use, Disclosure, and Privacy,* ed. Molla S. Donaldson and Kathleen N. Lohr (Washington, D.C.: Government Printing Office, 1994), 27–29.

32. Ibid.; Lawrence O. Gostin, "Health Information Privacy," *Cornell Law Review* 80 (1995): 451, 470–84.

33. Mark Siegler, "Confidentiality in Medicine—A Decrepit Concept," *NEJM* 307 (1995): 1518, 1519.

34. Beverly Woodward, "The Computer-Based Patient Record and Confidentiality," *NEJM* 333 (1995): 1419, 1420.

35. President's Commission for the Study of Ethical Problems in Medicine and Biomedical and Behavioral Research, *Screening and Counseling for Genetic Conditions: A Report on the Ethical, Social, and Legal Implications of Genetic Screening, Counseling, and Education Programs* (Washington, D.C.: Government Printing Office, 1983), 42–43.

36. Some of these tissue banks include samples taken from persons without the person's knowledge or consent, as with the case of blood samples taken from newborns. Jean E. McEwen and Philip R. Reilly, "Stored Guthrie Cards as DNA Banks," *NEJM* 331 (1994): 1167, 1167–68.

37. Institute of Medicine, *Health Data in the Information Age,* 190–213.

38. By 1993, managed care plans insured more than half of those in the United States who received their health insurance through employer-sponsored plans. Moreover, most traditional, indemnity plans were using such techniques of managed care as utilization review. John K. Iglehart, "Physicians and the Growth of Managed Care," *NEJM* 331 (1994): 1167–68.

39. Carol Hymowitz, "High Anxiety: In the Name of Freud, Why Are Psychiatrists Complaining So Much?" *Wall Street Journal,* Dec. 21, 1995, A1.

40. American Medical Association, *Code of Medical Ethics,* 22–23.

Chapter 5 A Clinical Geneticist Perspective of the Patient-Physician Relationship

Eugene Pergament

For more than two centuries, physicians have had a professional obligation to keep confidential all medical and personal information obtained from their patients during the course of practicing medicine. The Hippocratic Oath states that "whatsoever you shall see or hear of the lives of men which is not fitting to be spoken, you will keep inviolably secret." For, if a physician is to be able to "exercise . . . [his] art solely for the cure of [his] patients," then there must be unequivocal trust on the part of the patient to provide accurate and complete medical and personal histories. In an atmosphere of mistrust between physician and patient, patients will either not seek such services or will be wary of telling physicians the truth about themselves.

Clinical genetics, a relatively new medical specialty dating from the 1950s, relies heavily on patient trust, not only to obtain individual patient information, but also to secure detailed medical and family histories over three or more generations about siblings, parents, children, cousins, aunts and uncles, and more distantly related family members. How else are clinical geneticists to "exercise [their] art"? First and foremost, clinical geneticists are responsible for accurate diagnoses of genetic diseases and congenital malformation syndromes. Complete individual and family social, reproductive, and health history, exhaustive clinical examinations, and relevant laboratory tests are all essential components leading to accurate risk assessment. These efforts lead to the identification of individuals at reproductive risk because they are carriers of gene mutations; the provision of information about the medical implications of a genetic disease as to prognosis, disease severity, disease prevention, and family planning; and the medical management of genetic disease.

At the same time, the clinical geneticist is also responsible for assuring that patients comprehend the medical facts, understand how heredity contributes to a disorder and the risk of recurrence for themselves and their family members, and chooses the course of action that meets their needs, way of life, and moral standards. Further, clinical geneticists must assist a patient and his or her family adjust psychologically and socially to a genetic disease by providing emotional support and guidance on completion of the medical evaluation and genetic analysis. Meeting these responsibilities based primarily on intimate knowledge about a patient's genotype and that of his or her family places the clinical geneticist in a distinct position in medicine.

To fulfill these responsibilities, the clinical geneticist must also counsel the patient about the potential risks, benefits, limitations, interpretation, and psychological and economic consequences of genetic diagnosis and genetic testing. The challenge to the clinical geneticist is to explain all of this in ways that help resolve patients' concerns and contribute positively to their overall well-being. A tenet of clinical genetics is that accurate diagnosis and genetic testing enhance the opportunity of a patient to obtain information about personal health and reproductive risk and to make autonomous and noncoerced choices based on this genetic information.

Before the 1950s, explanations about genetic disease were framed in terms of genes, families, and populations. Genetic choices and risk-taking were restricted to predictions based on Mendelian inheritance, population genetics, and available biochemical testing, limited as it was.[1] The rapid expansion of genetic knowledge over the ensuing decades, principally through the development of chromosome analysis (karyotyping) and recombinant DNA technology, markedly has expanded the role of the clinical geneticist and dramatically altered the patient's choices. The focus has shifted from diagnoses based on phenotype alone and reproductive risks based solely on chance to molecular definition of genetic disease and defined reproductive and testing choices to prevent genetic disease.

From the beginning of modern medical genetics, there has been a clear sense of allegiance of the clinical geneticist to, and only to, the patient. The clinical geneticist premises all professional interactions with a patient on confidentiality and his or her role as a facilitator of medical and reproductive decision making in a nondirective fashion. The hereditary nature of genetic disease challenges the clinical geneticist because genetic disease places family members at risk, adds to the genetic load of humans, and can strike future generations. The patient-centered emphasis combines with the tradition of nondirective counseling to create the distinctive practices of the clinical geneticist.

Genetic counseling is characterized by complete disclosure of diagnostic and testing results, the explicit confidentiality of these results, and the unequivocal control by the patient of subsequent clinical and reproductive decisions. Three considerations have been proposed to explain why a patient's welfare is an "overriding priority" to the interests of family members, the community, and future generations.[2] These considerations have developed in reaction to the excesses of the eugenics movement during the early part of the twentieth century, a respect for reproductive autonomy and self-determination, and the prognostic uncertainty and lack of effective therapies that characterize most genetic diseases.

These considerations support the underlying philosophy and application of nondirective counseling by the clinical geneticist that ensures patient confidentiality. Nondirective counseling avoids value judgments on the part of the clinical geneticist about the social, medical, and economic consequences of the patient's choices. It ensures that the patient who bears the consequences of any medical and reproductive decisions has the opportunity and the responsibility to make such decisions. Nondirective counseling thus serves as a powerful rationale and a powerful impetus that confidentiality of a patient not be breached in any circumstance.

Nevertheless, over time, the obligation of physicians to keep confidential personal medical information has been challenged and even eroded. It is now well established that confidentiality can be breached in at least three circumstances: in the duty to report certain illegal acts, in court trials requiring medical testimony where the patient-physician privilege has been waived, and if it is determined that a patient presents a clear-cut danger to others. Whereas clinical geneticists have adhered rather rigidly to the principle of patient confidentiality, a relatively simple example will illustrate the challenge to this principle in medical practice.

A mother is diagnosed as a carrier of a mutant, X-linked gene causing deficiency of Factor VIII protein (hemophilia) through an affected son. The mother's sisters must then be considered at increased risk for having sons with hemophilia. If it can be established that they indeed are carriers, they have a 50% chance of also having affected sons (and carrier daughters like themselves). The accepted standard of care in clinical genetics is to limit genetic counseling to the mother about the potential benefits of informing her female siblings, for example, for purposes of prevention and family planning. The clinical geneticist is not expected to inform relatives of their potential reproductive risk as carriers of a mutant gene, even if the proband (in this case, the mother with the hemophiliac son) adamantly refuses to notify her at-risk siblings.

Does this case meet one of the three circumstances where patient confidentiality in a related medical setting has been previously breached—namely, a clear-cut danger to others, in this instance the mother's sisters and their offspring? Does the gene mutation for hemophilia in this family meet this criterion? A majority of clinical geneticists would not agree to this proposition, arguing that the patient's refusal to notify siblings should be respected despite nondirective counseling about the risk of occurrence and recurrence in specified relatives. The overriding responsibility of the clinical geneticist remains with the patient and not to any other family members and certainly not to society because of the public health effects of the mutant gene. Nevertheless, the question of whether a mutant gene present in one member of a family constitutes clear-cut danger to others in the family, thereby justifying warning family members regardless of a patient's preference, has not yet been answered satisfactorily. Arguments for a breach in confidentiality on ethical and moral grounds have been made,[3] but from the perspective of the clinical geneticist, such an approach would not only thoroughly undermine the patient-physician relationship but completely negate the basic approach and philosophy developed by clinical geneticists over the past four decades in the provision of patient services.

A number of legal cases in which physicians have been permitted to disclose otherwise confidential medical information could also be applied to the case of the mother carrying the gene mutation for hemophilia. To protect the health and safety of society (e.g., in cases of child abuse, gunshot wounds, and certain infectious diseases), it is considered a physician's duty to disclose what would otherwise be confidential information. A clinical geneticist might argue that there is a duty to inform female family members who also may be carrying the hemophilia gene mutation because their sister has an affected son. Can the argument be sustained that such a disclosure to potential carriers would be permissible in the legal system, even though it is not required under current practices in genetic clinics, because of a clear and present danger to their offspring? Evidence is now accumulating that when presented with the dilemma as to whether clinical geneticists have an obligation to inform relatives about their potential genetic risks, clinical geneticists, physicians in general practice, and patients themselves do not respond uniformly.

When health professionals (private practitioners, midwives, and residents) were interviewed concerning presymptomatic testing for Huntington disease, they were presented with a hypothetical situation involving the decision to breach confidentiality by informing an at-risk relative. A surprising 83% of health professionals felt that they should inform this relative even if the patient requested privacy.[4] When geneticists were presented with similar scenarios involving third-party disclosures, 32% said that they would maintain confidentiality, 34% would tell if asked, and 24% would tell even if not asked.[5] And when patients were queried about third-party disclosures in regard to Huntington disease, 65% believed that physicians should maintain patient confidentiality despite inquiries by at-risk individuals, whereas 22% believed that physicians should inform at-risk individuals only if specifically asked, and only 8% stated that physicians should seek out relatives at risk and inform them of their chances of carrying the mutant gene for the disease.[6]

The paradox is that although patients, physicians, and clinical geneticists operate on the premise that medical and personal information should be kept confidential and private, a significant proportion of each group appears willing to violate that privacy when presented with specific examples.

Is this willingness to breach confidentiality based on understanding of the serious implications of many genetic disorders and placing primacy on the concept of genetic danger to others? Or is such willingness based on failure to understand the implications and consequences of such a violation? If strict nondisclosure without patient consent fosters patient autonomy and self-determination while maintaining the professional integrity of the patient-physician relationship, how much of this distinctive ethos can the clinical geneticist afford to preserve in response to the remarkable advancements in genetic knowledge and DNA technology, products of the Human Genome Project? Have the rules of the game really changed because of these advancements?

Because genetic information is particularly sensitive and highly personal, protection of genetic privacy is warranted now and in the future.[7] The potentially volatile hazards of disclosure to third parties, whatever their relationship to the patient, are several and have been previously described. These include stigmatization and possible family ostracization; discrimination in school, the workplace, insurance coverage, the courts, and such daily activities as obtaining a loan.[8] Because genetic disorders are transmitted from parent to offspring, it is not surprising that privacy is sought as protection from familial and societal isolation as well as from a sense of unworthiness and inadequacy. Nor is it surprising that being publicly identified as a carrier of a disease-causing gene or being affected by a genetic disorder is frequently associated with withdrawal, depression, anger, and loss of integrity and self-esteem.

Both patients and physicians, including clinical geneticists, appear unaware of or unwilling to recognize the potentially catastrophic consequences of failing to maintain strict confidentiality when confronted with specific clinical genetic problems. For example, in a clinical study in which researchers attempted to define the gene for familial amyotrophic lateral sclerosis (ALS), confidentiality was not a concern to the overwhelming majority of participants and their married partners: only 8% expressed fear about disclosure to other family members.[9] Only 17% were concerned that participation in a study identifying whether they carried the mutant gene for ALS would adversely affect their health insurance coverage or that of their family.[10]

Concern about the sharing of personal patient information among clinical geneticists and genetic counselors has been minimal, but this possibility has not been formally investigated by any of the organizations of genetics professionals. Clinical geneticists have generally sought on a case-by-case basis to protect their patients from the societal and family stigmatization associated with being a carrier of a disease-causing allele or actually being affected by a genetic disorder. It is not unusual for many clinical geneticists to accede to the wishes of their patients in such situations. They will, for example, forgo submitting to insurance companies charges related to clinical evaluations, diagnoses, or laboratory analyses because they along with their patients mistrust the motives and intentions of organized medicine, employers, and insurance companies. Yet clinical geneticists put themselves at legal risk in concealing medical information, genetic or otherwise, including the potential for lawsuits initiated by the insured whom they were originally trying to protect.[11]

Because clinical genetics evolved apart from mainstream medical practice, the patient-physician relationship developed in a manner that is distinctive for its focus on patients' rights of autonomy, confidentiality, and nonjudgmental counseling. Medical genetics was recognized as a medical specialty by the American Medical Association (AMA) only in 1995, and the AMA determines and approves schedules for medical services and fees through Current Procedural Terminology (CPT) codes. In response to forces in the marketplace, medical geneticists formed the American College of Medical Genetics in conjunction with joining the AMA. Therefore, until the American College of Medical Genetics formally becomes part of the AMA, CPT codes for genetic services, including both clinical evaluation and laboratory tests, will continue to be established and fees set by nongeneticists.

THE FUTURE OF CLINICAL GENETICS

Three developments are likely to become serious hazards to maintaining patient confidentiality in the future. The first, beyond the control of the genetic establishment, relates to the "information highway." The second hazard is germane to the field of molecular medicine itself, a product of recombinant DNA technology. And the third hazard to patient confidentiality arises as a consequence of the rapid changes in health care delivery systems in the United States, specifically the role of physicians (including clinical geneticists) in managed care programs of HMOs (health maintenance organizations).

The sensitive nature of genetic information obtained from patients by clinical geneticists is recognized throughout the West, but the level and kind of protection of confidentiality varies from country to country. In the United States, privacy is not well protected in spite of laws protecting medical confidentiality in many states. Developments in information technology have markedly increased the likelihood that confidential information can be breached not only in the case of individual patients and families but at a broad societal level.[12] Past concerns about confidential information being overheard in hospital elevators and the selling of newborns' names to vendors of infant products seem petty when compared to the enormous potential for misuse through electronic communications and databases with enormous storage and retrieval capacities.

Given the public's general mistrust of institutions, patients and clinical geneticists may share a common sense of helplessness when confidential information is actively sought by either private or governmental agencies. The following developments well illustrate this sense of helplessness. First, individual medical records containing highly sensitive personal information are increasingly being gathered and stored in commercial data banks supported by hospital networks, HMOs, insurance companies, employers, public health agencies, researchers, and drug companies. Second, private medical information can be bought, sold, and transferred freely across state lines without patients' knowledge or consent simply by ignoring state laws. Third, only 28 states offer any rights to medical privacy, violations are difficult to monitor, and there is minimal remediation.[13] No federal law explicitly protects the confidentiality of a patient's medical record. In attempting to establish uniform federal rules for the use and disclosure of health information, congressional committees have been criticized concerning who may examine health records and under what circumstances they may do so. Public interest groups continue to claim that patient protection has yet to be achieved and that existing as well as proposed legislation actually both makes it easier for large computer, data bank, and telecommunications corporations to set up databases of medical records and in fact may authorize law enforcement agencies as well as health authorities and medical researchers to delve into patients' records without their consent.

Clinical geneticists have always had the responsibility of informing patients, in advance of providing genetic services, how their confidentiality would be protected. Developments in computer technology have made it urgent that a medical geneticist who assesses any patient's genetic risk, either of acquiring a genetic disease or of being at increased reproductive risk for affected offspring, must clearly enunciate each of the following: what kind of genetic information will be obtained and from whom; what genetic information will be recorded and in what form; who will have access to genetic information and under what conditions; and, finally, for what length of time will genetic information be retained and in what manner will it be disposed. There is currently no standardized approach to meet these responsibilities. In almost all cases when clinical genetic services are being provided, assurances that patients have control over the genetic information generated about themselves, when offered, are part of the verbal exchanges between patients and medical geneticists and are not recorded. At best, assurances about confidentiality are given piecemeal in most clinical settings, usually in response to a need to address an issue involving confidentiality. Interestingly enough, if similar genetic information is collected under a clinical research protocol, most institutional review boards require that each of these important aspects relating to confidentiality be considered and documented not only in the research proposal but in any consent form presented to prospective participants.

If clinical geneticists collect sensitive medical and personal genetic information, it would seem obvious that they have the responsibility of protecting that information from disclosure to third parties who are not part of the patient-physician contract and relationship. If clinical geneticists are counselors and advocates for patients, is it not their role as "ombudsman" to protect against genetic discrimination of any sort and in any setting? If clinical geneticists provide nondirective genetic counseling in discussing genetic alternatives and choices, should they guide and inform patients concerning issues of confidentiality and the possible consequences when confidentiality is not maintained? Is it not appropriate for clinical geneticists to discuss the possibilities of discrimination based on clinical findings, family history, and DNA testing? Is it not appropriate for clinical geneticists to inform patients about discrimination based on information to, and about, their relatives on their health status both present and future or on the health status of their offspring? Ultimately, is it not the role and responsibility of clinical geneticists to manage the medical care of patients with genetic disorders as effectively as possible? Most clinical geneticists would respond affirmatively to each question, yet these responsibilities and roles are being actively challenged because of changes in the practice of medicine.

Further, if the clinical geneticist identifies himself or herself as "ombudsman," is it then not appropriate for the geneticist to be the advocate of the patient in regard to such nonmedical matters as insurance and employment?[14] Does patient advocacy extend to anonymous testing, the keeping of separate medical charts apart from hospital charts so that they are not accessible to third-party payers, encouraging billing for patient services only in cash, or advising patients on strategies to obtain the maximum insurance coverage before genetic testing results are known? If there are no legal restrictions to the consequences of such advocacy, are there moral or ethical limits to such advocacy? Again, to each of these questions most clinical geneticists would answer in the affirmative, and precedence in regard to physician involvement with nongenetic diseases, for example, in the context of HIV testing, would support such an approach.[15]

Since the formal introduction of clinical genetics into medical practice nearly half a century ago, patients' genetic charts have been kept separate from standard hospital charts throughout the United States on the grounds that the information contained in them is the property of the patient alone and therefore that no other person or agency should have access to this information unless the patient so approves. In the context of patient-geneticist relationships, this practice is the quintessential expression of privacy and confidentiality and does not force the clinical geneticist to engage in misleading, deceptive, or fraudulent practices or to compromise the integrity of the genetic information.

And yet, is it morally and ethically justifiable for clinical geneticists to advise, even encourage, patients at considerable risk of developing a genetic disorder to secure maximum health and life insurance before genetic testing results are known? The rationale for such advice would be to permit the patient to obtain insurance coverage before such insurance would likely become unavailable or prohibitively expensive. Accordingly, it has been concluded that in the present U.S. health care system, the clinical geneticist would be "aiding and abetting the commission of fraud" by misleading the insurer.[16] Moreover, it can be argued that it is morally and ethically unjustifiable for relatives to benefit financially from life insurance benefits accrued because an insured family member has a fatal genetic disease. In the case of genetic disease, however, the question is whether health insurance and medical care are considered inalienable rights of the entire citizenry or limited to those for whom risk-taking on the part of insurance underwriters is minimized in order to maximize profits. Although most Western societies consider health insurance and comprehensive medical care to be inalienable rights, in the United States private health insurance plays a crucial role in health care access, thus creating the foundation for ethical and moral conflicts between the patient and clinical geneticist and the health care system.

One expected outcome of the Human Genome Project is that the playing field in health care will be leveled—that is, as a direct result of being able to sequence the entire human genome, it will be determined that every individual, hence every family, carries multiple gene mutations that place them and their offspring at risk for developing a spectrum of disorders. Another anticipated outcome of the Human Genome Project is the development of a multiplicity of highly expensive gene therapies to prevent and ameliorate the clinical expression of such disease-causing mutations. These two consequences of the Human Genome Project will lead either to a plethora of abstruse insurance policies or the eventual realization that reliance on the private sector for health care is no longer viable or acceptable. In short, from the standpoint of the clinical geneticist who serves as patient advocate, the current health and life insurance industries in the United States will have to be eliminated as unnecessary and counterproductive to the welfare of society and its members. Indeed, as the provision of health care shifts its focus from the individual toward a larger societal perspective, the clinical geneticist will face enormous challenges to maintain patient confidentiality and privacy.

A second challenge to patient confidentiality relates to the nature and type of genetic information generated through application of recombinant DNA technology to the human genome. A primary goal of the Human Genome Project is to sequence, by the year 2005, the 3 billion base pairs that constitute the 50,000–100,000 active genes of the human complement. This sequencing of human DNA is only a first step. Knowledge of the sequences of DNA that comprise the human genome will permit decoding the DNA message of each of the 50,000–100,000 human genes and, in turn, defining the primary structure of each protein specified by these genes. However, knowledge of the particular arrangement of these 3 billion base pairs may not necessarily provide insight as to how these genes function at the cellular level; this is critical if medical geneticists are to understand how gene mutations disturb normal biological processes. When and how human genes express themselves is a major focus in medical genetics, starting with studies of embryonic gene expression—that is, how does a human being come into being, and encompassing the effects of genes expressed throughout a person's lifetime. It is the nature of this gene expression that holds great risk to confidentiality and privacy, to insurability and employment, and to sense of self and family.

Recombinant DNA technology was until recently applied principally to Mendelian disorders. Mendelian disorders are caused by single gene mutations and are characterized by well-defined patterns of inheritance and, often, well-defined clinical effects that are not significantly influenced by the environment. Diseases such as sickle-cell anemia, Duchenne muscular dystrophy, and Tay Sachs disease, for example, were the first of a series of Mendelian disorders to be defined at the molecular level using the recombinant DNA technologies of cloning and gene sequencing. In the past decade, the application of recombinant DNA technologies has resulted in the molecular definition of hundreds of different genetic diseases in humans, for example, such hemoglobinopathies as thalassemia and hemophilia, such neurological disorders as Huntington disease and Alzheimer's disease, and such skeletal dysplasias as achondroplasia and Marfan syndrome. Two relatively new areas of genetic research have come to the attention of the general public and medical practitioners, for which clinical geneticists have yet to develop effective counseling strategies and for which issues about confidentiality will certainly exceed current concerns about discrimination, insurability, employability, and stigmatization following unauthorized disclosure to third parties.[17]

The first of these new areas of genetic research involves identifying genes predisposing to cancer and its clinical consequence, presymptomatic testing for cancer. Cancer is now widely held to be a genetic disease. Breast cancer can serve as a model, in which at least four different gene mutations have already been identified as associated with an increased propensity to develop malignancies of the breast, BRCA1 (breast cancer 1 gene), BRCA2, p53 (associated with various cancers), and the gene for ataxia telangiectasia in the heterozygous state. It is estimated that 5–10% of all breast cancers occur as a consequence of germline mutations (passed from parent to offspring), whereas the remainder occur as a consequence of somatic mutations (limited to tissues of the body, e.g., the breast). Whether the mutation is germinal or somatic, the molecular events leading from gene mutation to tissue pathology appear to be the same. Presymptomatic testing is estimated to become available soon for healthy persons where there is a concern for heritable forms of breast cancer.

The ability to identify carriers of mutated genes that predispose toward the development of breast cancer may at first appear to raise no new problems in confidentiality or privacy but rather variations on existing concerns in providing clinical genetic services and counseling. The clinical geneticist's obligations would still be exclusively to his or her patient, acting in the patient's best interest while respecting the patient's rights. This model of clinical practice of medicine continues to dictate nondisclosure to other family members unless the patient explicitly permits it, even if disclosure of the information is clearly in the best interest of relatives. This approach prevents the possible invasion of privacy and the elimination of free choice concerning information about one's future, the right not to know.

If all this fits the clinical geneticist's practice model, will it continue to be morally acceptable for the geneticist to withhold valuable information that would likely benefit others? Is it not a moral, and even a medical, duty to warn other family members? The identification of a breast cancer mutation in a patient clearly marks other family members as being at considerable risk. Such knowledge markedly increases the ability of carriers of a breast cancer mutation to make health-promoting lifestyle choices and to take steps to prevent the onset of the disease; if breast cancer does develop, early intervention and treatment is clearly advantageous with regard to clinical management and prognosis. A patient may nonetheless object strenuously to revealing this type of information to relatives, and unless clinical geneticists are willing (or mandated) to switch to a public health model of medicine—that is, justifying the breaching confidentiality because of probable harm resulting from nondisclosure—a patient's genetic information must continue to be held in strictest confidence.

As the practice and funding of medical care continues its rapid change, government and private insurance agencies will increasingly pressure clinical geneticists to alter their prevailing practice to that of a public health model. If this happens, the clinical geneticist–patient relationship will be disrupted, and the obvious concerns about insurability, job tenure and employment opportunities, stigmatization, and other negative consequences attendant to disclosure will increase.

BEHAVIORAL GENETICS

A more sinister consequence of the application of recombinant DNA technology relates to mapping genes for human personality, genes that predispose people to such complex behavioral traits as aggression, alcoholism, or drug abuse, and even toward novelty seeking, impulsivity, or thrill seeking as one of four temperaments (the others being persistence, avoidance of harm, and "reward dependence").[18] Brian Gladue of the Institute of Policy Research at the University of Cincinnati has termed this new field "molecular personality research." While newspaper editors and the media conjure up engaging titles describing research about genetic predisposition and genetic determinism (e.g., "At the Mercy of Our Genes" and "Is a Gene Making You Read This?"), health professionals are becoming increasingly critical of scientific studies that link genes to behavior. In addition to the conventional fears about stigmatization and discrimination, there is an even greater concern that a science based on molecular personality will lead to interventions based on a public health model—"soothe an impulsive personality, quell a rapist's tendencies or dull an alcoholic's cravings."[19]

What are the implications of studies on genes that may control aggression and intelligence, particularly with regard to potential abuses of patient confidentiality? Will the field of medical genetics expand to encompass personality disorders? If so, will information about alleles that predispose an individual toward a set of antisocial behaviors be treated as personal and confidential, or will the social implications of these studies encourage society to use such information as a basis for treating personality and behavioral disorders? The dilemma is the unresolved conflict between the ultimate good attributable to all knowledge and knowledge that can only be abused. Will a clinical geneticist be able to protect a patient's confidentiality as genetic testing for personality traits progresses in conjunction with the Human Genome Project?

MANAGED CARE

In an editorial entitled "Extreme Risk—The New Corporate Proposition for Physicians," Steffie Woolhandler and David Himmelstein of Cambridge Hospital in Cambridge, Massachusetts, portray HMOs as routinely limiting a physician's ability to talk freely with patients concerning treatment options that the HMO will not approve and the HMO's payment policies, including the awarding of bonuses for saving money by withholding care.[20] In their contracts with physicians, an increasing number of managed care organizations have what are termed, ironically enough, "confidential" clauses (frequently denigrated as "gag" rules). HMOs deny that these confidentiality clauses override the patient-physician relationship and assurances of confidentiality, but they have come under heavy criticism for imposing these rules on conversations between physician and patient and have even been accused of terminating physicians who tell their patients too much about diagnostic or treatment options. One AMA trustee believes that physicians are "ethically bound" to ignore contract clauses that limit their ability to share information with patients about relevant diagnostic tests and the full range of appropriate treatments.[21] In a recent notice to physicians employed by a nationally prominent HMO, physicians were directed not to discuss proposed treatments with patients before they received authorization from an outside company that sets guidelines for the treatment of patients, nor were they to discuss the authorization procedure. Such an approach would profoundly disturb the relationship between the patient and the clinical geneticist.

CONCLUSION

The current status of patient-physician relationships in clinical genetics is encountering significant challenges. The traditional client-centered approach, stressing patient confidentiality and counseling in a nondirective fashion, will increasingly confront the possibility of a shift to a public health model rationalized in terms of reducing health costs to society and based on genetic information generated from the Human Genome Project. Clinical geneticists will need to face the likelihood that patients will realize that a product of the "information highway" is the virtual loss of all medical privacy and as possible consequences, the loss of insurance coverage, employment opportunities, and credit. Clinical geneticists will also have to realize that as the populace continues to shift from individual health care providers to managed care companies, clinical geneticists' behavior will be regulated and monitored in ways similar to those of other health providers who work in the corporate medicine system. These dangers to the integrity of the patient-physician relationship based upon confidentiality and nondisclosure are real, and it is tenuous at best whether the U.S. legal system is willing to protect this relationship.

NOTES

1. Eric T. Juengst, "The Ethics of Prediction: Genetic Risk and the Physician-Patient Relationship," *Genome Science and Technology* 1 (1995): 21–36.
2. Ibid.
3. Marlene Huggins et al., "Ethical and Legal Dilemmas Arising During Predictive Testing for Adult-onset Disease: The Experience of Huntington's Disease," *American Journal of Human Genetics* 47 (1990): 4–12; M. Yarborough, J. Scott, and L. Dixon, "The Role of Beneficence in Clinical Genetics: Non-Directive Counseling Reconsidered," *Theoretical Medicine* 10 (1989): 139–49; Karen H. Rothenberg and Elizabeth Thomson, *Women and Prenatal Testing: Facing the Challenge of Genetic Technologies* (Columbus: Ohio State University Press, 1995).
4. S. A. Cummings, "DNA Testing: A Comparison of Opinions Between the Public and Health Care Providers" (M.S. thesis, Northwestern University, 1995).
5. Dorothy C. Wertz and John C. Fletcher, "Ethics and Medical Genetics in the United States," *American Journal of Medical Genetics* 29 (1988): 815–27.
6. Cummings, "DNA Testing."
7. Lori B. Andrews, "Genetic Privacy: From the Laboratory to the Legislature," *Genome Research* 5 (1995): 209–13.
8. Ibid.
9. J. L. Miller, "Participation in Human Genetic Research: The Subject's Viewpoint" (M.S. thesis, Northwestern University, 1995).
10. Ibid.
11. Ad Hoc Committee on Genetic Testing/Insurance Issues, "Genetic Testing and Insurance: A Background Statement," *American Journal of Human Genetics* 56 (1995): 327–31.
12. Jerome P. Kassirer, "The Next Transformation in the Delivery of Health Care," *New England Journal of Medicine* 332 (1995): 52–53; Beverly Woodward, "The Computer-based Patient Record and Confidentiality," ibid. 333 (1995): 1419–22.
13. C. Jouzaitis, "Americans Losing Medical Privacy; Data Banks Blamed," *Chicago Tribune,* Dec. 31, 1995.
14. Mark A. Rothstein, "Genetics, Insurance, and the Ethics of Genetic Counseling," *Molecular Genetic Medicine* 3 (1993): 159–77; Mark A. Rothstein, "The Use of Genetic Information for Nonmedical Purposes," *Journal of Law and Health* 9 (1994–95): 109–20.
15. Rothstein, "Genetics, Insurance."
16. Ibid.
17. Philip R. Reilly, "ASHG Statement on Genetics and Privacy: Testimony to United States Congress," *American Journal of Human Genetics* 50 (1992): 640–42.

18. J. Benjamin et al., "Population and Familial Association Between the D4 Dopamine Receptor Gene and Measures of Novelty Seeking," *Nature Genetics* 12 (1996): 81–84; R. P. Epstein et al., "Dopamine D4 Receptor (D4DR) Exon III Polymorphism Associated with the Human Personality Trait of Novelty Seeking," *Nature Genetics* 12 (1996): 78–80.

19. C. Siebert, "At the Mercy of Our Genes," *New York Times,* Jan. 5, 1996; Gina Kolata, "Is a Gene Making You Read This?" ibid., Jan. 7, 1996 (quotation).

20. Steffie Woolhandler and David Himmelstein, "Extreme Risk—The New Corporate Proposition for Physicians," *New England Journal of Medicine* 333 (1995): 1706–7.

21. D. Levy, "Docs Urged to Ignore 'Gag Rules,'" *USA Today,* Dec. 27, 1995.

Chapter 6 Privacy in Genetic Counseling

Barbara Bowles Biesecker

The individual's sense of identity and continuity is formed not only by the significant attachments in his [or] her intimate environment but also is deeply rooted in the biological family—in the genetic link that reaches into the past and ahead into the future.

Genetic counseling is a short-term psychotherapeutic relationship that incorporates the transmission of genetic information. As in any medical or psychotherapeutic relationship, the protection of the client's privacy is paramount to its success. The counselor has a fundamental responsibility to maintain the confidentiality of all information that is obtained or disclosed during the counseling process. This obligation includes protecting the client from inadvertent and intentional loss of privacy. Certain aspects of genetic counseling create obstacles to protecting privacy, including counseling entire families. Changes in health care delivery and an onslaught of new genetic tests will further challenge the protection of client privacy as aspects of genetic counseling move into mainstream medical practice.

Through genetic counseling clients come to understand the genetic contribution to a condition present in their family. Genetic counselors assist clients in making a decision about a genetic test or about a reproductive option. They may also help clients adjust to, or cope with, a child with special needs. In 1975, the American Society of Human Genetics adopted this definition of genetic counseling written by an ad hoc committee:

> Genetic counseling is a communication process which deals with the human prob-lems associated with the occurrence, or the risk of occurrence, of a genetic disorder in a family. This process involves an attempt by one or more appropriately trained persons to help the individual or family to 1. comprehend the medical facts, includ-ing the diagnosis, probable course of the disorder, and the available management; 2. appreciate the way heredity contributes to the disorder, and the risk of recurrence in specified relatives; 3. understand the alternatives for dealing with the risk of recurrence; 4. choose the course of action which seems to them appropriate in view of their risk, their family goals, and their ethical and religious standards, and to act in accordance with that decision; and 5. to make the best possible adjustment to the disorder in an affected family member and/or to the risk of recurrence of that disorder.[1]

This definition emphasizes the client's understanding of the genetic informa-tion and choice of an appropriate course of action. Other descriptions of genetic counseling have expanded the educational component to include the theory and practice of clinical psychology.[2] These comprehensive descriptions acknowledge the emotional obstacles clients face in assimilating new and anxi-ety-provoking information and the complexities of reproductive decision mak-ing. Broader descriptions also acknowledge the grief, shame, and guilt that genetic information may unleash. It is time for genetic counselors to develop a newer, more complete definition of genetic counseling that encompasses more fully the psychotherapeutic aspects of the counselor-client relationship.

The communication of risk information is a fundamental goal within the educational component of genetic counseling, yet in isolation it is insufficient to meet clients' needs.[3] Counselors report that persons in families affected by genetic conditions perceive genetic information as more personal, revealing, and stigmatizing than other medical information.[4] The client's experiences and perceived burden of risk dramatically affects his or her decisions, and the emotionally laden information often inhibits comprehension.[5] Those who seek to understand the contribution of heredity to a condition in their family do so in the context of other elements in their lives. Nongenetic issues thus become as critical as genetic information. A case of prenatal genetic counseling for amniocentesis, a procedure that should not be considered routine for any pregnant woman, highlights these issues.

If a woman is of advanced age for childbearing and is presented with the option of amniocentesis, she may seek to understand her chances for having a baby with Down syndrome. She may explore what life is like for a person affected with Down syndrome, available economic and social resources, her beliefs about abortion, her fertility, her desire to have more children, risks for other conditions, effects on siblings, the opinions of her family and friends, and so on. Genetic counseling for prenatal diagnosis is not limited to the recital of chromosome misdivision and risk statistics. It involves the communication and assistance that allow an individual or couple to make the best decision for themselves about an optional genetic test. The counselor explores the client's circumstance, values, and desires to help her to make an informed and autonomous decision about prenatal testing.

In this example, however, the decision about prenatal diagnosis involves the contributions of loved ones, friends, health care providers, cultural norms, and societal pressures, and so it is not entirely autonomous. In prenatal decision-making it is critical that professionals and the larger community of employers and insurers not dictate which pregnancies undergo testing or result in termination. Genetic counseling is therefore based on the principle of respect for autonomy rather than the paternalism of professional advice or recommendation. This respect for autonomy extends beyond making reproductive or testing decisions. It includes clients' ability to maintain control over information about their life and relationships and the privilege of secrecy.

Clients may seek genetic counseling services preconceptually, during pregnancy, after childbirth, and during adulthood. The informational content and priorities of genetic counseling sessions vary tremendously. Yet several basic moral tenets of genetic counseling remain relatively constant. These include respect for the cultural and social background of the client, voluntariness, autonomy, nondirectiveness, and confidentiality.[6]

RESPECT FOR CLIENTS' SOCIAL AND CULTURAL BACKGROUND

Genetic counselors have recognized for some time that their values may not be identical to those of their clients. A client-centered approach to counseling and an ethical framework that focuses on the relationship between the counselor and the client provides the basis for a nonjudgmental and supportive counseling relationship. This relationship requires that counselors are sensitive to their client's needs, health and spiritual beliefs, and cultural norms. Because most genetic counselors in the United States are Caucasian females, this often presents challenges. The National Society of Genetic Counselors (NSGC) recognizes the need for diversity in recruiting counselors into the field. Efforts are also under way to introduce greater cultural diversity into the psychological counseling training of counselors. Although counselors learn to adjust their practice to the educational and social background of their clients, improvement in this area is needed.[7]

VOLUNTARINESS

Voluntariness in genetic counseling is as central to good practice as it is in other types of psychotherapeutic relationships. Clients are unlikely to benefit from counseling if they are not seeking genetic understanding and support of their own will. No one can be mandated to be educated or counseled. Clients may discontinue the relationship at any time. Further, within the counseling process, voluntary disclosure of private information is within the client's purview. Clients are free to choose not to disclose private information or secrets as they desire. The accuracy of the information provided by the genetic counselor, however, thus depends on the truthfulness, knowledge, and disclosure of clients, as well as on medical records and physical examination. This needs to be understood by clients who may be weighing the costs involved in disclosing hidden information. The voluntariness so central to the process supports the important need for privacy.

CLIENT AUTONOMY AND NONDIRECTIVENESS

The practice of individualized counseling and the preservation of client autonomy (nondirectiveness) are the central dogmas of genetic counseling.[8] *Nondirectiveness* is a term appropriated from the clinical psychologist Carl Rogers, who coined it in 1942 to describe the therapeutic approach of not judging, advising, or guiding a client.[9] Rogers came to recognize, however, that his mere presence in the counseling relationship had directive components. He later modified his approach, terming it *client-centered,* referring to an unconditional acceptance and regard for the client.[10] In spite of these advances, the term *nondirectiveness* has persisted in genetic counseling, though not without controversy. Several scholars have pointed out the impracticability of nondirectiveness.[11] Confusion has been spurred by the use of the term *value neutrality* to describe nondirectiveness. All human therapeutic relationships are value-laden. It is counterintuitive to suggest that genetic counseling could ever be value-neutral. All counselors have biases and values. Those inherent to genetic counseling include the expectation that most clients can make decisions for themselves and can adjust to life-altering information. Clients are valued as able individuals striving to make sense of their lives in the face of genetic risk. Counselors acknowledge that their values may differ from those of their clients and thus strive to practice in a compassionate, supportive, and nonjudgmental manner. This is not, however, synonymous with the concept of value neutrality.

Further confusion has been generated by using nondirectiveness to mean not directing clients toward a certain reproductive outcome (specifically, non-eugenic practices). Rogers's client-centered approach provides a good working framework for the nonjudgmental stance of genetic counselors. True client-centered counseling does not involve imposing a professional bias toward certain reproductive outcomes and supports the avoidance of eugenic practices. It may help to clarify professional responsibilities by replacing the term *nondirectiveness* with *client-centered* in genetic counseling literature. Client-centered psychotherapy focuses on clients making the best decisions for themselves in light of their values and needs and allows for aspects that may be directive. The optional nature of most genetic tests and reproductive options coheres with a client-centered approach to genetic counseling. If there is no recommendation or "right" answer whether to undergo a genetic test or to have children, then the counseling interaction represents an opportunity to explore the options with a client. In doing so, trust and rapport are established with the counselor and private information is volunteered in confidence.

CONFIDENTIALITY

Genetic counseling strives to address clients' concerns about the inheritance of a condition in the family. In this process, highly intimate information may be disclosed. Assessing potential genetic risks commonly involves reviewing medical records, collecting family history (both biological and social), and undergoing physical examination or genetic testing of some type. In addition, discussion of matters of self, family, health, childbearing, employment, and economic and social resources may transpire. These activities require that clients relinquish information that they may consider to be private. In spite of this disclosure, clients expect to retain some control over the information that is discussed. This is true regardless of whether the counseling is provided primarily for diagnostic or psychotherapeutic purposes.

A client's innermost thoughts, emotions, and fantasies may be disclosed during the exploration of the impact of a genetic condition. The genetic counseling relationship is built on trust. Without the inherent promise that such intimacies will remain private, the therapeutic process would be thwarted. Clients rightly expect that their information will remain between the counselor and client and that their records will be protected from access by others. Only on rare occasions would a counselor be morally or legally justified in breaching confidentiality. Confidentiality is thus integral to the success of genetic counseling.

GENETIC COUNSELING PROFESSIONALS

Genetic counseling is provided by a master's level–trained counselor, a clinical geneticist, or by a team of genetics providers. Professional roles may overlap, but an important difference is that clinical geneticists make medical diagnoses. Master's level–trained counselors and clinical nurse specialists in genetics, in most cases, provide information about risks and short-term psychotherapeutic counseling. The training of these professionals includes awareness of the sensitive nature of genetic information and the importance of protecting the client's privacy.

The National Society of Genetic Counselors (NSGC) has more than 1,200 master's level–trained counselors.[12] A further 120 clinical nurse specialists comprise the International Society of Nurses in Genetics (ISONG).[13] The field of genetic counseling has remained small and focused primarily on prenatal diagnosis. In adult and pediatric settings discussions revolve around relatively esoteric or rare conditions. The field is presented with important challenges to expand in new directions. As the Human Genome Project expands genetic research, increasing numbers of genetic tests will diffuse into general medical practice. The disorders for which testing will become available include common diseases of complex origin, such as cancer, diabetes, and heart disease. This suggests that many more individuals in the general population will be aware of genetic testing and possible predisposition to disease and may seek genetic education and counseling.

The small and relatively new profession of genetic counseling is insufficient to meet the current needs for counseling services in the United States.[14] As more genetic tests arise and a larger portion of the population is genetically aware, primary care providers will provide certain aspects of genetic counseling services. There is reason to be concerned that the movement into clinical medicine will increase the opportunities for loss of privacy of genetic information. For example, there will be greater access by insurers and managed care administrators as more genetic testing information is entered into clinical charts. Also, more professionals involved with the client will have access to the information, as was demonstrated for an Institute of Medicine Committee on Privacy.[15] There is an urgent need for primary care providers to be educated about the sensitive and potent genetic information they will increasingly have access to and particularly how it differs from other medical information.

GUIDELINES FOR PROTECTING PRIVACY

In 1992 the NSGC adopted a code of ethics to guide its members' conduct. The code addresses counselors' responsibilities toward their clients' privacy: "The counselor-client relationship is based on values of care and respect for the client's autonomy, individuality, welfare and freedom. The primary concern of genetic counselors is the interests of their clients. Therefore, genetic counselors strive to maintain as confidential any information received from clients, unless released by the client."[16] Although this guideline addresses protection over the release of information, it should be interpreted broadly. Interpretation should include genetic counselors' responsibility to protect the privacy of: DNA samples obtained from their clients, medical records, intimate relationships, client secrets, and activities (such as research endeavors) in which clients may choose to be anonymous.

The Institute of Medicine Committee on Assessing Genetic Risks endorsed a similar NSGC policy statement on the confidentiality of test results. The committee concluded that the genetic counselor, as a messenger of devastating or discriminatory information, must honor the patient's desire and expectation for privacy except under rare circumstances when a breach of confidentiality may be necessary to avert serious harm. The committee recommended that any potential for disclosure of private information should be anticipated by the counselor and thus addressed with the client before services are rendered. On a broader scale, the committee recommended that codes of ethics of other professionals providing genetic services contain specific provisions to protect autonomy, privacy, and confidentiality.[17]

Genetic counselors are not licensed professionals. But they may be certified by the American Board of Genetic Counseling. This credentialing body strives to maintain a high standard of practice by requiring that counselors complete an accredited graduate program and participate in a broad range of clinical cases. Certification helps to ensure that counselors are trained to anticipate potential obstacles to the protection of privacy. Legal liability issues in the area of breach of confidentiality are uncertain for this new profession. A review of the history of litigation in mental health services would suggest that courts would not endorse a breach unless risk of serious harm to a third party could be shown unequivocally.[18]

OBSTACLES TO MAINTAINING CONFIDENTIALITY

Although genetic counselors aspire to protect the privacy of their clients in a manner similar to other psychotherapeutic professionals, unique situations in genetic counseling present peculiar challenges. The client in genetic counseling is often an entire family. Even if this is not the case at first, the counseling process may identify relatives at increased risk who later pursue services. Further, genetic information is potentially stigmatizing and can render clients vulnerable to employment or insurance discrimination. Discussion of genetic conditions or the risk for such conditions touches on issues of self-worth, self-identity, personal dignity, health, and vulnerability. Persons who view themselves at increased risk for disease or for having affected children because they carry a certain gene may have concerns about access to health or life insurance and about continuing or obtaining rewarding employment. The personal stigma and social risk for discrimination further substantiates the importance of maintaining confidentiality. The consequences of the loss of privacy of genetic information may be greater than that of other medical information.

Confidentiality may be infringed in two distinct ways: deliberate breach and inadvertent disclosure. Genetic counselors may be party to either. They may be responsible for a disclosure or involved with the consequences when a third party is responsible (including other family members, health care providers, insurers, and employers). Deliberate breach by genetic counselors is morally and legally justifiable only when averting serious harm to a third party. The risk of inadvertent disclosure is a risk of clinical practice, record keeping, and teaching and may be reduced by certain safeguards.

INADVERTENT INFRINGEMENT ON CONFIDENTIALITY

Although counselors' responsibilities are to honor their relationships with their clients, complicating factors may make the reality of protecting privacy difficult. The counselor's role includes the collection of family history. The process of collecting genetic information on the family requires extreme sensitivity. If a client is open and chooses to share private information with the counselor and a different family member seeks services from the same counselor but does not divulge similar information, the counselor must be careful not to disclose the information inadvertently. A counselor may learn that a particular family member is affected or at increased risk for a genetic condition through a relative. For instance, a counselor may wish to share a picture of the family history with a client in order to explain a mode of inheritance. If there is biological or medical information about others on the pedigree that the client does not know, use of the diagram would be a breach of confidentiality for the original client. Such an inadvertent mishap could result not only in a loss of professional trust but also in psychological harm if people learn undesired information. This is particularly true if the information affects a client's relationship with a relative. Counselors involved in family history collection have duties to protect the privacy of separate individuals whose lives are intertwined.

Genetic counselors may be involved in the collection of blood samples from several members of a family. (When a DNA test is performed using linkage analysis, samples from affected and unaffected relatives are required.) A family reunion may be scheduled and the counselor may be in the position of collecting private medical and family history information in the presence of other family members. Even when private counseling sessions are arranged, it may be difficult to conceal confidential information. If a family member prefers not to participate in the linkage analysis but requests that family members not be told, the counselor might have to tell the client (the person requesting the test) that the test cannot be performed without explaining why. Further, a family member who chooses to participate in order to make testing informative for a relative may choose not to learn his or her test result. The counselor must honor this request, even in circumstances when the status may easily be derived from other family members' results.

Genetic counselors have an obligation to consider who may have access to written documentation on a client and who else may create such information, thereby increasing the opportunity for loss of privacy. Counselors commonly put genetic information about relatives into their client's record. If the family members live near one another and have the same insurer, a loss of privacy may occur for the relative if the insurer obtains and reviews the client's chart. Genetic counselors also may share private information with other health care providers involved in the care of the same family. If that health care provider chooses to document the information in the patient's medical record, a loss of privacy could occur if it is not a disclosure the client authorized.

Because the client in genetic counseling may be an entire family, the counselor must maintain the ability to serve each family member responsibly. Relatives may be unable to receive services from a separate provider due to the esoteric subject matter and expertise of the counselor or simply because there are no other counselors in their geographical area. Should a loss of privacy occur, the remaining members of the family may feel that they have no genetic counselor they can trust or from whom they can obtain services. The voluntary nature of genetic counseling may be jeopardized, along with the professional integrity of the counselor.

A genetic counselor's inadvertent breach of privacy is illustrated in the following example: A family gathers to participate in genetic counseling about predictive genetic testing for breast cancer. Each family member undergoes individualized private counseling sessions to make a decision about testing. The timing of the sessions inadvertently reveals to those in the waiting room which family members have chosen to pursue predictive testing. Drawing blood adds 10–15 minutes to the length of the counseling sessions and "announces" the decision of the client to those in the waiting room.

At their clients' request, genetic counselors and nurses have been known to participate in subtle deceptions, such as placing a bandage on the arm of a family member who would like the family to think that he or she had a blood sample drawn. Such arrangements, if instituted thoughtfully, may minimize inadvertent professional disclosures. But without careful consideration on behalf of the counselors and nurses, even the circumstances surrounding a client visit can be an infringement on privacy.

Disclosure due to carelessness can occur if a counselor makes a note outside of the medical record and another health professional or insurer gains access to that information. Other examples of professional carelessness on behalf of counselors include discussing client information in a public place, presenting family history information at a seminar using proper names, or disclosing information to anyone who has no ethically justifiable reason to know it. These professional oversights should never occur.

Client confidentiality can be violated by a third party when other medical professionals discuss clients' circumstances in public; administrators involved in managed health care review and discuss private information or enter it into a database through which others may gain access; family members reveal one another's private information; other health care providers document genetic information about one person in the record of another (usually a family member); or an insurer obtains information the client did not request or was not given permission to obtain. Loss of privacy by a third party may happen simply as an accident or oversight. It can also occur from deliberate disclosures by others, such as family members or health care providers, who do not mean to cause harm but lack appreciation of the potency and privacy of the information they disclose.

The following is a common example of a case in which another professional inadvertently violates the privacy of a client's family. An oncologist who learns of a client's negative test results for a hereditary predisposition to breast cancer writes in good faith to the client's insurance carrier (at her request) announcing her negative test status to assist her in obtaining lower rates. The insurer might realize that other family members may have been tested. The insurer might assume that those who have not requested lower rates may have received positive test results and accordingly increase their premiums or drop them altogether. This is a serious infringement on the privacy of family members who tested positive. Further, the insurer may mistake those who chose not to be tested for those who tested positive and discriminate against them based on no reasonable information.

Further threats to confidentiality arise when a team of providers is involved or when the institution is a training center, because of the number of professionals and their trainees who have potential access to client information. In their excitement to learn a new field, trainees may discuss a case they participate in with their loved ones or fellow students. Although they can protect the identity of the client by disguising various facts, they may also reveal sufficient information for the client to be recognized. This is particularly true when a client is counseled for a rare disorder; in such cases the diagnosis and time of the visit alone can be enough to identify the client. Names may also be inadvertently left on family histories during teaching presentations or mentioned by trainees or their instructors. An important aspect in professional training of all providers involved in genetic counseling is maintaining the confidentiality of the counseling sessions.

BREACHES OF CONFIDENTIALITY

In rare instances a genetic counselor may purposefully breach confidentiality. This can be considered only in situations where it is indisputable that the withholding of confidential information would harm a third party. One such

area is when a breach of confidentiality would avert life-threatening consequences of a genetic condition in a client's relative.[19] Another justifiable case
would be if a client is basing life-threatening decisions on inaccurate assumptions about a risk or the lack of a risk. For instance, if a relative is unaware that
he or she is at increased risk for Huntington disease and has a job that involves
public safety (e.g., an airline pilot), the counselor may feel compelled to breach
the confidentiality of a client. Sufficient cause to justify a breach is rare. The
therapeutic nature of the relationship is at stake, as is the moral responsibility of
the counselor to the client. An unjustifiable breach would also render a genetic
counselor legally liable for any harm to the client that results.

COLLUSION IN DECEIT

Genetic counselors may be challenged morally and legally when they are asked
to collude in family deceit to protect a client's privacy when doing so would
amount to medical risk or insurance fraud. During genetic counseling sessions,
clients volunteer private information to facilitate the therapeutic process. In
discussing family and medical history information, clients may disclose secrets.
These secrets may bear on their genetic history and lead to inaccuracies in
estimating risk or a prognosis. Secrets may also be pertinent to a client's
emotional status, hence the success of the therapeutic relationship. Private
information discussed in genetic counseling ranges broadly from what is asked
of the client to what is unexpected (such as secrets) and may be considered
private to an even greater degree by the client. Such secrets raise issues of the
limits of protecting confidentiality, and the responsibilities to partners, parents,
children, and third parties who either do not know the information or from
whom it has been kept. The professional integrity of the counselor may be
jeopardized when clients ask counselors to collude in a deception that would
result in documenting inaccurate information or in misleading others. These
deceptions can involve misidentified biological relationships or secrets parents
harbor about their children.

SECRETS OF BIOLOGICAL RELATIONSHIPS

A classic ethical dilemma in genetic counseling is disclosure by a client of
misattributed paternity due to an adoption or infidelity. Risk estimates are
based on assumptions that biological relationships in the family are correct.
Thus a person's misunderstanding about his or her biological relationship to

other family members could determine whether he or she is at increased risk for an inherited condition. Beyond the estimates of genetic risks, secrets may also have psychological ramifications that are significant to the counseling relationship. Serious psychological issues may underlie a decision not to disclose an adoption. Incest or teenage pregnancy, for example, may have resulted in the child being adopted within an extended biological family. A child may have been protected from learning of his or her true parentage. Counselors face conflict when knowledge of an individual's actual biological identity would change the risk status of a family member and the client requests that the family member not be told.[20] In some cases, the disclosure of a family secret may cause harm even when the revealing of true biological relationships would not influence genetic risks. Based on the counseling interaction, the counselor may feel that the client or a family member would benefit from unveiling the secret. Psychotherapeutic techniques may be used to support the client's recognition of such benefits. Yet if the client chooses not to reveal the secret, the counselor is unlikely to breach the confidence. Participating in a delusion about paternity, however, raises an issue of professional integrity for the counselor.

These issues are raised in the following example: A young woman, a married Caucasian graduate student, seeks genetic counseling because of concerns about alcohol ingestion and its potential effects on her developing fetus. She is early into an unplanned pregnancy. She comes to the counseling session alone but describes herself as happily married with a very involved husband who is enthusiastic about the pregnancy even though it was unplanned. She has had several episodes of binge-drinking that she is concerned may have damaged the baby and is contemplating terminating the pregnancy. After carefully determining when she conceived the pregnancy, the counselor determines that she ingested the alcohol before implantation and so the fetus was not exposed. The counselor reassures the client that her baby is not at increased risk for any alcohol-related injury. A thorough family and medical history reveals no other risk factors to suggest the pregnancy is at any increased risk.

In spite of this information, the client demonstrates no relief. On the contrary, she becomes increasingly anxious. Further into the session, she tells the counselor that she had extramarital sex but does not want her husband to find out. She is interested in pursuing an abortion and wants to use potential damage to the fetus due to the alcohol use as the reason. She explains that this was a one-time infidelity and that she has no plans to leave her husband. The counselor pursues the possibility for disclosure in the marriage and the ramifications of the client's reproductive options. The client believes that her husband would not be able to tolerate the infidelity and that her marriage would be destroyed. Eventually, she reveals that the father was of a different race so that paternity would be apparent at birth. She feels that she can neither tell her husband nor continue the pregnancy. Her husband opposes terminating the pregnancy unless there are substantial risks of harm to the baby. The client asks the counselor to support her deceit, in the name of preserving her relationship with her husband, by documenting in a letter an increased risk for birth anomalies as a result of drinking alcohol.

This case illustrates the potent information that may be revealed in the short-term therapeutic relationship of genetic counseling. The client's concerns were complex despite the outward appearance of a straightforward medical question about the risk of alcohol ingestion early in pregnancy. To facilitate such sensitive disclosure, the client must feel that the information remains confidential with the counselor. What is the counselor's responsibility toward the client's husband and toward the developing fetus? To what degree, if any, should the counselor participate in the deception in the name of preserving the therapeutic relationship?

Consider another example: A pregnant woman seeks prenatal testing to determine if her developing fetus is predisposed to Huntington disease. Her husband is at 50% risk for developing Huntington disease later in his life and has chosen not to undergo predictive testing. The woman is seeking testing without her husband's knowledge. She tells the counselor that if the fetus is positive, she will terminate the pregnancy and will tell her husband she had a miscarriage.[21] Should the counselor assist the client in pursuing testing under these circumstances?

These examples suggest a limit to the responsibilities of genetic counselors to uphold the privacy of clients' secrets. When a counselor is asked to collude, the counselor risks potential harm (psychological and medical) to others, inaccurate documentation of medical and psychological information, and a jeopardizing of professional integrity by lowering the standards of practice. Harboring a client's secret may be easier than participating in the deception of others. Yet when a counselor concedes and places a bandage on the arm of a client who chose not to have a test performed, is this not also collusion? The limits to collusion must be determined by evaluating the potential harm to others. If the client simply wants to encourage relatives to undergo testing by setting an example (if he or she is affected, relatives may be hesitant unless the client is tested), the risk of harm may be little. Or perhaps the client is feeling pressured by relatives to undergo testing and would like to consider the options further in a more private setting. The accuracy of other family members' information and their access to genetic services are not jeopardized. However, if the interpretation of others' test results depends on the client's participation, then to collude in the deception would be to impose potential harm on others.

A more common example of genetic counselors colluding in secrets relates to clients' efforts to obtain health or life insurance. In some testing programs, counselors may advise their patients to obtain insurance coverage before undergoing genetic testing. Although counselors may view this as client advocacy, it leads to adverse selection. Adverse selection occurs when insurance applicants know more about their risk of illness than does the insurer. Those at higher risk end up buying more insurance while paying the same as those at low risk. Although this may seem to be fair to some counselors, it runs counter to the principles on which our insurance system depends. Further, counselors who advise their clients not to disclose known test results when applying for insurance may be colluding in insurance fraud. In spite of counselors' desires to protect their clients from insurance discrimination, participating in fraud risks rendering a client uninsured and is both unethical and illegal. Counselors' efforts may be better spent in advocating for insurance reform.

SECRETS ABOUT CHILDREN

Few things are more personal than people's feelings about child-bearing. These feelings involve the choice to bear children and the intimate nature of the relationship between parent and child. Parents may seek genetic counseling for advice about revealing a diagnosis to their child, such as a diagnosis that was made in in the first months after birth. This is not uncommon when the condition is mild, such as most cases of Turner syndrome or Klinefelter syndrome, both of which result from anomalies of the sex chromosomes and commonly cause learning disabilities without mental retardation or other serious medical problems. The parents may choose not to disclose the diagnosis to the child when there is no educational or medical need to do so. They may rationalize their decision by maintaining that there are no relatives at risk nor is there anything they can do to undo the child's medical diagnosis. Certainly young children are incapable of understanding information about their condition, and there are no clear guidelines about when and how to disclose such news to a child. But once a child reaches adolescence, he or she may have questions about perceived differences. Parents are often unaware of potential psychological harms that may be rendered even when their actions are well-intentioned. An inadvertent message is that the diagnosis was withheld because it is such bad news. The child may become angry and resentful of the protectiveness of his or her parents if the information was disclosed later than when the child was first capable of understanding and accepting it.

Genetic counselors may struggle with participating in the parents' deceit of the child if the parents choose to delay disclosure, particularly if it has been withheld well into adulthood. Yet the client encompasses the parents as well as the child. For the sake of all family members it is critical that the parents be supported, not judged (particularly because most often they simply want to protect their children). They may need to be helped to discuss the diagnosis with their adolescent or adult child. Only under extreme circumstances when parents may choose never to tell an adult child of a condition and a counselor anticipates a serious health threat might a counselor go against the wishes of the parents and reveal the secret. To do so is to risk additional harm to the parent-child relationship. In most circumstances counseling the family means that in the counselor's discussions with the child, the secret must be upheld even when it is against the counselor's professional opinion and values.

Another example of a genetic secret is ambiguous genitalia, in which gender selection and surgical alterations are made shortly after birth. In these situations parents commonly choose to keep the diagnosis hidden from the child during genetic counseling. Whose best interests does the secrecy serve? Is it to protect the child, or is it a result of the stigma of sexual identity or the discomfort of the parents? If the child asks a direct question, should the counselor lie? Beyond the counseling relationship, there is also a medicolegal issue of the accuracy of the medical record. If the record states a secret, the child may gain access to it at a later date. The record would indicate that the counselor colluded with the parents. The adult child may feel betrayed, not only by his or her parents, but by the entire health care system. Further interest in counseling may also be thwarted due to a lack of trust. The counselor's collusion may add to the harm engendered. As much as possible, limits to participating in family secrets should be spelled out with parents before genetic counseling begins.

CONCLUSION

Genetic counselors must protect client privacy, but not at the expense of their professional integrity or to the serious detriment of a third party. It behooves these professionals to outline the limits on maintaining privacy with their clients before they provide services. Counselors must preserve privacy even within families and consider a breach of that confidence only under extreme circumstances. The unintentional loss of privacy that may result from the actions of colleagues, trainees, or family members can be minimized by establishing careful practice guidelines. Further, an important aspect of the counseling interaction is to address with clients the potential ramifications of a loss of privacy. These include the possibility of insurance and employment discrimination, social stigmatization, and adverse health outcomes for relatives or in relationships with relatives. Clients themselves should have control over the genetic information that they consider private. Genetic counselors are in a critical position to advocate for clients in maintaining that control.

NOTES

Note to epigraph: Joan Laird, "An Ecological Approach to Child Welfare: Issues of Family Identity and Continuity," in C. Germain, ed., *Social Work Practice: People and Environments, An Ecological Approach* (New York: Columbia University Press, 1979).

1. Charles J. Epstein et al., "Genetic Counseling: Statement of the American Society of Human Genetics Ad Hoc Committee on Genetic Counseling," *American Journal of Human Genetics* 27 (1975): 240–42.
2. Barbara B. Biesecker, "Genetic Counseling: Settings, Providers and Goals, Current and Future," in Jane Fullarton, ed., *Proceedings of the Committee on Assessing Genetic Risks* (Washington, D.C.: National Academy Press, 1992); Seymour Kessler, ed., *Genetic Counseling: Psychological Dimensions* (New York: Academic Press, 1979); Seymour Kessler, "A Psychological Paradigm Shift in Genetic Counseling," *Social Biology* 27 (1980) 167–85; Steven Targum, "Psychotherapeutic Considerations in Genetic Counseling," *American Journal of Medicine Genetics* 8 (1981): 281–89.
3. Marc Lappé, "The Limits of Genetic Inquiry," *Hastings Center Report* 17 (August 1987): 5–10; Abby Lippman-Hand and Clark Fraser, "Genetic Counseling: Provision and Perception of Information," *American Journal of Medical Genetics* 3 (1979): 113–27.
4. Clair Leonard, Gary Chase, and Barton Childs, "Genetic Counseling: A Consumer's View," *New England Journal of Medicine* 287 (1972): 433–39.
5. Abby Lippman-Hand and Clark Fraser, "Genetic Counseling-the Postcounseling Period I: Parents' Perceptions of Uncertainty," *American Journal of Medical Genetics* 4 (1979): 51–71; James R. Sorenson, Judith P. Swazey, and Norman A. Scotch, *Reproductive Pasts, Reproductive Futures: Genetic Counseling and Its Effectiveness* (New York: Alan R. Liss, 1981); Diane Beeson and Mitchell Golbus, "Decision Making: Whether or Not to Have Prenatal Diagnosis and Abortion for X-linked Conditions," *American Journal of Medical Genetics* 20 (1985): 107–14.
6. Lori B. Andrews et al., eds., *Assessing Genetic Risks: Implications for Health and Social Policy* (Washington, D.C.: National Academy Press, 1994), chaps. 4, 6, 8, 9.
7. Rayna Rapp, "Chromosomes and Communication: The Discourse of Genetic Counseling," *Medical Anthropology Quarterly* 2 (1988): 143–57; Rayna Rapp, "Amniocentesis in

Sociocultural Perspective," *Journal of Genetic Counseling* 2 (1993): 183–96; Vivian Wang, "Cultural Competency in Genetic Counseling," *Journal of Genetic Counseling* 3 (1994): 267–78.

8. Sheldon Reed, "A Short History of Genetic Counseling," *Social Biology* 21 (1994): 332–39.

9. Carl Rogers, *Counseling and Psychotherapy: Newer Concepts in Practice* (Boston: Houghton Mifflin, 1942).

10. Carl Rogers, *Client-Centered Therapy: Its Current Practice, Implications, and Theory* (Boston: Houghton Mifflin, 1951).

11. Arthur L. Caplan, Dianne M. Bartels, and Bonnie S. LeRoy, "Neutrality Is Not Morality: The Ethics of Genetic Counseling," in Caplan, Bartels, and LeRoy, eds., *Prescribing Our Future: Ethical Challenges in Genetic Counseling* (New York: Aldine de Gruyter, 1993); Angus Clarke, "Is Non-Directive Genetic Counseling Possible?" *Lancet* 338 (1991): 998–1001.

12. National Society of Genetic Counselors, NSGC Membership Directory, 1996.

13. International Society of Nurses in Genetics, ISONG Membership Directory, 1996.

14. Andrews et al., eds., *Assessing Genetic Risks.*

15. Tom L. Beauchamp and James F. Childress, *Principles of Biomedical Ethics,* 4th ed. (New York: Oxford University Press, 1994).

16. National Society of Genetic Counselors, "NSGC Code of Ethics," *Journal of Genetic Counseling* 1 (1992): 41–43.

17. Andrews et al., eds., *Assessing Genetic Risks.*

18. Tarasoff v. Regents of Univ. of Cal., 551 P.2d 334 (Cal. 1976).

19. See Eugene Pergament, "A Clinical Geneticist Perspective of the Patient-Physician Relationship," Chap. 5 in this volume.

20. Ibid.

21. Wendy R. Uhlmann, University of Michigan case, personal communication, 1996.

Chapter 7 Informed Consent and Genetic Research

Ellen Wright Clayton

Risks to privacy and confidentiality may arise in two contexts in genetic research. The first is the setting in which an individual is invited to participate in a specific protocol. The ethical and legal issues posed by this type of research have been considered at length for many years. The second context is the use of stored tissues for genetic research, a form of investigation that until recently has received far less scrutiny.

THE CHOICE TO PARTICIPATE IN RESEARCH

Individual choice regarding participation in research is usually but not always required. Research affects the interests of subjects, investigators, and society at large. These interests are largely congruent in that a fundamental tenet of our society is that advances in knowledge are beneficial. But in spite of these general benefits, research subjects are exposed not only to the potential for good but also to the possibility of harm. Individuals may perceive the costs and benefits of participating in research differently from the investigator. For this reason, people are not conscripted to become research subjects despite the benefits that might result from their participation. Instead, in most instances, the informed consent of the individual is required.

Other interests also underlie the general policy of seeking the consent of research participants. One is the need to promote access to the health care system. Many individuals already fear that they will become "guinea pigs" if they seek medical care, particularly at teaching institutions. As a result, some delay seeking attention until their needs are more pronounced, delays that often increase the cost of health care. Making clear that participation in research is voluntary and is not part of becoming a patient decreases this undesirable reluctance to seek care in a timely fashion.

In the debate that led to the rules that currently govern research, the need to protect individual autonomy and to make clear the distinction between research and health care, though deemed important, were not considered sufficient reasons to require informed consent in all cases. Some research projects proceed without informed consent or even review of protocols by institutional review boards (IRBs). The usual justification for giving the final decision-making authority regarding participation with people other than the prospective subject is a judgment that the individual's interests at stake are relatively small.

THE DECISION TO PARTICIPATE IN RESEARCH

Individuals who are considering participating in research face an array of issues in making a decision. Individuals' concerns about the information revealed by genetic research often extend beyond worries about their privacy and confidentiality. Genetic research reveals information not only about the subject but also about his or her relatives and even his or her kinship and ethnic group. In some instances, this information may pose risks of harm. One of the harms most often considered in current discourse is the loss of access to health, life, or disability insurance.[1] Stigmatization is also possible, particularly for individuals who have mutations that predispose them to develop undesirable behavioral or mental traits. The risk of stigmatization may extend beyond the particular individuals who carry these mutations. The conclusions by Richard Herrnstein and Charles Murray in *The Bell Curve* that blacks are genetically less smart than whites have raised serious concerns among the African-American community, for example, that such conclusions will be used to justify devoting fewer resources to educating blacks.[2] Similarly, American Indians might be concerned if research showed that a mutation prevalent in their ethnic group predisposed carriers to become alcoholic. This is not to say that genetic information necessarily leads to punitive or discriminatory responses; such information could also lead to the devotion of more resources to those who for whatever reason, genetic or environmental, are in greater need of them. But the experience of individuals who come from groups in which a relatively high prevalence of HIV infection has been documented, such as Haitians and gay males, demonstrate that fears of punitive responses to those who are associated by ethnicity or sexual orientation with a disfavored condition are not groundless.[3]

Because of these concerns, some individuals may wish to prevent certain research from being undertaken altogether. The pressure that led to the cessation of research on men who had an extra copy of the Y chromosome (once thought to predispose individuals to violence) demonstrates the power of such concerns.[4] Short of preventing certain projects from proceeding, a course appropriately undertaken only rarely, some individuals simply may wish not to participate in research that may generate information that could harm their family or kinship group. The question is how much deference should be given to these desires. For guidance, we may observe that for years individuals have been encouraged to participate in research that may benefit others even when there is no chance that the they will receive any medical benefit from taking part and may even suffer some harm. Such altruistic behavior clearly is praiseworthy. Society benefits both from the knowledge gained and from the individual affirmation of commitment to the public good and the needs of others. But no matter how great the benefit may be, the investigator does not have the right to force the individual to take part. Moreover, to require participation rather then permitting voluntary enrollment would itself be costly because it would eliminate the social benefits of altruism.

By analogy, then, potential subjects ought also to be informed of the risks that research may cause others and to weigh those potential harms for themselves as they decide whether to participate in a study. This is not to say that individuals must always act to prevent harm from befalling others; for the most part, the law does not require this. It is also the case that different people may weigh harms differently. In the end, however, investigators must not be permitted to withhold from subjects the full array of potential harms or to limit the concerns that subjects may wish to consider.

PROBLEMS POSED BY PARTICIPATION IN RESEARCH

At first glance, it would appear that research poses few risks to subjects' interests in privacy and confidentiality. Many investigators promise to preserve the subjects' confidentiality, although some, exhibiting a degree of realistic humility, acknowledge that they will provide protection only to the extent permitted by law. Some say that they will keep results in locked files or in "secure" computers. It is noteworthy, however, that a study conducted in 1995 in which 23 consent documents from different projects were analyzed, only 4 discussed plans for either physical security of data and samples or coding information or removing identifiers. Five others simply asserted that confidentiality would be maintained, while the remainder (14) contained no language about these issues.[5]

Anecdotal evidence reveals that some consent forms state that they will provide specific research results to the subjects' health care providers only with the written permission of the subjects. In addition, most consent forms include statements that results will not be published in a way in which individuals can be identified. Where statements regarding privacy and confidentiality do appear in consent forms, they demonstrate at least some awareness of the potential problems. Often, however, closer analysis reveals that these provisions promise more than they can provide.

STRENGTHS AND LIMITATIONS OF CERTIFICATES OF CONFIDENTIALITY

Great enthusiasm has been expressed in recent years about the utility of certificates of confidentiality to prevent compelled revelation of research records, even though they have rarely been used in practice.[6] The relevant statute provides that the holder of such a certificate, which can be obtained from the United States Department of Health and Human Services (DHHS), may not be compelled to reveal the names or identifying information about research subjects in "any Federal, State, or local civil, criminal, administrative, legislative, or other proceedings."[7]

Some caveats regarding the availability and utility of these certificates must be considered. First, the interim guidance provided by DHHS states that this protection is to be granted "sparingly" and directs the assistant secretary, the only person empowered to issue these certificates, to do so "only when the research is of a sensitive nature where the protection is judged necessary to achieve the research objectives." The guidance does state that research can be considered sensitive if it involves the collection of information in any of the following categories: . . . (d) Information that if released could reasonably be damaging to an individual's financial standing, employability, or reputation within the community; (e) Information that would normally be recorded in the patient's medical record, and the disclosure of which could reasonably lead to social stigmatization or discrimination; . . . Information in other categories, not listed here, might also be considered sensitive because of specific cultural or other factors, and protection can be granted in such cases upon appropriate justification and explanation.

The guidance also empowers various personnel within DHHS to advise the assistant secretary about requests for protection they feel are not warranted.[8]

On balance, then, the guidance does not envision the easy availability of such certificates that some commentators have advocated. In addition, the criteria set forth to guide the assistant secretary's decisions leave room for great discretion. One can argue, for example, that loss of insurability would "reasonably be damaging to an individual's financial standing," but that interpretation is not required. Nor is it clear that preventing the risk of losing insurance would be "necessary to achieve the research objectives." People may well be willing to take part in a particular project in spite of this risk. Moreover, the guidance purports only to protect investigators and their institutions from being compelled to provide identifying information; although certificate holders are to be directed to use the certificate to resist compulsion, they remain free to reveal such information voluntarily even when they may be ill advised to do so. Finally, the guidance recognizes that certificates provide limited protection and requires that subjects be informed of these limitations.

PROBLEMS FOR INDIVIDUALS WITH RARE DISORDERS

Research on extremely rare disorders may pose additional problems of privacy and consent. It may not be possible, for example, to publish research results without including private information regarding identifiable individuals. In particular, family members may be able clearly to identify which relatives carry a particular mutation and which do not. One solution is to alter the pedigree, but such actions may undermine the integrity of the results. If identifiable information is to be published, permission must be sought, but from whom? Will the subject plus or minus his or her immediate family do, or must everyone in the pedigree agree? On occasion, some individuals within the family object to publication or even decide that they no longer wish to participate in the project. Questions then arise regarding their ability not only to decline to take part in the future but also to withdraw the information and samples they have already provided. In some instances, withdrawal of results may not be possible.

THE PROBLEM OF THE SUBJECT'S KNOWLEDGE

The farthest-reaching threat to the ability of subjects to control who obtains access to their private information lies with the subjects themselves. When individuals apply for health, life, or disability insurance, insurers generally can ask them whether they have ever had genetic testing. For purposes of answering this question, it does not matter whether the tests were performed in the course of clinical care or as part of a research protocol. If former subjects say that they have been tested, and particularly if they then disclose, perhaps in response to a follow-up question, that they were found to have a possibly deleterious mutation, they will likely find themselves denied insurance or at least charged higher rates. Yet if they answer such questions falsely, they may later be denied coverage or held liable for defrauding the insurer.

Insurers are most likely to obtain the results of research not by directly asking either researchers or subjects but rather by reviewing the subjects' medical records. In many instances, subjects will believe that the results of testing conducted during the course of research may be relevant to their clinical care and so may wish to share these results with their health care provider. Although subjects may often be mistaken about the clinical utility of the results of genetic testing, this sort of disclosure by patients to physicians appropriately is promoted in the health care system. After all, open communication of information and concerns by patients generally improves the health care they receive. But the cost of such conversation may be high, for once the results are entered into the medical record, whatever protection is provided to research data is lost, and numerous entities and individuals may gain access to the information.

In response to this dilemma, some commentators have suggested the creation of "shadow charts" in which to enter the results of genetic testing, paralleling those used in psychiatry and to a lesser extent, more recently, in the care of patients infected with HIV. This solution, however, is becoming less tenable as health care providers move toward the creation of detailed, integrated electronic records. Moreover, reliance on shadow charts has always created problems. Because they are almost never accessible to all the patient's health care providers, the patient may receive care without the benefit of this information, leading to fragmentation and conflicts that can compromise the patient's care. The use of shadow charts to avoid access to information by insurers also creates an ethical conundrum for the clinician, who then becomes involved in what may be seen as deception.

At present, few statutes attempt to avert the risks that knowledge poses for research subjects, and none are completely successful in their efforts. For the most part, the best that can be done is to inform prospective subjects before they decide to enroll in a project that the mere fact of participation and more particularly the information they receive may compromise their access to insurance. In some instances, subjects may be given information that they dare not share with their physician, regardless of their desires. In others, subjects may decide that they are better off not receiving any results at all.

IS ANONYMOUS TESTING AN APPROPRIATE SOLUTION?

Citing concerns about confidentiality and discrimination, Max Mehlman and his colleagues proposed in 1996 that anonymous genetic testing be made available, particularly for tests to detect mutations that predispose individuals to develop untreatable late-onset diseases. This proposal, however, is flawed in numerous ways. A central problem lies in the authors' attempt to rely on recent experience with anonymous testing for HIV to support a similar approach to genetic testing. Although genetic testing may indeed raise "some of the same issues as HIV testing with regard to the rights of others 'at risk' to gain access to test information," the differences in the implications of the two types of testing are far more pertinent.[9] The most important public health justification for anonymous testing for HIV—namely, the chance that a person found to be infected would alter his or her behavior to avoid infecting others who are not yet infected—does not apply to anonymous testing for genetic disorders. Finding a mutation in one person may have implications for his or her relatives, but the risks those relatives face already exist, whether or not they are aware that they may have the mutation. Because people do not have to share their test results with relatives, and indeed should not if they wish to maintain confidentiality, the main benefit of making available anonymous testing for untreatable late-onset genetic disorders is to relieve the anxiety of the person at risk.

Differences also exist in the degree of consensus regarding the appropriateness of preventing the appearance of disease in others. Almost everyone agrees that it is desirable to prevent the spread of HIV, whether by transmission to another individual (horizontal transmission) or to a later-born child (vertical transmission). By contrast, there is substantial agreement among geneticists that using prenatal diagnosis and selective abortion to avert the birth of children with untreatable disorders that would become symptomatic only in adulthoood (the diseases for which anonymous genetic testing is proposed) is inappropriate.

Given these different implications, there is no reason to suspect that public or private funding will or should be made available to support anonymous testing for mutations that predispose individuals to develop late-onset disorders. As a result, these tests would be available only to relatively wealthy individuals. In the absence of insurance reform, the risks of sharing results with health care providers and of obtaining testing and later seeking insurance without disclosing results remain. Finally, in proposing that a mechanism be developed to permit long-term follow-up by genetic counselors the authors demonstrate that even they are made squeamish by the prospect of truly anonymous testing in which consumer-patients decide for themselves exactly what sort of care and information they wish to receive and are then left to sort things out on their own. In short, the potential benefits of making anonymous genetic testing available cannot justify the complications such a policy would almost surely entail.

RISKS POSED BY THE USE OF STORED TISSUE SAMPLES

Biological samples from which DNA can be obtained, including blood, pathological specimens taken at surgery, and even hair, are frequently collected in the course of clinical care and research. Although many samples are destroyed after analysis, others are stored either as a matter of custom or as a result of legal requirements enacted primarily to promote quality assurance and improve patient care. Questions regarding the use of such samples for purposes other than those for which they were originally collected, though present for many years, have become much more urgent in light of recent and potential developments in genetics.

Any research in which samples can be linked with individuals from whom they were obtained poses the risks, such as loss of insurability, outlined earlier, albeit probably to a lesser degree. The recognition of such risks underlies the current regulatory provisions that (1) exempt from institutional review board oversight only those protocols using samples from which identifiers have been removed, and (2) impose limits on the ability of IRBs to waive or limit the requirements that informed consent be sought in protocols that use identifiable samples.[10] It appears, however, that these regulatory provisions are often honored in the breach, evidenced in part by the creation of data banks containing identifiable information about and tissue samples from large numbers of individuals without review by IRBs or informed consent. Similar problems are raised when samples collected for use in one research project are then used to investigate a completely separate issue without the subjects' knowledge.

This disparity between requirements and practice, as well as the greater recognition of the potential consequences of genetic research, has raised questions that are only now being addressed.[11] Foremost is whether the current regulations appropriately balance the interests of individuals and of society. Some researchers argue that these rules, if applied, unduly restrict research, whereas others urge that individuals' interests receive insufficient protection at present.

Within this larger debate there is widespread, though not unanimous, agreement that use of identifiable tissue samples for research requires review by an IRB or other similarly constituted body and usually the consent of the person from whom the sample was obtained. Substantial change will be required simply to bring practice into conformity with this position. Other contentious issues include defining what type of review and perhaps consent are required before samples collected in routine clinical care are used with or without removal of identifiers and deciding what removal of identifiers means—must linkage be irretrievably destroyed so that no one is ever able to identify the person from whom the sample was obtained or does preventing the investigator from making the connection suffice? This last question is particularly important in light of the suggestion that new techniques will soon make any sample that contains DNA uniquely identifiable.

THE SPECIAL PROBLEMS OF USING NEWBORN SCREENING SAMPLES

The temptation to use newborn screening samples for genetic research is strong. After all, such samples are collected from almost every child born in the United States and so represent a comprehensive population-based sample that could be of great value for research to determine such information as allele frequencies. Yet the use of such samples for research without review or consent is not appropriate. It must be recognized that state-mandated collection of blood samples from newborns, almost always without the parents' consent and usually without their knowledge, represents a substantial deviation from the usual norms of health care for children in which parental permission is required. Moreover, the justification for newborn screening is the detection of treatable serious disease in children, not research, a purpose with quite different justification and goals. The use of these samples for research is not mentioned to parents, has not been the subject of public debate, and raises the specter of conscription that generally has been rejected in the context of research. There is also evidence that some samples have been distributed for research by state laboratory directors with little oversight and in ways that could be particularly risky for children.[12]

If, after public debate, it is decided that newborn screening samples should be available for use in research, at a minimum states must develop policies to determine when newborn screening samples can be used for anonymous research. The development of such policies should encourage opportunity for public participation. In no circumstances should newborn screening samples be used for linkable research without meeting the stringent requirements for research on children.[13] Serious consideration should also be given to informing parents in the future about the potential use of newborn blood samples for anonymous research and giving them the opportunity to opt out of such research without forgoing newborn screening.

CONCLUSION

Much genetic research, like other efforts to expand knowledge, holds out the promise of substantial benefits for individuals and for society. At the same time, subjects who participate in such research often risk loss of privacy and confidentiality. In addition, efforts to obtain certain types of genetic information harm not only the subjects themselves but their larger kinship and ethnic groups. The issue now, as it has been for the past fifty years, is to balance the general desirability of obtaining new knowledge, particularly in those projects that the government has chosen to fund, with the need to honor individuals and their concerns. Although the interests of society and the individual are often congruent in the research setting, they are not always so.

Federal regulations for the protection of human subjects from research risks provide substantial guidance for resolving these conflicts, focusing on defining the need to inform and obtain consent from subjects for their participation. The first step, in which much progress has been made, is to determine precisely what these regulations mandate in the context of genetic research. The next step is to meet these requirements. At the same time the benefits and risks presented by the prospect of greater understanding of genetics have opened up for reexamination the roles that research and individual choice play in society.

NOTES

1. NIH-DOE Working Group on Ethical, Legal, and Social Implications of Human Genome Research, *Genetic Information and Health Insurance: Report of the Task Force on Genetic Information and Insurance* (Bethesda, Md.: National Center for Human Genome Research, National Institutes of Health, 1993).

2. Richard J. Herrnstein and Charles Murray, *The Bell Curve: Intelligence and Class Structure in American Life* (New York: Free Press, 1994). These concerns are considered in Steven Fraser, ed., *The Bell Curve Wars: Race, Intelligence and the Future of America* (New York: Basic Books, 1995).

3. Loretta M. Kopelman, "Informed Consent and Anonymous Tissue Samples: The Case of HIV Seroprevalence Studies," *Journal of Medicine and Philosophy* 19 (1994): 525–52.

4. Philip R. Reilly, *Genetics, Law, and Social Policy* (Cambridge: Harvard University Press, 1977).

5. Robert F. Weir and Jay R. Horton, "DNA Banking and Informed Consent, Part 1," *IRB* 17 (July–August 1995): 1–4; Robert F. Weir and Jay R. Horton, "DNA Banking and Informed Consent, Part 2," *IRB* 17 (September–December 1995): 1–8.

6. Charles L. Easley and Louise C. Strong, "Certificates of Confidentiality: A Valuable Tool for Protecting Genetic Data," *American Journal of Human Genetics* 57 (1995): 727–31.

7. 42 U.S.C. § 241(d) (1994).

8. Department of Health and Human Services, "Research Confidentiality Protection—Certificate of Confidentiality—Interim Guidance," May 22, 1989.

9. Maxwell J. Mehlman et al., "The Need for Anonymous Genetic Counseling and Testing," *American Journal of Human Genetics* 58 (1996): 393, 395.

10. 45 C.F.R. §§ 690.101(b)(4), 46.116(d) (1996).

11. American College of Human Genetics Storage of Genetic Materials Committee, "Statement on Storage and Use of Genetic Materials," *American Journal of Human Genetics* 57 (1995): 1499–1500; George J. Annas, Leonard H. Glantz, and Patricia A. Roche, *The Genetic Privacy Act and Commentary* (Boston: Boston University School of Public Health, 1995); Ellen Wright Clayton et al., "Informed Consent for Genetic Research on Stored Tissue Samples," *Journal of the American Medical Association* 274 (1995): 1786–92; Bartha M. Knoppers and Claude M. Laberge, "Research and Stored Tissues: Persons as Sources, Samples as Persons?" *Journal of the American Medical Association* 274 (1995): 1806–7; Nuffield Council on Bioethics, *Human Tissue: Ethical and Legal Issues* (London: Nuffield Council on Bioethics, 1995).

12. Jean E. McEwen and Philip R. Reilly, "Stored Guthrie Cards as DNA 'Banks,'" *American Journal of Human Genetics* 55 (1994): 196–200.

13. 45 C.F.R. § 46.401–8 (1996).

Chapter 8 Genetic Screening from a Public Health Perspective: Some Lessons from the HIV Experience

Scott Burris and Lawrence O. Gostin

Science has produced a powerful new technology in genetic screening, and the medical and biotechnology industries have been quick to find diagnostic and therapeutic uses for it in the care of individual patients. If one assumes that medicine is the same as public health—that public health is simply the sum of millions of individual outcomes—it is natural to assume that genetic screening technology will also be useful to public health. The main questions for public health users of the technology, then, would be how effective are the individual interventions following testing and how may we overcome the various problems posed by the socially dangerous quality of genetic information. On this view, the proper topic for this chapter would be the efficacy of genetic treatment and the adequacy of privacy and antidiscrimination law.

That, however, is not to be this chapter. If we have learned one lesson from the HIV epidemic, it is that disease and our responses to it are constructed of more than microbes (or genes). Much of the discussion of the human genome has been in a scientist, positivist mode, stitched without a seam to a construction of health and health care as a medical commodity. The discourse has focused on issues in the therapeutic relationship between physician and patient—such as reproductive counseling, informed consent to treatment, confidentiality of genomic information, and the "right to know" certain information. The literature seldom addresses the issue of the benefits of genetic screening and interventions for whole populations. What aggregate health benefits accrue to discrete populations and at what aggregate cost? From a public health perspective, emphasizing the health of a population and seeking determinants of health in the population's ecology, we are not ready to assume that genetic screening invariably has public health benefits that outweigh its costs. In spite of the enormous long-term potential of genetic research, a critical evaluation of the public health interest in genetic screening must be equally wary of the zeal of those who aspire to do good and those who wish to do well.

Putting aside the assumption that widespread collection of genetic data is both desirable and inevitable sets a very different genetic agenda for public health law. As a preliminary matter, we are required to ask, what criteria need to be satisfied to justify a particular genetic intervention in public health terms and to what extent have they been satisfied? Our experience with HIV teaches that these are not purely epidemiological questions. Any use of government authority to collect and use sensitive information reflects often controversial assumptions about whose health counts and how. It entails the potential for abuse. It requires social negotiation to ensure voluntary compliance—it must be sold, that is, both to those in society who write laws and budgets and to those in society whose information is to be sought. We consider these issues later in this chapter.

The HIV epidemic has also taught us yet again how difficult it is to do public health work and how little we know about many important questions of method. The experience of HIV testing illustrates the social and political potency of testing technology. As public health lawyers asking first and foremost about the role of law in genetic public health policy, we focus on how state authority can be wielded to promote the health of the community and to protect, or avoid harming, those whose health data will be sought in that cause. Without revisiting in detail the legal analyses of antidiscrimination and privacy law found in other chapters, we turn our gaze to the protective ambit of law in the HIV epidemic. This critical view reveals problems with the use of privacy as a proxy for discrimination and, indeed, with the antidiscrimination paradigm itself, not to mention that we know less about how to use this sort of law to influence behavior than we might at first admit.

ASSESSING THE PUBLIC HEALTH INTEREST IN GENETIC SCREENING

Genetic data are collected for discrete purposes and in different forms. A taxonomy of genetic screening provides a foundation for our subsequent assessment of the benefits and risks of genetic screening from a population-based perspective. First, we distinguish between genetic testing and screening. Testing represents a method of identifying disease or the potential for disease in an individual patient. Typically, and preferably, testing is accomplished through a careful process of discussion, nondirective counseling, and informed consent between a physician and a patient. Screening, by contrast, involves the systematic application of a testing instrument to a defined population. Its purpose is often to assess the prevalence or incidence of disease, or the potential for disease, within the population.

The objectives of testing and screening include clinical treatment, epidemiological assessment and intervention, and research. Clinical testing is often intended to prevent (e.g., reproductive counseling) or treat (e.g., somatic gene therapy) disease in the individual or his or her family. Screening, however, is usually intended to determine the prevalence or incidence in the population and, if possible, to intervene to reduce the overall burden of disease (e.g., through changes in behavior, diet, or environment).

Genomic data are collected in several forms, often in large databases held by government agencies like the Department of Defense[1] and the Centers for Disease Control and Prevention,[2] or such research institutions as the University of Utah. In addition to DNA, researchers, health care providers, and health departments frequently collect and store human tissue such as serological samples. Because human tissue is remarkably stable over a long period, stored tissue samples may be regarded as inchoate databases, given the technology to extract from the samples a vast amount of current and future genomic data. The public health and research communities have shown increasing interest in using existing tissue samples for genetic testing and for creating new genetic databases. In some cases genomic information is being extracted from large collections of tissue samples that were stored well before the advent of genetic testing; any consent that may originally have been obtained for tissue samples did not envisage future genetic applications. The most prominent example of an inchoate genetic database is the testing program for phenylketonuria (PKU, an inherited metabolic disease), whereby blood spots are taken from almost all newborns throughout the United States and stored in a dry condition on cards.[3]

For some conditions, genetic factors seem to be the sole or predominant cause of illness. In these instances, genetic testing may detect a carrier state, a current illness, or a marker indicating the likelihood of future illness. In most instances, however, genetic testing will identify only one factor among many other possible determinants of illness in the individual and his or her environment. Such information may help specify the individual's relative risk, as well as shedding light on the etiology of the condition generally. Any information from a genetic test is subject not simply to the limits of its predictive power in relation to illness but also to the reliability of the test itself. This is limited by the sensitivity and specificity of the test instrument and by the proportion of the known mutations in a target population the test is capable of detecting. For example, early screening programs could detect only about 75% of cystic fibrosis mutations in the white population of the United States.[4]

Testing for health conditions may be conducted with various degrees of coercion. Testing may be compelled by the state. For example, PKU screening is mandatory for newborns in almost every state. Testing, when not actually required, may be a condition precedent for the receipt of benefits or privileges. For example, testing requirements for a marriage license are in some sense coercive because the individual cannot obtain a state-issued license absent the test result. "Routine screening" refers to a program of systematically testing everyone who satisfies certain criteria.[5] Depending on the criteria, such screening may or may not have much to do with the subject's personal characteristics; compare, for example, PKU screening, conducted of all newborns, with amniocentesis, which is triggered by the age and health history of the mother.

Routine screening may be conducted with prior informed consent or may be done unless the patients affirmatively "opts out" of the test. Such a patient veto may have to be exercised without the information sharing that, ideally, is part of the process of informed consent, so it may be less than "voluntary." Even where informed consent is required, testing may not be completely voluntary because of the absence of adequate information and understanding. Merely signing a form does not assure genuine informed consent. HIV testing is the prime example of a form of testing generally subject to a higher level of informed consent, both in terms of the information presented and in the documentation of the patient's consent. Finally, screening may be done anonymously or with identifiers that lead more or less easily back to the subject.

THREE PRINCIPLES OF PUBLIC HEALTH SCREENING

The discourse on genetic screening in bioethics and health law has focused on the individual patient's right to information and hope of therapy. Without discounting either that debate or the value of genetic information to patients, the analysis of genetic screening is very different for public health than for health care. Indeed, the differences between the justifications for genetic testing in health care and genetic screening for public health purposes underline the importance of analyzing potential public health uses of genetic screening in public health terms. To that end, we offer the following three principles as useful in assessing the costs, benefits, and political prospects of particular screening programs to public health.[6]

Principle 1. Screening should enhance the health of the population. Much of the impetus for using genetic testing comes from the health care sector, but public health and health care aspire to complementary but meaningfully different ends. Public health aims to improve the health of the group, as measured by aggregate outcomes. Medicine aims to improve the health of the individual, as measured largely by the individual's satisfaction with his or her own outcome. Any number of differences follow from this basic distinction, among them: population health depends more on the causes of incidence of disease in populations than the causes of illness in individuals, and from the population standpoint, it is the distribution of cases rather than the accidental fate of any particular person that matters. Individual risk factors, which seem to explain why certain people get sick, do not tend to explain why certain ills are prevalent in certain populations. Thus, genetic differences may help to explain why people exposed to the same environmental co-factors differ in their health, but environmental factors provide the chief explanation of health differences between populations living in different environments. Because health risks constituted in a population are different than those expressed in individuals, even a very powerful individual risk factor may not constitute a public health priority if the prevalence of the marker is low.[7]

The breast cancer 1 gene (BRCA1) for breast cancer is an example. As Caryn Lerman and Robert Croyle observe, "Much of breast cancer is not caused by inherited susceptibility at all, but results from somatic events that produce genetic changes in a woman's breast cells during her lifetime. Moreover, the majority of women who develop breast cancer have no known major risk factors."[8] To find a genetic screening measure "ethical" in the public health sense, then, we need to determine that it has a reasonable probability of leading to information that can be used to reduce the incidence of genetic illness or mortality in the society as a whole or in a significant population facing a special threat. If it does not, the measure, however useful to individuals, may not be an important public health priority and may not be worthy of significant public sector resources.

Principle 2. The measure should be an efficient and just use of resources. Although rationing may be ethically problematic for many doctors, in public health it is a "moral imperative . . . in the face of scarce resources."[9] Ideally, each public health dollar will be spent to achieve the greatest marginal increase in the level and distribution of well-being in the population. Although the problems of comparing incommensurate values quickly burst any illusions about the objectivity or mechanical quality of this analysis, this principle is nevertheless a useful reminder to build waterpipes and sewers before cholera wards and to bear in mind the relative costs and benefits of oral rehydration kits and heart transplants. The high cost of health care accentuates the resource problem. Although doctors can often do miraculous things for individual patients, such care not only does not help the public health but has a price that may drive out nonmedical forms of prevention.[10] Even assuming that an expensive regimen of screening and treatment might be worthwhile in purely theoretical terms, there is always the problem that our current health care payment system will not provide equitable access. Even counseling, which is often the only intervention of consequence in genetic testing, depends on the deployment of thousands of well-trained counselors throughout the health care system, a cadre of professionals who exist largely in the hopes of genetic optimists.[11]

Screening programs often illustrate the significance of marginal cost in public health planning. There is an impulse in medicine to routinize the use of a test or treatment that seems to work for the individual, an impulse that is often quicker off the mark than the validation of the measure's efficacy on a large scale.[12] Making a useful test routine sometimes carries with it in turn the impulse to make it "mandatory," which the HIV experience has shown is a highly problematic move. Decreeing that an entire population shall be tested has a superficial logic when a test seems to promise health benefits to each and all, and it allows politicians to underline their concern and their toughness with one and the same vote. Yet apart from the difficulties of enforcing compliance, which we shall discuss next, the move to routine or mandatory testing makes a more fundamentally faulty assumption: that the cost-benefit ratio of reaching hard-to-find or resistant targets is comparable to that of reaching the compliant and eager. For example, the medical benefits of prenatal HIV screening of pregnant women may be great; it hardly follows, however, that the reduction of HIV transmission to newborns will be maximized by testing every pregnant woman regardless of the cost.[13] Indeed, particularly in the instance of tests that offer the patient useful information about relative risks or even therapeutic options, one might most logically start with the assumption that most people at risk will accept the test without intervention from public health authorities.

Both the efficiency and fairness of a public health intervention should be evaluated in more than just monetary terms. Indeed, in this case efficiency demands what justice requires. Genetic conditions may often be stigmatizing, leading to ostracism and discrimination. The problem tends to be greater when a particular condition is linked to other disfavored traits. Stigma is thought to increase resistance among the targets of health measures, raising their cost and reducing their effectiveness. Social dispute about the meaning of conditions is a serious and constant friction on the workings of health and prevention programs and can render utterly impractical measures that seem wonderful in theory.

The morality of public health's utilitarianism is rooted in the imperative to improve the distribution as well as the level of health. Were there truly a mechanical formula for achieving the greatest good for the greatest number, ethics would be largely self-executing, for the marginal gains of measures to help a large number of those in need would almost always be greater than the benefits of helping the fortunate few.[14] In fact, nothing could be more complicated and controversial than deciding who is needy and should get what help. In a politicized world of scarcity, there is a constant danger that health expenditures will reflect existing distributions of wealth and influence. Ill health follows and reflects social disadvantage; social differences create different health problems.[15] Spending money to address the leading killers of the population as a whole may exclude expenditures on the leading killers of subgroups in the population. Although cancer is the leading cause of death in the population as a whole, spending to find its genetic causes must be seen in light of such facts as the toll of violence and HIV on young African-American men. We believe that a just health policy requires recognition of the pernicious synergies of socioeconomic disadvantage and the problematic nature of existing social entitlements. To the extent that disease is a social product, public health ought to act as a conscience.[16]

Principle 3. The measure should be as acceptable as possible to its targets. This principle has roots in both practicality and morality. Public health depends largely on voluntary compliance with its guidelines. This is equally true of "voluntary" advice, like wearing a bike helmet in most states, and of "mandatory" rules, like wearing seat belts. Resistance can raise costs enormously, the more as prevalence of the condition rises. It has proven possible, with a fair amount of money and talent, to impose directly observed therapy on a few hundred recalcitrant tuberculosis patients in a few major cities;[17] it is unlikely ever to have been feasible to isolate and monitor the sex lives of tens of thousands of people with HIV. Even most "mandatory" measures are either largely voluntary in effect (e.g., premarital screening) or are so broadly acceptable that they are not resisted (like screening for PKU). The success of a public health intervention and its cost therefore depend significantly on the degree to which its targets perceive it to be more beneficial than costly.

Resistance to health measures is rarely as irrational as it might seem to the paternalistic professional observer. A measure that leads to immediate and short-term health benefits for targeted individuals is obviously more desirable than one that does not; there is the difference between PKU screening and HIV testing (at least before the advent of effective combination therapy). Monetary or other incentives may increase the benefits of compliance, as is sometimes done with directly observed therapy (DOT). The costs of compliance are often in something like inverse proportion to the treatability of the condition: the less we can do for a trait, the more social costs screening is likely to entail. Being marked as having a dangerous, untreatable condition may be costly in psychological terms and may expose the subject to the risk of social stigma. These sorts of costs may be addressed to some extent through counseling and the legal protection of social status, but this, as we will see, is difficult and problematic in its own way. In moral terms, this principle emphasizes the fairness of allocating both the benefits and burdens of a disease that threatens public health or the public generally rather than placing them primarily on the shoulders of those who have the illness.

In the HIV epidemic, resistance to public health rules has taken on a perhaps unprecedented but now widely followed political dimension. Legal and advocacy organizations, capable of generating grass-roots action and of effectively lobbying and litigating, have demonstrated their capacity to influence the development of public health policy.[18] In many respects this has been a boon to public health, facilitating the social negotiation necessary to design broadly acceptable measures. It has also, however, added even more complexity to the rich symbolic politics of health and disease. A final caution under the heading of the principle of acceptability thus is that measures may not always be judged for their intrinsic merits, or even their objective likelihood of causing harm to the target population. The example of HIV reporting typifies a measure that has in many states been strongly opposed by advocates, despite the excellent record of health departments in protecting the confidentiality of their records. In this instance, the fear of what government might someday do with an "AIDS list" outweighs health departments' excellent track record.[19]

GENETIC SCREENING INITIATIVES AND PUBLIC HEALTH

It is well beyond the purpose of this chapter to apply these principles to any genetic screening initiative. Nevertheless, an overview of genetic screening shows the need for caution in designing large-scale screening programs in the name of improving the public's health.

Genetic illness is an important threat to public health. Historically, genetic disease has been seen both as a major source of ill health and premature mortality and as largely intractable.[20] With its significant impact on the population as a whole as well as on distinct subpopulations, genetic illness is obviously an important challenge to public health.[21]

Some level of pure research would surely be a wise and just use of resources for population health, provided always that information about the impact of genetic factors on health is integrated into a broader examination of the determinants of health.[22] There is good historical evidence that the facts of the germ theory had a greater impact on the decline in mortality in the United States in the past century than did the medical interventions derived from them.[23] Research may help identify important co-factors for illness in the environment or help provide behavioral guidance. Likewise, epidemiological research, including formal surveillance, is justified precisely because of the difficulty of assessing the potential of genetic knowledge on public health. Some commentators have lamented the state of genetic-related data collection in public health. James Hanson argues that

> for the most part, public health officials are not well-informed on birth defects or on medical genetics in general and have tended to view birth defects surveillance as a private responsibility rather than as a part of a broader public health agenda. There is also the general perception that birth defects and genetic conditions are rare events, and not subject to prevention or intervention. Yet recent advances in genetics (through the Human Genome Project and other genetics research programs), molecular biology and teratology offer substantial evidence to the contrary, and have

extraordinary implications for preventive health care, including birth defects prevention.[24]

Public health data collection is a prerequisite for according genetic illness greater public health priority.

The value of screening individuals in medical care depends from a public health point of view on such elements as the extent and severity of the condition in the population, the cost of detecting it, and the availability of some intervention to cure or prevent the expression of the condition. In those relatively few instances in which the identification of a genetic trait leads to effective, life-sustaining therapy at a reasonable cost—PKU, for instance—screening evidently has real public health value. More controversial but comparably effective at the population level is prenatal screening to which the preventive response is contraception or abortion. Chorionic villus sampling (CVS) and amniocentesis, for instance, have led to a substantial reduction in the prevalence of Down syndrome at birth, although some racial and ethnic differences may reflect unequal access to prenatal diagnostic services.[25] As the complexity and cost of the response increases—as might happen in the area of prenatal surgery—both the public health cost-benefit ratio and the problem of access increase.

This is all fairly obvious, as is the observation that the most problematic use of genetic screening, from both the medical and the public health standpoint, is in cases when little or nothing can be done to prevent an illness or its intergenerational transmission or where the genetic factor is but one among many individual or environmental co-factors to a higher relative risk of an illness. The psychological value of knowing about something one cannot alter may be positive or negative for the individual,[26] and likewise may make for a net increase or decrease in the sum total of public well-being. Stigma and stress add to the social costs of screening for risk factors, as does an increase in the prevalence of that most modern of ills, being "at risk." In the case of illnesses with behavioral co-factors, there has been some support for the proposition that personalized relative risk information can enhance the chances of behavior change, but the impact may be slight and short-term, and in any event must be placed in the context of the overall difficulties of changing behavior.[27] In a larger sense, genetic screening threatens to be a readily commodifiable, culturally powerful approach to dealing with disease that will complicate the discovery and alteration of the pathogenic elements of the ecology. Angus Clarke argues that "the focus on genetic factors may distract attention from 'the real challenge of the future which appears to be the behavioral and social issues of risk reduction.'"[28]

Although the potential costs of genetic screening are high, they are not uniformly distributed across all uses of the technology. Genetic databases collected by the state, or under its auspices, for research purposes can be reliably protected, even in an environment consisting largely of electronic records, because there is no need to allow access for medical care or payment purposes. Such programs could move as much as possible to blinded collection or storage and can maintain rigid barriers to access without significantly burdening bona fide research.

Various populations are also likely to accept genetic screening to varying degrees, reflecting the different social and medical impacts genetic information can have and the level of access different populations have to those benefits, as well as their confidence in the legal protection of their social status. Resistance on the general ground of state intrusion into privacy is likely, including spill-over from efforts to gather and use genetic information for purposes of identification and law enforcement. Markers of serious future or inheritable diseases are likely to be stigmatizing, particularly insofar as insurers and employers use them to avoid health care costs. As genetic factors have more and more influence on individual social status, we can expect more principled resistance to screening. The popularity of prenatal screening, for example, is giving rise to concerns about the perceived value of disabled lives.[29]

The use of genetic screening for public health purposes will tend to be most effective when it serves a clear population goal, has a healthy ratio of overall economic and social benefits to costs, entails a just use of resources, and is acceptable to the populations it targets. We recognize that the public health agenda is never written by fully autonomous, fully informed rational actors on a clean slate.[30] Yet precisely because social and political factors influence public health policy so heavily, it is important to seize the opportunity for reflection before the time for action arrives and to at least aspire to rationality in the heat of action.

Given the unresolved issues of social cost and the limited promise of population health benefits, we remain skeptical that there is a clear basis for organized public health intervention on genetic matters. We are not arguing that screening is never useful, rather that the current ethical and legal implications of screening do not justify implementation of population-based screening for genetic conditions until there is for each intervention a clearer public health rationale and a strategy to win the acceptance of the targeted population.

LAW, POLITICS AND PUBLIC HEALTH: INSIGHTS FROM HIV SCREENING

The Rush to Testing and Screening

Screening tends to be powerfully attractive: the diagnostic gold standard for the physician, the key to accurate surveillance for the epidemiologist, and, for the worried citizen, the magic marker of the sick. Screening is feasible, tangible—if not the link to a cure, then the first step toward it. And there is money to be made. Commercial companies, for example, are quick to market "home tests" for BRCA1, even absent an established intervention.[31] It is precisely because testing can be so attractive, on so many levels, that there is a danger of investing in it too much, too soon. The HIV experience suggests that a major public health investment can be made under pressure, with enormous political consequences, simply because the technology exists. The adoption of counseling and testing by the Centers for Disease Control and Prevention as the centerpiece of its prevention program reflected the considerable political pressure to identify carriers, a medicalized view of public health, the control practices applied to sexually transmitted diseases and tuberculosis, even a desire to find ways to allow explicit education without offending the public or Senator Jesse Helms (R-N.C.). The strategy was chosen before basic decisions had been made about the use of the result, in reporting and partner notification, and before laws protecting testing privacy and prohibiting discrimination were solidly in place. Although the counseling and testing protocols of the CDC reflected the input of advocates, the program was launched with little data about how people would react to testing. Assessment of its probable impact on sexual or other risk behavior was almost entirely theoretical, to the degree there was a theory. A decade and several billion dollars later, there is still room to dispute its effectiveness.[32] Even the CDC's Advisory Committee on the Prevention of HIV Infection questioned the agency's excessive reliance on testing as the centerpiece of HIV prevention activities.[33]

In spite of the resources thrown into testing, its acceptance has not been overwhelming. Millions of tests have been performed, but there are still concerns that people at high risk are not taking the test as much as public health officials would like. Though screening programs and other associated measures like reporting and partner notification have been seen by some as "traditional," they have traditionally been problematic.[34] If large numbers of people are unhappy or worried and the requirement is avoidable, the HIV experience reminds us yet again that the rules can be frustrated.[35]

The experience with HIV sheds special light on the problem of using antidiscrimination and privacy law to reduce the social costs of screening and increase its acceptability. The passage of state privacy laws and, indeed, the extension of disability discrimination laws and their application to HIV were heavily influenced by the public health importance given to testing. The practical concern of encouraging compliance and avoiding stigmatization is mentioned explicitly in leading cases like School Board of Nassau County v. Arline and in statutes themselves.[36] This "antistigma project" in the law should by no means be taken to have succeeded, much less to be a model for use in the context of genetic screening.

Using Law to Reduce the Social Consequences of Screening

The most significant sociolegal experiment in HIV control has been the widespread use of privacy and confidentiality law to protect the social status of persons living with HIV and AIDS and to encourage them to comply with health advisories. When applied to genetic screening, this becomes problematic on several levels: the social construction of genetic "inferiority," the practical difficulties in extending meaningful protection to genetic status, and the lack of data on how law affects stigma-related behavior.

It is common to speak of health and illness as being socially constructed, meaning that these states depend for their definition on a web of social and cultural meanings of which we are commonly unconscious.[37] Law, too, is a social construct, but it is also a meaning-creating activity. Indeed, on some accounts, the main function of law is to normalize certain social arrangements and render others "deviant" or even unthinkable.[38] Law, on this view, both reflects and influences the social construction of those things to which it pertains.

People with HIV have been protected by privacy and disability discrimination laws, but from a critical standpoint, these laws have also contributed to the stigma associated with the disease. The price of having a refuge against discrimination has been acceptance of the label of "disabled," a source, at least, of cognitive dissonance for anyone "living with HIV." More fundamentally, as Wendy Parmet explains, there is a basic problem with the discrimination paradigm: in seeking to ensure "equal" treatment of people with HIV, it sets as the norm the status of those who do not have it, thus validating the very difference it purports to make suspect.[39] Similarly, the right to be left alone is the mirror image of the secrecy of stigma, so that, in the HIV epidemic, protection of privacy has been justified because "society's moral judgments about the high-risk activities associated with the disease, including sexual relations and drug use, make the information of the most personal kind."[40] Thus does law "protect" the silence of the love that had better not dare speak its name.

Carrying these arguments into the genetic field, Susan Wolf has argued the dangers of what she calls "geneticism":

> Like racism and sexism, it is a long-standing and deeply entrenched system for disadvantaging some and advantaging others. It can be seen in the pervasive individual and institutional use of genetic information and concepts to disadvantage people whether singly or by creating groups. It predates any accurate understanding of genetics, and now refers to social structures, practices, beliefs, and predispositions that together support disadvantaging based on a mixture of accurate and inaccurate genetic ideas.[41]

In her view, "antidiscrimination analysis cannot deal adequately with the pressing issues of genetic labeling and disadvantage . . . . [C]linging to 'genetic discrimination' . . . actually does damage by creating a false genetic 'norm,' frustrating structural reform, obscuring the deep psychological roots of genetic stereotyping and prejudice, and isolating genetic from other harms."[42] If we believe that law is supposed to influence attitudes and behaviors, we have to be worried about the content of the message, which not only supplies information but structures how we think about the issue. By "protecting" those with genetic "differences" from stigma and discrimination, we are actually reinforcing the belief in their inferiority or otherness. Although this may be a necessary evil, it ought not to be an unrecognized one.

Not that protection is easy. There are real practical problems to using the law for these purposes. The legislative response to genetic privacy concerns is following much the same track as the HIV experience: failed attempts at a national standard but widespread passage of state laws.[43] Providing for both efficient access and adequate privacy protection for health data are enormously complicated problems that we have not solved.[44] The patchwork protection of specific kinds of information, such as we have seen in both the HIV and genetic realms, is a response in avoidance of the problem. Such legislation is more politically "do-able"[45] and may have the advantage of sending a particularly strong message of the importance of privacy to the holders and users of records (though, as we discuss next, we know little about the effects of such laws), but in the end it cannot escape the larger privacy problem. A narrow definition of the protected information fails to provide adequate security, whereas broadly written provisions may impose unnecessary burdens on the proper use of data.[46]

Patchwork protection in and of itself is faulty on several grounds. Special rules require holders and transmitters of data, who seldom hold only those relating to HIV or genetic information, to apply different standards to different bytes of information in their possession. The practical burdens of segregating data or subjecting different quanta of data to different standards is probably substantial. Patchwork protection also accentuates the idiosyncratic quality of individuals' privacy concerns. Many people do indeed see secrecy as shame and are "out" about their HIV or genetic differences. For others, a diagnosis of venereal warts or genital herpes is as sensitive as one of HIV.

One of us has suggested elsewhere that "a more thoughtful solution would be to adopt a comprehensive federal statute on health information privacy, with explicit language applying privacy and security standards to genomic information. If genomic data were insufficiently protected by these legal standards, additional safeguards could be enacted."[47] Several bills providing a national privacy standard, including genetic privacy, are pending in Congress.[48] Passing individual statutes at the state or even the federal level will provide some protection, as it has for people with HIV, but even more than in the case of HIV it will leave loopholes, which will themselves reflect the political difficulties of securing protection as well as the problems inherent in protecting one kind of health data. We do not argue against privacy protection but do note the likely limits on its efficacy.

Of course, the fact that our health care and public health systems function reasonably well without strong privacy protection may suggest that privacy is more valued in theory than in practice. Americans, in spite of their strong expressions of concern to pollsters, may not frequently make health-related decisions based on privacy concerns.[49] We have already noted the corollary of this, that privacy can be a potent political issue even absent evidence of a breach. One of the conundrums of privacy law is that it may both fail to protect privacy in ways that hurt people, but of which they are unaware, and fail to reassure them in areas where it is, in fact, effective.

In both the HIV and genetic realms, privacy has been used as a proxy for antidiscrimination protection, particularly in insurance. That is, the role of the law is not to prevent the collection or proper use of the information but rather to prevent its falling into the wrong hands and being used to deprive the subject of a job, a service, or insurance. This is proving problematic. Absolute privacy cannot be guaranteed, particularly in the context of insurance. Insurers and self-insured employers, as the payers, have a claim on some information about what they are paying for that is not only reasonable but backed by considerable political clout. In both the HIV and genetic realms, it has often been difficult to place strong limits on insurers' access to records through state law. Even when limits are in place, insurers, whose business is built on discrimination, have a strong incentive to deduce information from other factors (like behavior in the case of HIV or family history in the context of genetics). As Parmet notes, "Substantive law allows—and public policies which encourage market-driven health insurance may even encourage—the precise types of discrimination that procedural privacy seeks to thwart."[50] In spite of the adage about the ounce of prevention, trying to control records in the hands of the good to forestall misbehavior by the bad could prove both burdensome for the good and ineffective against the bad.

This takes us to a final concern: the notion that public health policy makers can count on privacy and antidiscrimination law to regulate behavior and attitudes toward persons with genetic disease rests on two barely tested assumptions—that people know about the law and that it influences their behavior in desired ways. Our experience with HIV would suggest that the wish is not father to the deed. Although we rely on federal laws like the Americans with Disabilities Act and state statutes protecting confidentiality to influence the attitudes of the masses and the behavior of both those who might discriminate and those who might suffer discrimination, we have little evidence that any of these populations know about or understand the rules. Many public opinion polls have asked respondents about their views on matters such as isolation and screening and a patient's right to know his or her doctor's HIV status,[51] but they have not asked people if they are aware of or approve the legal rules relevant to these policies. Indeed, a review of 32 national opinion surveys between 1988 and 1991 reported only one asking respondents whether they supported the passage of the Americans with Disabilities Act.[52] Thus, even though we know a great deal about how the public feels about fair treatment and privacy, we do not know whether the attitudes reflect the law, the law reflects the attitudes, or the two are entirely unconnected. Without better data, we cannot begin to measure the influence of the antistigma project on public attitudes or predict with confidence the effect of genetic discrimination and privacy laws.

Similarly, studies of particular populations in a position to discriminate against people with HIV—employers, providers of public accommodations, and holders of medical information—shed little light on people's level of awareness of the law, how closely their understanding of its behavioral commands matches the prevailing views of lawyers and judges, how other attitudes influence their comprehension and interpretation of legal rules, and their attitudes toward the rules and the legal system generally. In fact, the only study we know of that probes this question, an attitude study of residents and house staff at a Pennsylvania medical center, found that most were unaware of a recently passed state HIV privacy and testing law.[53]

As for people subject to stigma and discrimination, the studies that have come closest to examining legal knowledge and attitudes have been those of people seeking the HIV test.[54] This literature supports the idea that privacy matters to people who are considering taking an HIV test but not whether they are aware of privacy and antidiscrimination laws and whether these laws influence their attitudes and behavior. Indeed, we know very little about the actual level of discrimination and breach of confidentiality. Although there are some reliable data on frequency of claims, litigation is not a good indicator of frequency of the underlying behavior.[55] "Testing" data are rare, so generally we must estimate the extent of HIV discrimination either by reference to self-reports by people with or at risk of HIV or from attitude studies of potential discriminators.[56]

Even less information is available about the relation of law to behavior of people with or at risk of the disease. The claim that legal protection against discrimination and release of private information will encourage people to be tested and, in a larger sense, provide a social context that supports positive changes in behavior, remains the most important and least studied policy argument in the HIV epidemic. It is notable that Tamara Hoxworth and colleagues found that only 1% of respondents indicated fear of reporting as their main reason for choosing anonymous testing.[57]

All this is not to suggest that the efforts to protect people with HIV have been unjustified and that no such effort should be made to protect those with disease of genetic origin. It does claim, however, that we can and should know more about both the extent of the problem and its nature in various contexts as we begin to craft sweeping policies to handle it. Above all, our claim is that the best protection against discrimination and invasions of genetic privacy lies in rigorous examination and justification for collection and use of genomic data, particularly on a population basis.

CONCLUSION

We do not oppose genetic screening and research, nor do we dispute that these pursuits hold important promise for public health; rather, we assert the critical value of the null hypothesis as a check on policy enthusiasm. We believe that much good has come from the use of law to protect people living with HIV and AIDS from the social consequences of the disease, but that is difficult to prove, and even if we could prove it, we would surely find that the blessings were not unmixed. We challenge proponents of public health interventions in genetics to address the issues we and others have identified in the hopes not of impeding technological progress but in using advancements in genetic understanding to enhance the health of the population.

NOTES

1. The Department of Defense's Registry and Specimen Repository for Remains Identification was authorized in 1991 to serve as an improved method for identifying soldiers' remains. Deputy Secretary of Defense memorandum no. 47803 (Dec. 16, 1991). See Information Management and Technology Division, General Accounting Office, CHCS Deployment Strategy, GAO/IMTEC-91-47 (1991), 1.

2. U.S. Department of Health and Human Services, *National Health and Nutrition Examination Survey III* (Washington, D.C.: Government Printing Office, 1994).

3. Jean E. McEwen and Philip R. Reilly, "Stored Guthrie Cards as DNA 'Banks,'" *American Journal of Human Genetics* 55 (1994): 196, 196–97.

4. Benjamin S. Wilfond and Norman Fost, "The Cystic Fibrosis Gene: Medical and Social Implications for Heterozygote Detection," *Journal of the American Medical Association* 263 (1990): 2777, 2779.

5. See Allan M. Brandt, Paul D. Cleary, and Lawrence O. Gostin, "Routine Hospital Testing for HIV: Health Policy Considerations," in Lawrence O. Gostin, ed., *AIDS and the Health Care System* (New Haven: Yale University Press, 1990).

6. In this we follow the model of Allan M. Brandt and colleagues.

7. For discussions of the differences between medicine and public health goals, upon which we have relied, see Geoffrey Rose, "Sick Individuals and Sick Populations," *International Journal of Epidemiology* 14 (1985): 32; Bernard Lo, "Ethical Dilemmas in HIV Infection: What Have We Learned?" *Law, Medicine, and Health Care* 20 (1992): 92; Mary Northridge, "Public Health Methods: Attributable Risk as a Link Between Causality and Public Health Action," *American Journal of Public Health* 85 (1995): 1202; and Ralph L. Keeney, "Decisions About Life-Threatening Risks," *New England Journal of Medicine* 331 (1994): 193.

8. Caryn Lerman and Robert Croyle, "Psychological Issues in Genetic Testing for Breast Cancer Susceptibility," *Archives of Internal Medicine* 154 (1994): 609.

9. Richard H. Morrow and John H. Bryant, "Health Policy Approaches to Measuring and Valuing Human Life: Conceptual and Ethical Issues," *American Journal of Public Health* 85 (1995): 1356.

10. See, e.g., Robert M. Kliegman, "Neonatal Technology, Perinatal Survival, Social Consequences, and the Perinatal Paradox," ibid., 909.

11. See Philip R. Reilly, "The Impact of the Genetic Privacy Act on Medicine," *Journal of Law, Medicine and Ethics* 23 (1995): 378, 380.

12. For a recent example, see Dermot MacDonald, "Cerebral Palsy and Intrapartum Fetal Monitoring," *New England Journal of Medicine* 334 (1996): 659; and Karin B. Nelson et al., "Uncertain Value of Electronic Fetal Monitoring in Predicting Cerebral Palsy," ibid., 613.

13. See discussion in Charles F. Clark and Michael D. Knox, "The Effectiveness of Condoms: An Individual versus a Societal Perspective," *AIDS and Public Policy Journal* 8 (1993): 193.

14. See Morrow and Bryant, "Health Policy Approaches."

15. See Paul Sorlies, Eric Backlund, and Jacob Keller, "U.S. Mortality by Economic, Demographic, and Social Characteristics: The National Longitudinal Mortality Study," *American Journal of Public Health* 85 (1995): 949; David Blane, "Editorial: Social Determinants of Health—Socioeconomic Status, Social Class, and Ethnicity," *American Journal of Public Health* 85 (1995): 903; Thomas A. LaVeist, "Segregation, Poverty, and Empowerment: Health Consequences for African Americans," *Milbank Quarterly* 71 (1993): 41; and George D. Smith and Matthias Egger, "Socioeconomic Differences in Mortality in Britain and the United States," *American Journal of Public Health* 82 (1992): 1979.

16. See Mervyn Susser, "Health as a Human Right: An Epidemiologist's Perspective on Public Health," *American Journal of Public Health* 83 (1993): 416.

17. See Thomas R. Frieden et al., "Tuberculosis in New York—Turning the Tide," *New England Journal of Medicine* 333 (1995): 229.

18. See Ronald Bayer, *Private Acts, Social Consequences: AIDS and the Politics of Public Health* (New York: Free Press, 1989); and Robert M. Wachter, *The Fragile Coalition: Scientists, Activists, and AIDS* (New York: St. Martin's Press, 1991).

19. For data on the fears of gay men with regard to data collection, see K. Siegel et al., "The Motives of Gay Men for Taking or not Taking the HIV Antibody Test," *Social Problems* 36 (1989): 368.

20. See Thomas McKeown, *The Role of Medicine: Dream, Mirage, or Nemesis* (Princeton, N.J.: Princeton University Press, 1979).

21. See Centers for Disease Control and Prevention, "Surveillance for and Comparison of Birth Defect Prevalences in Two Geographic Areas—United States, 1983–88," *Morbidity and Mortality Weekly Report* [SS-1] (1993); Centers for Disease Control and Prevention, "Surveillance for Anencephaly and Spina Bifida and the Impact of Prenatal Diagnosis—United States, 1985–1994," *Morbidity and Mortality Weekly Report* 44 [SS-4] (1995).

22. See Angus Clarke, "Population Screening for Genetic Susceptibility to Disease," *British Medical Journal,* July 1, 1995, 35.

23. See Samuel H. Preston and Michael R. Haines, *Fatal Years: Child Mortality in Late Nineteenth-Century America* (Princeton, N.J.: Princeton University Press, 1991).

24. James W. Hanson, "Birth Defects Surveillance and the Future of Public Health," *Public Health Reports* 110 (1995): 698.

25. Centers for Disease Control and Prevention, "Down Syndrome Prevalence at Birth—United States, 1983–1990," *Morbidity and Mortality Weekly Report* 43 (1994): 617.

26. See Sandi Wiggins et al., "The Psychological Consequences of Predictive Testing for Huntington's Disease," *New England Journal of Medicine* 327 (1992): 1401; Lerman and Croyle, "Psychological Issues in Genetic Testing"; and Paul R. Marantz, "Blaming the Victim: The Negative Consequence of Preventive Medicine," *American Journal of Public Health* 80 (1993): 1186.

27. See Rose, "Sick Individuals and Sick Populations."

28. Clarke, "Population Screening" (quoting Roger R. Williams, "Nature, Nurture and Family Predisposition," *New England Journal of Medicine* 318 [1988]: 769).

29. See Lois Shepherd, "Protecting Parents' Freedom to Have Children with Genetic Differences," *University of Illinois Law Review* (1995): 761.

30. Geoffrey Vickers, "What Sets the Goals of Public Health?" in Alfred H. Katz and Jean S. Felton, eds., *Health and the Community: Readings in the Philosophy and Sciences of Public Health* (New York: Free Press, 1965).

31. Tim Beardsley, "Vital Data: Trends in Human Genetics," *Scientific American* 274 (March 1996): 100.

32. For a review of the effectiveness of testing and counseling, see Jeff Stryker et al., "Prevention of HIV Infection: Looking Back, Looking Ahead," *Journal of the American Medical Association* 273 (1995): 1143. On the development of HIV testing policy, see Ronald Bayer, *Private Acts, Social Consequences;* and Scott Burris, "Testing, Disclosure, and the Right to Privacy," in Scott Burris, Harlon L. Dalton, and Judith Leonie Miller, eds., *AIDS Law Today: A New Guide for the Public* (New Haven: Yale University Press, 1993).

33. Centers for Disease Control and Prevention, Advisory Committee on the Prevention of HIV Infection, *External Review of CDC's HIV Prevention Strategies* (June 1994).

34. Scott Burris, "Public Health, 'AIDS Exceptionalism,' and the Law," *John Marshall Law Review* 27 (1994): 251.

35. Bernard J. Turnock and Chester J. Kelly, "Mandatory Premarital Testing for Human Immunodeficiency Virus: The Illinois Experience," *Journal of the American Medical Association* 261 (1989): 3415.

36. School Board of Nassau County v. Arline 480 U.S. 273 (1987); see Pa. Stat. Ann. tit. 35, § 7602 (1995).

37. See Elizabeth Fee and Nancy Krieger, "Thinking and Rethinking AIDS: Implications for Health Policy," *International Journal of Health Services* 23 (1993): 323.

38. Robert Gordon, "New Developments in Legal Theory," in David Kairys, ed., *The Politics of Law: A Progressive Critique,* 2d ed. (New York: Pantheon, 1990).

39. Wendy E. Parmet, "Discrimination and Disability: The Challenges of the ADA," *Law, Medicine and Health Care* 18 (1990): 331.

40. Doe v. Borough of Barrington, 729 F. Supp. 376, 384–85 (D.N.J. 1990).

41. Susan Wolf, "Beyond 'Genetic Discrimination': Toward the Broader Harm of Geneticism," *Journal of Law, Medicine and Ethics* 23 (1995): 345, 349–50.

42. Ibid.

43. Compare Scott Burris, "Testing, Disclosure, and the Right to Privacy," with Karen H. Rothenberg, "Genetic Information and Health Insurance: State Legislative Approaches," *Journal of Law, Medicine and Ethics* 23 (1995): 312.

44. Lawrence O. Gostin, "Health Information Privacy," *Cornell Law Review* 80 (1995): 451.

45. Usually, but not always. See Neil A. Holtzman, "The Attempt to Pass the Genetic Privacy Act in Maryland," *Journal of Law, Medicine and Ethics* 23 (1995): 367.

46. The depth of this problem is attested to by several of the contributors to a recent symposium on genetic screening and the law. See Lawrence O. Gostin, "Genetic Privacy," ibid., 320, 322; Reilly, "Impact of Genetic Privacy Act"; Rothenberg, "Genetic Information and Health Insurance"; and Wolf, "Beyond 'Genetic Discrimination.'"

47. Gostin, "Genetic Privacy"; accord Scott Burris, "Healthcare Privacy and Confidentiality: The Complete Legal Guide (Review)," *Journal of Legal Medicine* 16 (1995): 447.

48. See, e.g., S. 1360, 104th Cong., 2d Sess. (1996).

49. Gostin, "Health Information Privacy," 454.

50. Wendy E. Parmet, "Legislating Privacy: The HIV Experience," *Journal of Law, Medicine and Ethics* 23 (1995) 371, 372.

51. For example, Gregory M. Herek and John P. Capitanio, "Public Reactions to AIDS in the United States: A Second Decade of Stigma," *American Journal of Public Health* 83 (1993): 574; Robert J. Blendon, Karen Donelan, and Richard A. Knox, "Public Opinion and AIDS: Lessons for the Second Decade," *Journal of the American Medical Association* 267 (1992): 981; and Barbara Gerbert et al., "Physicians and Acquired Immunodeficiency Syndrome: What Patients Think About Human Immunodeficiency Virus in Medical Practice," *Journal of the American Medical Association* 262 (1989): 1969.

52. Blendon, Donelan, and Knox, "Public Opinion and AIDS."

53. Margaret Hoffman-Terry, Luther V. Rhodes, and James F. Reed III, "Impact of Human Immunodeficiency Virus on Medical and Surgical Residents," *Archives of Internal Medicine* 152 (1992): 1788. The literature on dental health care workers' attitudes, which one of us has recently reviewed, is more typical. Two studies of dental health care workers suggest the potential for law-related questions, but also the pitfalls for the legally unwary. See Scott Burris, "Dental Discrimination Against the HIV-Infected: Empirical Data, Law and Public Policy," *Yale Journal on Regulation* 13 (1995): 1.

54. Laura J. Fehrs et al., "Trial of Anonymous Versus Confidential Human Immunodeficiency Virus Testing," *Lancet* 1988 (2): 379; D. Hirano et al., "Anonymous HIV Testing: The Impact of Availability on Demand in Arizona," *American Journal of Public Health* 84 (1994): 2008; Tamara Hoxworth et al., "Anonymous HIV Testing: Does It Attract Clients Who Would Not Seek Confidential Testing?" *AIDS and Public Policy Journal* 9 (1994): 1982; S. M. Kegeles et al., "Many People Who Seek Anonymous HIV-Antibody Testing Would Avoid It Under Other Circumstances," *AIDS* 4 (1990): 585; Siegel et al., "Motives of Gay Men"; Pamela A. Meyer et al., "Comparison of Individuals Receiving Anonymous and Confidential Testing for HIV," *Southern Medical Journal* 87 (1994): 344.

55. Lawrence O. Gostin, "The AIDS Litigation Project: A National Review of Court and Human Rights Commission Decisions, Part I: The Social Impact of AIDS," *Journal of the American Medical Association* 263 (1990): 1961; Gostin, "The AIDS Litigation Project: A National Review of Court and Human Rights Commission Decisions, Part II: Discrimination," ibid., 2086; B. Friedland and R. Valachovic, "State Dental Boards' Policies on a Practitioner's Duty to Care for HIV Seropositive or AIDS Patients," *Journal of the American College of Dentists* 62, no. 3 (1995): 37.

56. Herbert M. Hazelkorn, "The Reaction of Dentists to Members of Groups at Risk of AIDS," *Journal of the American Dental Association* 119 (1989): 611; see Burris, "Dental Discrimination."

57. Hoxworth et al., "Anonymous HIV Testing."

Part Three **The Effect of New Technology**

Chapter 9 Confidentiality, Collective Resources, and Commercial Genomics

Robert Mullan Cook-Deegan

Information about genes has potential value not only for science but also in commerce. Patents and trade secrets are at root an extension of property rights into the realm of information, based on control of data. The Human Genome Project, conceived initially as a public infrastructure initiative for human genetics, has since 1993 been joined by private commercial genomics. Commercial genomics is funded through private investments intended to generate new information, usually as part of a strategy to expedite the discovery of new drugs and diagnostics. The prospect of profit infuses genome research with private dollars in addition to public ones, but it also introduces incentives to bind genetics researchers into agreements that constrain the flow of information. These agreements raise issues about confidentiality quite different from those addressed in other chapters of this book.

The launching of commercial genomics in 1993–94 has brought with it several important consequences. The evolving strategies for drug discovery in private firms have placed constraints on confidentiality of data, and rules governing industry-university-government relations in the national innovation system have changed. Such issues as privacy, confidentiality, and regulation of new technologies, discussed in other chapters, are also critical to commercial genomics. Unfair use of genetic data in insurance underwriting, harms that follow from unauthorized disclosure of genetic information, genetic discrimination in the workplace, premature introduction of genetically based products that the public perceives as motivated by profit, and other problems could well stymie research and application. Policy failure in those arenas would predictably lead to public backlash against genetics in general, and commercial genomics in particular. The primary focus here, however, is on confidentiality constraints within the context of genomics research and how commercial interests might modify current practices.

The commercial potential of genetic technologies has been discussed since the first discussions of the Human Genome Project. The initial prospect of commercial interest was more rhetorical and theoretical than real—the dollars did not follow the words. The advantages of having a robust domestic project for the nascent biotechnology industry was linked to an active debate about national economic competitiveness during the mid- to late 1980s, when the genome project was conceived and launched. For the most part, however, commercial interests were framed in terms more of enabling technology—DNA sequencing and mapping instruments and methods—than of the informational results of genomic research. The 1988 National Research Council and Office of Technology Assessment (OTA) reports on the genome project focused mainly on the infrastructural elements of the project (maps and sequence data) and technology development, not private investment in the research and all that might imply.[1] The initial five-year plan that emerged from the National Institutes of Health (NIH) and Department of Energy (DOE) contained a short, general section on technology transfer.[2] These policy reports and the initial government plan implicitly assumed that most of the investment for research and development would come from federal sources, with potential private users, such as major pharmaceutical firms or instrument manufacturers, plucking the fruits of federally funded research as they began to ripen. The focus was on a clean hand-off from publicly available and federally funded research to privately funded research and development for commercial applications. What has actually emerged is far more complex, with some firms privately funding infrastructure of use to academic researchers in their quest for genes and many private firms doing work that closely parallels work done in federally funded research laboratories—performed in universities, federal laboratories, and other private firms.

Commercial genomics began to attract substantial private funding in 1993 and 1994, as investors began to appreciate the scientific potential of genomic analysis to provide advantages of lead time in drug discovery. The theoretical prospect of commercial relevance gave way to a tide of actual investments in private firms dedicated to genomic research. A number of companies were started or reconfigured from existing firms to focus on genomics. New companies included Darwin Molecular, Human Genome Sciences, Mercator Genetics, Millennium Pharmaceuticals, and Sequana Therapeutics.[3] Genome Therapeutics (formerly Collaborative Research), Incyte Pharmaceuticals, and Myriad Genetics transformed themselves into dedicated genome research firms.[4] Existing pharmaceutical houses also launched substantial research efforts. This included some first-generation biotechnology companies, such as Amgen and Genentech, some very large U.S. and multinational pharmaceutical firms, such as Merck, Pfizer, and SmithKline Beecham, and some Japanese firms and private research institutes, such as Sagami Chemical Research Institute and Ohtsuka Pharmaceuticals in Japan.[5]

The dedicated genome research firms fell into two general groups, positional cloning firms and cDNA sequencing firms, and a third category of variants. The positional cloning firms proposed to hunt for single genes or oligogenic complexes (groups of genes that function in concert) by using genetic linkage and other pedigree-based approaches. The positional cloning companies—Sequana, Mercator, Millennium, Myriad, and to some extent Darwin—started with families or animal models of a disease (including cancers, diabetes, heart disease, and Alzheimer's disease) or another character (such as baldness or obesity) and attempted to identify regions of the genome that were statistically correlated with inheritance (genetic linkage or other methods), followed by structural analysis of genes in those regions in search of specific mutations. This was a tried-and-true method for finding individual genes and a promising method for finding gene clusters associated with polygenic and multifactorial traits. They started with a known function or disease and hunted for the underlying genes.

The firms based on cDNA sequencing began with structural analysis of DNA and progressed to hunt for functions and uses. The starting points generally were libraries of "complementary DNA" constructed from messenger RNA transcripts. Messenger RNA is the transcript that is transported from the cell nucleus to the cytoplasm and decoded by ribosomes and transfer RNAs into protein. Many introns, binding domains, regulatory regions, and modulatory sequences in native nuclear (genomic) DNA have been edited out. This biological editing from genomic DNA to cDNA reduces the amount of DNA roughly tenfold. It focuses on DNA known to code for a protein—that is, a gene that is actively expressed in the relevant cell type. It is difficult to be sure that all genes are contained in such libraries—indeed, "normalizing" such libraries to ensure that most genes are captured is a major technical focus—but those DNA fragments that appear in such libraries are quite likely to be active genes and are thus of biological interest. The cDNA sequencing strategy is, in essence, a shortcut to the "juicy bits" of the genome. Each gene uncovered is a potential diagnostic, therapeutic agent, or target for modulation by small molecules—all possibly steps toward products with commercial value.

Most firms performed both sequencing and positional cloning to some extent, but different companies deployed their resources to emphasize one strategy or the other. Positional cloning moves from known function toward unknown genes; cDNA sequencing scans the genome for genes and works toward finding a function for those genes. Some firms added a technological spin. Darwin Molecular, for example, took pains to explain that it was not just another genomics company but that it proposed to follow positional cloning and sequencing with directed molecular evolution, aiming to find small drugs to affect the genes in question.[6] Genome Therapeutics used a particular DNA sequencing method and focused on regions of known interest as well as disease-causing microorganisms, alone among the small genomic firms in vigorously pursuing federal grant and contract research.[7] Genome Therapeutics had agreements with Astra (related to sequencing of *Helicobacter pylori,* the organism associated with peptic ulcer disease) and Schering-Plough (for unspecified microbial sequencing efforts).

Genome Therapeutics also pursued positional cloning and cDNA sequencing related to several human diseases, along with mapping chromosomes 4 and 10 and sequencing the bacteria associated with tuberculosis, leprosy, and staphylococcal infections. Genset, a French firm best known for producing synthetic DNA, announced intentions to shift toward large-scale sequencing and gene discovery early in 1996. It hired French scientist Daniel Cohen as its "chief genomics officer," presumably the first position with this title in the world, and established a "high throughput sequencing laboratory" using a capital infusion of $19.2 million from a group of its shareholders.[8]

Dedicated Genome Research Firms, 1993–94

Type of Firm	Genome Research Firm	Large Pharmaceutical Partners
Positional Cloning		
	Mercator Genetics	
	Millennium Pharmaceuticals	Hoffmann–La Roche, Lilly, Astra
	Myriad Genetics	Lilly, Ciba-Geigy, Bayer
	Sequana Therapeutics	Wellcome Glaxo, Corange, Boehringer Ingelheim
cDNA Sequencing		
	Human Genome Sciences	SmithKline Beecham, Takeda
	Incyte Pharmaceuticals	Upjohn, Pfizer, Hoechst, Novo Nordisk, Abbott, Johnson & Johnson
Hybrid		
	Darwin Molecular	Rhone Poulenc Rorer
	Genome Therapeutics	Astra, Schering-Plough
	Genset	

The private investment in these dedicated genomic research firms, excluding internal investment by existing and large pharmaceutical houses, approximated $150 million in 1993,[9] and roughly comparable amounts were invested in 1994, followed by an increase in 1995 and 1996.[10] The new investments came from diverse private sources. The startups were mainly financed by one or a few private investors, often later supplemented by modest capital (from a few million to tens of millions of dollars) from either a venture capital firm or a large pharmaceutical firm. The next wave of larger investments (tens of millions to over $100 million) came from agreements with established pharmaceutical firms. Most of the small genomics research corporations issued initial public offerings of common stock (Human Genome Sciences, Incyte, Millennium, Myriad, and Sequana; Genome Therapeutics had been publicly traded as Collaborative Research for many years and issued new stock early in 1996). Human Genome Sciences linked with SmithKline Beecham (and, subsequently, Takeda); Sequana with Wellcome Glaxo (on noninsulin-dependent diabetes), Corange (for osteoporosis), and Boehringer Ingelheim (for asthma); Millennium with Hoffmann–La Roche (obesity and noninsulin-dependent diabetes), Lilly (atherosclerosis), and Astra (inflammatory bowel diseases); and Darwin with Rhone Poulenc Rorer (for novel thymidine kinase genes).[11]

Myriad expanded its agreement with Lilly (breast cancer) and found additional partners with Ciba-Geigy (cardiovascular disease) and Bayer (obesity, osteoporosis, and asthma); and Incyte signed separate agreements with Pfizer (July 1994), Upjohn (December 1994), Novo Nordisk (August 1995), Hoechst (October 1995), Abbott (December 1995), and Johnson & Johnson (January 1996).[12]

The complex corporate deals introduce novel issues that directly affect the flow of information. Conflicts may arise between the best interests of private firms, on one hand, and the best interests of those who originally contributed information about themselves and often also donated blood or tissue samples from their bodies, on the other. Such conflicts are not inevitable, but neither are they unlikely. As genomic research progresses into areas of potential commercial application, the risks increase. At the least, the world is a more complicated place.

CASE STUDY OF A GENE HUNT

A concrete case study of the hunt for one of four Alzheimer's genes isolated to date—the gene for presenilin 2 located on chromosome 1—well illustrates a successful gene hunt related to a disease that has devastating social impact and high commercial interest.[13]

In 1976, Emma Ross contacted the neurology department at the University of Colorado in Boulder.[14] Her husband, Robert Ross, had Alzheimer's disease, as did many other members of his family stretching back more than 70 years through three generations. Constructing the Ross family pedigree took several years. Many people within the family and from the university gathered clinical data on those affected; took blood, saliva, and other samples from several hundred people in the family; and even conducted skin biopsies and elaborate clinical examinations of several key individuals. The pedigree was published in 1979,[15] and the last of the University of Colorado studies involving the Ross family was published in 1981, but the pedigrees remained scientifically valuable.

In 1983 or 1984, I copied the pedigrees and relevant clinical data and sent them to investigators at the University of Washington, Seattle; the Familial Alzheimer's Disease Foundation in Tulsa, Oklahoma; and the Laboratory for Central Nervous System Studies at the National Institute on Neurological and Communicative Disorders and Stroke (as it was then called) in Bethesda, Maryland. The initial purpose of constructing the pedigree was to confirm autosomal dominant inheritance, as well as to enable genetic linkage studies.

We proposed to attempt genetic linkage of Alzheimer's disease in this and other smaller families, using the 70 or so protein, biochemical, and other genetic markers available at the time. This was before the advent of restriction fragment length polymorphism (use of markers that vary among individuals in a family and can be used to trace inheritance of chromosome regions), as proposed in 1980 by Botstein and colleagues.[16] It was unlikely to work then, but with the elaboration of much denser and more polymorphic markers during the 1980s, and especially as the Human Genome Project made tools for genetic linkage vastly more powerful, these studies became quite practical and likely to succeed.

The Seattle group, funded by NIH and the Veterans Administration, did considerably more work with the Ross family, gathering more clinical information and samples. They pursued linkage studies in the Rosses and many other families. In 1995, they found genetic linkage to chromosome 1.[17] At about the same time, Rudolph Tanzi's group at Massachusetts General Hospital, Cambridge, contacted them about a cDNA that might be related (because its sequence was similar) to the presenilin 1 gene located on chromosome 14. The presenilin 1 gene, whose mutation was associated with early onset Alzheimer's disease in other families, had first been discovered by Peter Saint George-Hyslop and his group at the University of Toronto.[18] Tanzi was a coauthor of the presenilin 1 discovery paper with Saint George-Hyslop. Tanzi had found a DNA sequence similar to the presenilin 1 gene in a collection of cDNA fragments derived from brain and sequenced at the University of Colorado.[19]

The Massachusetts General group thus had a promising candidate gene, and the Seattle group had a region likely to contain an Alzheimer gene. The two groups quickly formed a collaboration, and within weeks they confirmed that the candidate gene did indeed map to chromosome 1 and that mutations of that gene correlated with Alzheimer's disease in some families, including the Rosses. The groups jointly prepared papers published in the August 18, 1995, issue of *Science*.[20] The sequencing work to identify the mutations was performed by Darwin Molecular in collaboration with the Seattle group and by the Massachusetts General group. The *Science* papers reported the linkage of Alzheimer's disease in the Ross and other so-called Volga German families (named for their distinctive migratory history) to chromosome 1, correlated with mutations in the presenilin 2 gene located there. Two weeks later, a paper from the Toronto group appeared in *Nature*, describing the presenilin 2 gene.[21] This work, initiated in Toronto before Tanzi knew of the presenilin 1 sequence, was based on using that sequence to identify similar ones in various databases, identifying a cDNA, mapping it to chromosome 1, and finding mutations in the few individuals from Volga German families with tissue samples in public repositories.

A third independent effort also turned up a chromosome 1 gene. A Harvard team from the laboratory of Huntington Potter of Harvard University found a sequence similar to the presenilin gene on chromosome 14 and mapped this to chromosome 1.[22] The investigators suggested it might be another Alzheimer's gene, which was confirmed by the other groups whose papers were published soon after this independent discovery paper was submitted for publication.

Finding the chromosome 1 gene culminated the first phase of genetic research started by the Ross family before 1976, when the pedigree was first presented to a biomedical research group. The successful discovery of the presenilin 2 gene involved considerable effort by investigators at a half-dozen major research institutions, augmented by a private corporate firm collaborating with one of the academic groups. This work paralleled similar work going on elsewhere, entailing several collaborations focused on Alzheimer's genes and including one between the University of South Florida, Tampa, and Human Genome Sciences.

The scientific history of this discovery is punctuated by a related series of patent applications.[23] The University of Toronto filed patent applications on its discovery of the presenilin 1 and 2 genes. The Seattle group filed a patent application in 1992, based on chromosome 14 linkage in some early onset Alzheimer's families. In 1995 (reportedly a few weeks after the independent Toronto application), another patent application on the presenilin 2 gene was also filed, listing members of the Massachusetts General, Seattle, and Darwin teams. Use of the EST fragment sequenced at the University of Colorado, the one used to fish out the presenilin 2 gene, was not encumbered by patent rights, as the University of Colorado team did not file a patent application, in contrast to the action taken by NIH for similar work.[24] There are thus potentially competing claims for patent rights on discoveries related to genetic linkage of early onset familial Alzheimer's disease to chromosomes 14 and 1, as well as both the presenilin 1 and 2 genes themselves.

The hunt for presenilin 1 and 2 genes for early onset familial Alzheimer's disease was only part of a larger story that is still unfolding. Similarly complicated stories could be told about the earlier discovery of an Alzheimer's gene on chromosome 21, or about the risk factor association between late onset Alzheimer's disease and different forms of the apolipoprotein E gene on chromosome 19. Both these scientific discoveries were likewise accompanied by patent applications that potentially overlap and whose ultimate scope and significance are now highly uncertain. And the Alzheimer's story is just one of many disease-gene hunts. There have been hotly contested races for breast cancer genes, colon cancer genes, the cystic fibrosis gene, and many others. Scientific races have been attended by patent applications in some of these stories as well. But the theme of relevance here is that in all cases, hundreds of people beyond those finally listed as inventors set the stage for gene discovery. Beyond the major research centers lie countless hospitals and clinical services and hundreds of family members who contributed blood and tissue samples and clinical information. Those who crossed the finish lines in these gene races would be the first to acknowledge the complexity of the task and the futility of trying to recognize all those who contributed. But the patent system is a "winner take all" reward system, vesting all rights in those listed as inventors or those to whom they assign their rights. Second-place finishers and background supporters do not generally secure rights, although the inventors can choose to reward their contributions through royalties, licenses, or in other ways.

Linkage maps are becoming much better and easier to use so that relatively less effort is expended on genotyping, which used to be a significant bottleneck. The time and effort needed to construct a pedigree and confirm clinical data are substantial, and family resources may now become the rate-limiting step in some gene hunts that employ the positional cloning strategy. If so, the relative value of family resources will rise, increasing the opportunities for a moral foul and reinforcing the need for an agreed set of rules.

EFFECTS ON FLOW OF FAMILY DATA

This case illustrates several complexities of information flow and the role of commercial interests in governing that flow. First, the transfer of the Ross pedigree from the University of Colorado to other research groups was possible in part because it was not considered a valuable financial asset. It had scientific value, but only if considerable further work were done. A pre-existing agreement with a commercial firm would at least complicate such sharing and might preclude it. If the same situation arose now, the university office of technology transfer might request a formal transfer agreement, which might specify future rights or require an option to negotiate such rights should commercial potential become apparent. Some institutions impose few constraints on future use, whereas others might entirely block a transfer. The viability of a deal hinges critically on the perceived value of the information, which is relatively low when so much work is necessary to enable subsequent discovery. The ultimate commercial value is often highly uncertain, and investigators may have visions of the Cohen-Boyer patent (a patent covering recombinant DNA techniques owned by Stanford University and shared with the University of California, San Francisco) dancing in their heads, while corporate negotiators play Scrooge, recounting countless expensive trips down blind alleys of drug discovery.

When information is deemed likely to attract commercial interest—and Alzheimer's genetics now surely qualifies—constraints built into material transfer agreements are more likely. At the least, exchange is slowed by adding paperwork and introducing more people into the decision; it might well get scuttled. Incentives are already low for sharing data when no publication is in prospect. At the time the Ross pedigree and clinical files were copied and distributed, Alzheimer's genetics swam outside the research mainstream and few pharmaceutical firms had relevant attachments to academic research groups. Were the same search to happen in 1997, the situation would likely be different. The pedigree and files might still be transferred, but the transfer would probably follow a formal agreement and surely would entail many more phone calls.

Commercial interests are far weaker constraints on information flow than scientific competition, at least to date. The standards for sharing data are far less open in human genetics than in nematode, yeast, or bacterial genetics. Those fields are smaller, do not contend with the complexities of pedigree construction intrinsic to human genetics, and have long research traditions that encourage openness. In the long run, those other fields may produce information that is more fundamental and perhaps even more practical, but the findings are not as obviously related to dread diseases and they produce fewer stories in the pages of the *New York Times* and *Wall Street Journal*. Searches for conspicuous disease-related genes have for the past decade loomed large as a pathway to prominent research careers that attract legions of competitors. Given the considerable premium on first discovery in science, the incentive to restrict sharing introduced by commercial interests is overwhelmed by these much stronger forces in the sociology of science that already encourage data hoarding. But the solutions for dealing openly with contending career interests parallel those for commercial interests. Indeed, the fact that pharmaceutical firms must be sensitive to their public image and desire to keep their intellectual property holdings clean and secure could actually clarify the proper rules of conduct. Investigators could, through a public statement formulated by the American Society of Human Genetics or some other scientific organization, pledge to share family-based information and resources when it is in the families' interests to do so, subject to reasonable "first investigator" advantages. This could rein in the groups pushing the ethical envelope, holding family data hostage to their career aspirations and commercial interests, while encouraging the research community to set a reasonable standard for the duration and scope of rewards for those who construct pedigrees.

COMMERCIAL USE OF DONATED INFORMATION, DNA SAMPLES, AND TISSUES

Commercial uses of donated information, DNA samples, and tissues are often not in mind when the donations are made. This can raise questions about how to deal with the introduction of commercial interests, the just distribution of rewards, and who should control the information. How do families fare under these arrangements? On one level, their interests are very well served. Private research funds increase the resources devoted to understanding and managing disease. Commercial interest intensifies the vigorous competition among different groups hunting down disease-associated genes and focuses attention on practical applications, goading faster and better research efforts as more groups with greater resources vie for leadership. If the main goal is to improve diagnosis and devise new treatments, then private investment is a welcome addition. Private firms can make products and provide services that universities and government laboratories cannot. Moreover, the private research and development investments do not come from taxpayers, at least not directly.

New private sources of funding could also add diversity to the mix of possible ways to advance science. Private firms or privately funded academic groups may choose a research path that is too venturesome to secure federal funding through peer-reviewed competitive grants. Or new sources of funding may enable sufficient concentration of equipment and expertise that is not otherwise available yet is crucial to the success of a capital-intensive research strategy. From the perspective of the companies involved, the gene would not be discovered at all, or at least not as quickly, but for the efforts of the scientific workers. Any rewards that flow from selling products and services derive from a desired end—the discovery of a treatment or diagnostic that did not exist before. The reward from any patents or trade secrets is earned through innovation and can be reinvested to make new discoveries.

On another level, however, families may be left out of the picture. The privately funded research investment may contribute to the discovery, but so do the tissues and clinical information from afflicted families. The family contributions are decidedly not public data but rather very private information and materials held in trust by investigators. In the financial allocation of rewards, the current system redounds solely to the benefit of the companies who seize rights by crossing the finish line with a gene in hand, who make some other discovery protected by patent or trade secrecy, or who license from the groups who control such intellectual property. Families benefit by having a treatment available.

This state of affairs conflicts with an intuitive sense of just rewards, at least on its face. There are several arguments, however, that it may reflect a pragmatic balancing of interests. First, although the contributions of family members are indeed crucial, their interests may be restricted to discovering the knowledge and new technologies, not to reaping the financial rewards. We could decide that as a matter of policy, we are all better off if we divvy up rewards so that innovators are richly rewarded financially so that families ultimately get the technologies they desire. The quid pro quo here is conferral of intellectual property rights in return for technological advance.

Second, the process of accounting for individual (or even worse, collective) contributions to an ultimate product or service is liable to prove hopelessly expensive and complex. One way to ensure fair distribution would be to assert property rights over the information and tissue samples, so that control by family members is never fully relinquished. But this invites a litany of accounting problems. Just whose DNA was most important? Should affected relatives get a bigger share than those unaffected? Should those whose family shows a genetic crossover event and contributes a disproportionate share of information about gene location get more than those with no such crossover? What will be the costs of tracking the sometimes thousands of individuals involved? Attempting to allocate financial benefits according to material contribution to a discovery invites internecine fights over the relative magnitude of those contributions. Should one include only those families with a particular mutated gene, excluding those with other mutations? What about any contributions by those with Alzheimer's disease, for example, but no clear inheritance pattern? What about other conditions that closely resemble Alzheimer's disease? Even if one believes that the current system is unfair, the costs and complexity of making it fair might well overwhelm the benefits of doing so.

Some human geneticists have become uncomfortable, however, with the possibility of granting exclusive or privileged access to clinical resources (including pedigree, diagnostic, and genotype data plus DNA and biological samples) to private firms in return for research funding, future proprietary rights, equity shares for the investigators, or other benefits. They call the practice "selling families" and fear it could engender a backlash that would affect all human genetics. Family members may knowingly donate materials as proprietary assets for a particular firm because this brings new funds or new lines of inquiry. Problems are likely to arise, however, if pedigree and clinical information originally donated to academic or other nonprofit institutions are subsequently and without the donors' knowledge converted to trade secrets through commercial agreements and treated as the property of the investigators or institutions.

In the vast majority of cases financial returns from pedigree studies will be minimal, since most protocols do not produce commercially relevant information. Even when results prove lucrative, this will not be apparent until long after participants first enter a gene-mapping study. Many studies, therefore, may not entail disclosure of commercial relationships. But where family resources are material to an agreement—that is, when access to family resources is an important reason why a commercial firm chooses a particular group of investigators—then those investigators should be held to account for the interests of family participants. Full disclosure of every potential commercial transaction is probably impractical, but this does not preclude a commitment on the part of investigators and their host institutions to serving as guardians of family interests and evolving a community standard within human genetics that outlines how to do so.

The commercial interests of investigators could be treated as a matter to be disclosed in the informed consent process. Families involved in the studies could sign waivers of their commercial rights, stipulate a benefit, or reserve the right to later negotiations. In Moore v. Regents of the University of California, John Moore went to UCLA Medical Center for treatment of his hairy cell leukemia.[25] His treating physician recommended a spleenectomy. After surgery, without Moore's knowledge or consent, his treating physician and others developed and patented a cell line from Moore's spleen and licensed it commercially. The Supreme Court of California held that the failure of Moore's physician to disclose his research and economic interests gave rise to a legal action for failing to obtain informed consent before the medical procedures or breach of fiduciary duty.

Many medical facilities have reacted to the Moore case by requiring all those seeking medical services to sign away commercial rights in a blanket waiver. Unconstrained blanket waivers, however, cut donors off from all subsequent interests, including some that may be legitimate, such as wanting assurance that further research on the condition of interest is pursued further or not conceding to treatment of data as trade secrets. In the context of specific studies outside routine medical care, disclosure of commercial interests would be possible only when commercial relevance is foreseeable. Commercial interests are often not apparent at the outset, but if commercial interests arise later, universities and other institutional sponsors could pledge good faith efforts to ensure that interests of families are pursued, if only through such indirect means as royalty streams devoted to similar research. If informed consent is used only to keep family interests away from the bargaining table when money begins to change hands, this may clarify the rules, but it will not promote fair distribution of benefits.

As I have argued above, there is something special about family materials and information as they contribute to gene discovery. The discovery process draws on family contributions that go well beyond the expertise and industry of those doing the science. This truly is different from synthesizing new chemical compounds, writing a new software program, or building a computer. Although some lines of clinical research, such as clinical trials, share this feature, potential research subjects can more easily foresee any potential commercial implications linked to a treatment or diagnostic advance. As genetics becomes more closely linked to commercial interests in the public mind, the need to flag commercial interests when seeking consent of prospective research subjects might diminish. And yet, genetics differs from other fields in another respect, at least in degree—in the sense that the human genome is finite and precious.

GENES AS A COMMON RESOURCE

A pharmaceutical firm can synthesize any number of chemicals in its storehouse, keeping them as trade secrets until they prove useful, at which time the firm can disclose them in a patent. Or it can screen compounds purified from soil fungi or exotic plants. This does not hinder others from similar acts. In the case of synthesis, the new chemical entities exist only because of the firm that paid to make them. In the case of screening, there may be a shared resource argument, but it will hinge on control of the source material (perhaps a rare tropical plant) rather than a shared sense of ownership among all members of the species. But the number of human genes is limited, and genes are found, not created. The question is whether this matters.

A claim that the human genome is our "common heritage," as embodied in the draft declaration on the protection of the human genome by the United

Nations Educational, Scientific, and Cultural Organization (UNESCO), invites this line of analysis.[26] Indeed, documents explaining the UNESCO draft refer explicitly to the seabed outside national waters, the moon, cultural goods, and biological diversity as other areas of common heritage. Yet these are quite different senses of our heritage, and it is not clear that they may be analogous to the human genome. Common heritage may preclude declarations of national sovereignty over new territory, the terra incognita of the human chromosomes, but such national territoriality was not being contemplated. Public policy has often given substantial rewards to the discoverer who first makes a common resource useful. American law, for example, has historically rewarded risk-taking and exploration, giving individuals financial rewards as an incentive to achieve national goals. The Homestead Act of 1862 gave land to those who would tend it. Those who found gold or silver on public lands obtained mineral rights or exploitation rights for minimal fees. Whole bodies of law (in some cases dated and imperfect) deal with the conferral of rights over minerals, oil, water, ranching, logging, and so on. Generally, these laws deal with circumscribed rights to physical property. To what extent is the human genome a precious scientific and technical resource, a common intellectual property?

The common heritage argument is often taken to argue against patenting of any human genes. Of itself, as the examples make clear, the fact that a resource is shared precludes neither private property rights nor, by extension, intellectual property rights. Most of the elements in our shared environment are subject to patents. But they are also subject to additional guidance—inducements to private actions consonant with collective goals. How well the precedents of natural resource law can guide policy on the human genome is far from obvious. It seems likely, however, that some directives will be necessary beyond patent and trade secret law, the main body of law now applied to genetic discovery.

Patents are limited-term monopoly rights granted by the government to inventors in return for public disclosure of their invention sufficient for others to replicate it. Inventors must demonstrate in a patent application that the invention is new, not obvious to others skilled in the art, and useful. In return, the government confers a right to prevent others from making, using, or selling the patented invention. An inventor can destroy the chances of securing patent rights by advance public disclosure,[27] and so patents do require a period of secrecy until a patent application is filed. Once an application is filed, however, the invention can be disclosed without endangering issuance of a patent.

The legal strictures of trade secrecy require firms to take active steps to protect them, conflicting with the academic ethos of openness. Trade secrets are often fully intended to slow the scientific and technical progress of others. If a company keeps secret information it has discovered at its own expense, it does no harm. But public concerns are legitimate if that zone of secrecy expands into resources derived from publicly funded research. Public policy may still encourage private conversion, similar to patents, although the tit-for-tat exchange of proprietary advantage for public disclosure no longer holds. The argument for private conversion may be a judgment about the superior efficiency or effectiveness of the private sector in pursuing linkage or genes or products and services. Yet the interests of research subjects are also at stake if trade secrecy encumbers information and materials they have contributed. Family resources should not be held as trade secrets unless family members who contribute their data and materials understand the terms. Specifically, this suggests that genetic information initially gathered at academic centers that subsequently becomes relevant to a commercial agreement needs to be treated with special care. That special care would surely include, as part of informed consent, disclosure of known commercial interests in studies not yet started.

In connection with conversion of family data to proprietary use, two options spring to mind, and there are no doubt others. Individual family members could be contacted anew and given a chance to opt out of the collaboration, if they do not wish to be party to the commercial agreement. Academic and nonprofit groups that collect the data could evolve such collective mechanisms as the "soft regulation" of published voluntary guidelines. Or institutions that ultimately receive financial rewards could plow some fraction of the proceeds into research that furthers the interests of the populations who contributed data. One solution will not work, for the reasons stated above—an accounting system that traces individual contributions is usually impractical.

Several events might trigger these mechanisms. New restrictions on access to information relevant to a commercial collaboration, especially any period of secrecy that extends beyond the filing of a patent application, would be the most common trigger. This will require either exempting material and information contributed by research participants from the general restrictions or obtaining the consent of those who first contributed the materials and information.[28] As noted above, this is a burdensome and sometimes impossible task. One way around this is for institutional review boards to begin formulating standard language that would separate information and materials contributed by research subjects from those contributed by the investigators negotiating an agreement. If this proves too troublesome, and family resources cannot be extricated from the other contributions of investigators, then the agreements are unlikely to fare well when exposed to the full light of day. That is, it suggests that the investigators are mainly selling, not their expertise and technology, but access to family information and resources without consultation.

This line of argument should not be taken as inimical to any private conversion of public resources. Doing good by making money is a cornerstone of our culture, albeit within constraints. The history of the telegraph, telephone, railroads, aviation, microelectronics, and virtually any other "high technology" activity reveals instances in which benefits generated at public expense were turned over to the private sector. Public interest can indeed be served by transferring rights to the private sector, resulting in better, cheaper, or more widely accessible technology. Indeed, such private conversion underlies the Bayh-Dole Act of 1980 and many other technology transfer laws that govern federally funded research in all fields, including genetics. Under Bayh-Dole and similar acts pertaining to federally owned or federally owned, contractor-operated laboratories, institutions that receive federal funds take title to inventions that result, with limited exceptions. The sponsoring agency enjoys a royalty-free license, but the institution that receives the funds and performs the work owns the resulting patents. Such private conversion is generally, if not universally, regarded as serving the long-term public interest, reaching public goals through private means. The question facing policy makers now is whether human genetics requires constraints on the unfettered pursuit of profit. The answer could be no, or it could be yes, but legislation or regulation need not necessarily follow if voluntary mechanisms were credible.

Whatever we decide about transfer of publicly funded research to commercial application, this may not extend samples and information donated by private individuals. Government can choose to confer rights in work it funds to private interests, but that is a different matter from converting contributions made by one group of private parties to benefit another private interest. The conversion is particularly suspect if it entails a fundamental change in the rules and expectations of those who contribute information and materials for research and that rule change is not known by the donors.

Commercial genomics introduces distinctive issues regarding the conversion of genetic information to private intellectual property. Two conclusions have emerged that appear in tension: first, that private conversion of communal resources may be more efficient at reaching collective goals, and second that the only practical way to treat individual contributions to genomics is as donations, except when they meet the criteria of patentability. In this framework, there is room for a conflict between judgments of what is fair and what is most efficient or most effective.

Open disclosure of the relations between investigators and private firms combined with guidelines that prevent family resources from becoming trade secrets (unless fully acknowledged through informed consent) can address the problem of converting collective family resources into proprietary assets. But it does not address the problem of just distribution, which cries out for a collective solution. Several models for dealing with this problem are at hand.

POSSIBLE SOLUTIONS

When clinical trials to treat symptoms of dementia using tetrahydroamino-acridine (tacrine, now marketed by Parke-Davis as Cognex) began, investigators and the sponsoring company, Warner-Lambert, agreed to disclose their financial interests in that company or others that might directly benefit from sale of the drug. They also agreed that a fraction of net sales would be set aside in the event that the drug proved useful (5% for the first five years, declining to 2% for the next five years; figures are lower if another manufacturer begins to distribute the drug and captures 10% of the market).[29] The drug was approved for marketing by the Food and Drug Administration in September 1993.

An ethics panel that met in 1989 stipulated that the royalty funds from this drug should be used "for patient care, teaching and research in Alzheimer's disease and related disorders."[30] If the fund exceeded $1 million, it was to be directed by an independent advisory board and given a permanent administrative home at an existing foundation or organization. In 1994, the fund appeared likely to exceed the $1 million threshold, and the ethics panel selected the Alzheimer's Disease and Related Disorders Association to administer the funds. The association then appointed an advisory board. Tacrine is not a patented drug, because it was synthesized early in the century, but Warner-Lambert (and Parke-Davis, its subsidiary) agreed to manufacture it and helped fund clinical trials. A similar arrangement could be used in conjunction with a patented drug, however, or for that matter, any product.

The arrangement has been criticized for compromising the neutrality of the Alzheimer's Disease and Related Disorders Association regarding a particular treatment modality. The committee that administers the fund is separate from the association, but lack of objectivity is always a risk with close association. One main impact of the arrangement is that the interests of family members, as well as biomedical and health services researchers, have been brought to the table as a matter of deliberate policy. The tacrine royalty fund is essentially a tax on the successful innovation of a new treatment. It was crucial to the ethics panel that the special fund be set up "only if the royalties could be sequestered for Alzheimer's disease and related disorders."[31] The basic idea was to create a funding pool to benefit the class of people who contributed to the study. It is innovative in this respect, as well as in giving family members a voice in deciding on distribution of its benefits. The inventors listed on a patent for diagnostic or screening use of apolipoprotein E testing in Alzheimer's disease have agreed that a fraction of any royalties they receive from their license to Athena Pharmaceuticals will go to the Alzheimer's Disease and Related Disorders Association and other nonprofit research support groups that have contributed to scientific advance.

Berkeley economist Paul Romer has suggested the possibility of self-organizing industrial investment boards.[32] His concern is funding innovative activities that benefit collectives of firms rather than individual companies—a private sector approach to the problem of the commons—but the same general principles could be used also to solve the problem of "somewhat focused" distribution of royalty streams or private contributions (whether from pharmaceutical firms or other sources). Such modified "Romer boards" could redistribute benefits to comport with the contributions of groups by ensuring their proportionate representation on the boards deciding on the use of resources at their disposal. A network of such boards, into which private firms could flexibly opt in and out, would permit an alignment between supporting research to the benefit of all while ensuring shared control by the contributing firms and families and others who made progress possible.

Regarding claims that the human genome is a collective resource, additional options present themselves. Senators Mark Hatfield and Tom Harkin introduced a bill directing that a small fraction of health insurance premiums (initially 1%, but later reduced) be set aside to boost NIH appropriations. That bill would have been incorporated into most of the proposed health care bills contemplated in 1993, but its prospects died with reform. (The same senators have since introduced a bill to tax tobacco products, with resulting funds going to NIH.) In the past, congressional staffers have proposed using royalties that result from U.S. patents to create research funding streams, although these ideas have not been translated into bills. These mechanisms are intended to solve a somewhat different problem, that of finding additional sources of funding for research. Similar mechanisms have been suggested to serve a redistribution function. If genetics research is truly distinctive, based on exploitation of a common resource, then royalties spun off from patents of human genes could be used to promote genetic research. This tax on innovation would channel funds back into research intended to benefit these individuals with the mutated genes. Because we are all at risk of developing some genetic disease and we are all among the collective owners of the genome, it is not clear what introducing this mechanism achieves, unless it results from a pragmatic political judgment that it is needed to obtain an appropriate share for research. Such funding could be channeled through self-organizing Romer Boards, through a private quasi-governmental corporation, or through existing NIH structures.

Another option is to use natural resource law as a model. This is not a collection of fully successful policies, however. Mining law and ranching law have saddled the nation with many benefits that redound to the few, initially pursued for the benefit of all but frozen in place and politically difficult to change despite the passage of decades and even centuries. Mining rights are sold for a pittance, and private grazing on public lands costs far more than it brings in. So opening a new line of statutory law should give us pause. There is indeed a danger that biomedical research could join the ranks of suspect groups undeservedly feeding at the public trough. Moreover, most natural resource law has been primarily concerned with inducing sufficient private investment to exploit the subject resource. This is clearly not the first-order problem for commercial genomics, which seems to be attracting significant private funds with no apparent need for a further policy boost. Rather, the problem is distribution of benefits so that inventors and private firms that sell products share the benefits.

Several options present themselves to organizations that concern themselves with the conduct of human genetic research. They can begin to craft policies to achieve consensus on handling informed consent and private conversion of pedigree data and family resources donated for research. Constraints on confidentiality of genomic information regulating the use of genetic information, discussed in other chapters in this volume, will likely loom larger in the public eye, and they surely affect far more people in more dramatic fashion. But the fair collection and allocation of collective resources may also need attention, perhaps first by private professional and scientific organizations, or related issues could flare up at any time. Scandal may breed legislation. In the case of defined populations that contribute disproportionately to a class of discoveries, arguments in favor of a redistribution mechanism that channels benefits back to those groups are appealing. For arguments about the communal nature of the human genome, however, the redistribution is to all of us and is best left to our existing system of governance without the addition of further inefficiencies.

NOTES

1. National Research Council, Committee on Mapping and Sequencing the Human Genome, *Mapping and Sequencing the Human Genome* (Washington, D.C.: National Academy Press, 1988); U.S. Congress, Office of Technology Assessment, *Mapping Our Genes—The Genome Projects: How Big? How Fast?* (Washington, D.C.: Government Printing Office, 1988).

2. National Institutes of Health, National Center for Human Genome Research, and U.S. Department of Energy, Human Genome Research Program, *Understanding Our Genetic Inheritance—The U.S. Genome Project: The First Five Years, FY 1991–1995* (Springfield, Va.: National Technical Information Service, 1990).

3. Robert M. Cook-Deegan, *Survey of Genome Science Corporation* (1994; available through the National Reference Center for Bioethics Literature, Kennedy Institute of Ethics, Georgetown University, and the National Center for Genome Resources, Santa Fe, N.Mex.).

4. Ibid.

5. Ibid.

6. Darwin Molecular, *Darwin's Objectives in Brief; Company Background; Scientific Goals; and Combinatorial Library Strategy for Drug Candidate Identification—Public Information Documents* (Bothell, Wash.: Darwin Molecular, 1996).

7. Genome Therapeutics, *Commercializing Genome Expertise; Corporate Profile, Prospectus for Common Stock (Feb. 15, 1996) and Annual Report for 1995—Public Documents* (Waltham, Mass.: Genome Therapeutics, 1996).

8. Genset, *Corporate Overview, and High Throughput Sequencing Laboratory—Public Documents* (Paris: Genset, 1996).

9. Cook-Deegan, *Survey of Genome Science Corporation.*

10. The figures are inexact because financial data for 1993 and 1994 were openly available only for publicly traded firms, supplemented by such information as the firms financed by venture capitalists, or "angels," chose to make public. By the end of 1994, only Human Genome Sciences, Incyte, and Genome Therapeutics (then called Collaborative Research) were publicly traded. Myriad, Millennium, and Darwin went public in 1995.

11. Millennium Pharmaceuticals, *About the Company, and Press Statement* (Cambridge, Mass.: Millennium Pharmaceuticals, 1995); Sequana Therapeutics, *Prospectus for Common Stock* (La Jolla, Calif.: Sequana Therapeutics, 1996); William Haseltine, president, Human Genome Sciences, Annual meeting, University of Maryland, Rockville, May 15, 1996; Human Genome Sciences, *Genes: From Our Past—Our Future: Annual Report* (Gaithersburg, Md.: Human Genome Sciences, 1995); Darwin Molecular, *Darwin's Objectives in Brief.*

12. Incyte Pharmaceuticals, *Stock Prospectus* (Palo Alto, Calif.: Incyte Pharmaceuticals,

1995); Incyte Pharmaceuticals, *Press Statements, December 20, 1995 (re Abbott); January 2, 1996 (re Johnson & Johnson); and February 22, 1996 (re fourth quarter year-end results);* Myriad Genetics, *Prospectus for Common Stock* (Salt Lake City, Utah: Myriad Genetics, 1995).

13. A lively and much more detailed account of the quest for genes in Alzheimer's disease is available in the revised paperback edition of Daniel A. Pollen, *Hannah's Heirs: The Quest for the Genetic Origins of Alzheimer's Disease,* expanded ed. (New York: Oxford University Press, 1996).

14. The facts of this case are real, but the names of the donors and family members are pseudonyms.

15. Robert H. Cook et al., "Studies in Aging of the Brain. IV. Familial Alzheimer's Disease: Relation to Transmissible Dementia, Aneuploidy and Microtubular Defects," *Neurology* 29 (1979): 1402–12.

16. David Botstein et al., "Construction of a Genetic Linkage Map in Man Using Restriction Fragment Length Polymorphisms," *American Journal of Human Genetics* 32 (1980): 314–31.

17. E. Levy-Lihad et al., "A Familial Alzheimer's Disease Locus on Chromosome 1," *Science* 269 (1995): 970–73.

18. R. Sherrington et al., "Cloning of a Gene Bearing Missense Mutations in Early-Onset Familial Alzheimer's Disease," *Nature* 375 (1995): 754–60.

19. The University of Colorado brain cDNA sequencing project was funded by DOE and was entirely unrelated to the original Colorado studies of the Ross pedigree, which had long since terminated.

20. Levy-Lihad et al., "Alzheimer's Disease Locus"; E. Levy-Lihad et al., "Candidate Gene for the Chromosome 1 Familial Alzheimer's Disease Locus," *Science* 269 (1995): 973–77.

21. Eugeniy I. Rogaev et al., "Familial Alzheimer's Disease in Kindreds with Missense Mutations in a Gene on Chromosome 1 Related to the Alzheimer's Disease Type 3 Gene," *Nature* 376: 775–78.

22. Jinhe Li et al., "Identification and Expression Analysis of a Potential Familial Alzheimer Disease Gene on Chromosome 1 Related to AD3," *Proceedings of the National Academy of Sciences* 92 (1995): 1180–84.

23. Patent applications are not public documents. If there are conflicts among the claims, these would be resolved through "interference" proceedings initiated by the U.S. Patent and Trademark Office, based on dates of conception and reduction to practice, as well as due diligence in pursuit of the invention. The dates that patent applications were filed would be decisive outside the United States and may or may not play a role in determining the first inventors for the U.S. patent.

24. By the time the presenilin 2 gene was found on chromosome 1, however, NIH had abandoned its patent application. C. Anderson, "NIH Drops Bid for Gene Patents," *Science* 263 (1994): 909. For a much more complete analysis of patenting cDNA fragments, see Rebecca S. Eisenberg and Robert P. Merges, "Opinion Letter as to the Patentability of Certain Inventions Associated with the Identification of Partial cDNA Sequencing," *American Intellectual Property Law Association Quarterly Journal* 23 (Winter 1995): 1–52.

25. Moore v. Regents of the University of California 793 P.2d 479 (Cal. 1990).

26. UNESCO, "Declaration on the Protection of the Human Genome," *Eubios Journal of Asian and International Bioethics* 5 (1995): 97–99, 150–51.

27. The United States grants a one-year "grace period" to file a patent application after public disclosure. European nations and Japan do not permit advance public disclosure. Until recently the period of patent protection was 17 years from date of issue for most inventions in the United States. Some pharmaceutical patents are eligible for term extensions to compensate for the time needed for regulatory approval. The patent term has changed to 20 years from date of application, following the Trade-Related Aspects of Intellectual Property Rights recently agreed under the General Agreement on Tariffs and Trade.

28. Some agreements with commercial genomic firms do extend periods of secrecy beyond the filing of a patent application. One standard agreement extends secrecy for the full duration of the agreement plus five years. This is reasonable for information solely generated by the firm before the agreement. It is less clear that the company should have the right to bind investigators to secrecy in the subsequent collaboration if such work involves resources drawn from public funds or private parties not recognized in the agreement. Once a patent application is filed, the patent is theoretically not endangered by disclosure. But the invention is not disclosed publicly until the patent is issued in the United States (often several years later in the case of biotechnology) or 18 months after applying for foreign patent rights under the Patent Cooperation Treaty or at the European Patent Office. This amounts to a period, often several years in the case of gene patents, when public disclosure is optional. This is another area where universities and nonprofit centers could develop voluntary norms to discourage retention of "patent pending" information.

29. D. Blumenthal, letter to Edward Truschke, executive director of the Alzheimer's Disease and Related Disorders Association, inquiring whether the association would be interested in administering the royalty funds, on behalf of the 16-center tetra-hydro-amino-acripine (THA) trial funded in part by the National Institute on Aging, administered by the Department of Psychiatry, Mount Sinai Medical Center, New York, 1990.

30. THA Ethics Committee, minutes of the April 6, 1989, Executive Session, Mount Sinai Medical Center, New York.

31. Ibid.

32. Paul M. Romer, "Implementing a National Technology Strategy with Self-Organizing Industry Investment Boards," *Brookings Papers on Economic Activity,* vol. 2 (Washington, D.C.: Brookings Institution, 1993), 345–90, 398–99.

Chapter 10 Biomarkers—Scientific Advances and Societal Implications

Paul W. Brandt-Rauf and Sherry I. Brandt-Rauf

The broad term *biologic marker* (or *biomarker*) encompasses biochemical, molecular, genetic, immunologic, physiologic, or other signals of events in biologic systems.[1] By this broad definition, the use of biomarkers to study human disease processes is clearly not new. In recent years, however, interest has increased tremendously in the use of molecular biomarkers spurred by the explosion of knowledge of the mechanisms of disease at the molecular level. Much of this interest has focused on the detection of inherited defects in specific disease-related genes, which has been accelerated by the Human Genome Project.

In the area of occupational and environmental health, attention has focused on the detection of acquired molecular defects produced by exposures to exogenous toxic agents. A major rationale for this approach has been to attempt to open up the "black box" between the presence of the toxin in the environment and the occurrence of disease. Biomarkers can be used to delineate more precisely how a given ambient toxic exposure causes disease by tracing the "molecular footprints" as the toxin passes through the body, interacts with critical target molecules in the body, and produces the molecular and cellular

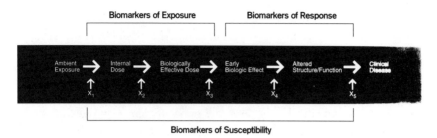

Figure 10.1 The use of biomarkers to measure the progression of disease from exposure to clinical expression

effects that eventually manifest as pathology. Along this continuum there can be biomarkers of exposure (internal dose, biologically effective dose) and biomarkers of response (early biologic effect, altered structure or function) (fig. 10.1). In addition, for a given exposure, different individuals vary in terms of their likelihood of developing a disease. This variability can be attributed to metabolic differences among individuals that operate at various levels of the exposure-disease continuum and can be represented by biomarkers of susceptibility (fig. 10.1). Although these divisions are somewhat arbitrary and can overlap, in this chapter all biomarkers are considered to represent one of the three divisions: exposure, response, or susceptibility.

Biomarkers are being used in occupational and environmental health to investigate the molecular mechanisms of exposure, response, and susceptibility for many of the common chronic diseases that account for the bulk of contemporary morbidity and mortality in Western culture. This field is expanding so rapidly that it would be impossible to cover all the latest developments in this chapter. Much research has focused on biomarkers of environmental carcinogenesis. Because the highest exposures to exogenous toxins typically occur in the workplace, biomarkers related to occupational exposures and their contribution to the development of disease have received particular attention. In addition, the potential application of these biomarkers on a larger scale in the workplace has probably raised the most concerns about issues of information transfer and control. This chapter therefore focuses on the use of molecular biomarkers to study the effect of occupational exposures and their relation to the development of chronic diseases, particularly cancer.[2]

BIOMARKERS OF EXPOSURE

Estimates of exposure of individuals to toxins in the workplace or general environment relied in the past on ambient monitoring. However, because people vary in their rates of absorption, distribution, metabolism, and excretion of toxins, individuals who have the same ambient exposure will retain different amounts of toxins in their bodies (internal dose). This variability in the strength and degree of an association impeded researchers' attempts to relate ambient exposure levels to increases in risk for the occurrence of disease. For this reason, researchers now measure the internal dose itself. This involves the direct measurement of a toxin or its known metabolite in body tissues or fluids by biochemical or other well-established analytic methods.[3]

Many of these biomarkers of internal dose are now widely accepted and used. As techniques have become increasingly sophisticated, it has become possible to make such measurements at exceedingly low levels (one part in 10^{18}).[4] These advances have raised the issue of our ability to measure internal doses of toxins for which the biologic significance, if any, is unknown.

In the case of carcinogens, an alternate approach to estimating internal dose has been to determine the presumed functional effect of biologic significance of carcinogens in body fluids, the mutagenic activity of biologic samples. Based on the premise that many carcinogens are known to have mutagenic activity, the mutagenic activity of these samples is attributed to the presence of carcinogens or their active metabolites. For occupational or environmental exposures, most testing has been done using the Ames assay (detection of a reversion to a normal metabolic phenotype in certain bacterial mutants due to their exposure to mutagenic agents) or a variant.[5]

All markers of internal dose, because of individual differences in the route and rate of metabolism, suffer from the shortcoming that they do not necessarily represent the amount of toxin that has actually interacted with the target molecule critical for the production of pathogenic changes. For genotoxins (including many carcinogens and reproductive toxins) the biologically effective dose is considered to be the amount of metabolite that forms adducts (chemical addition products) with the target cell DNA. The carcinogenic ability of many carcinogens correlates with this ability to bind to DNA. The formation of DNA adducts can lead to mutations that represent a critical step in the initiation of tumors, which in conjunction with subsequent epigenetic processes of promotion and progression, can ultimately lead to cancer. In some cases, DNA adduct formation at the target cell can be shown to correlate with DNA adduct formation in nontarget cells or with adduct formation with other macro-molecules such as proteins. Thus, adducts in easily accessible biological mate-rials (DNA adducts in white blood cells, protein adducts in hemoglobin or serum albumin) can sometimes serve as a surrogate biomarker for such adducts in the target tissue.

The presence of DNA adducts (though not specific identification) can be detected with a high degree of sensitivity.[6] Specific identification of adducts in DNA or proteins can be achieved by several techniques.[7] These approaches have been used to monitor biologically effective doses of carcinogens in exposed workers, cigarette smokers, chemotherapy patients, and individuals with envi-ronmental exposures from air pollution and diet.[8]

These studies have had limitations. For example, current monoclonal anti-body techniques are at best sensitive to the level of detecting one adduct in 10^8 DNA bases. However, recent developments in linking immunochemical tech-niques to DNA amplification technology based on the polymerase chain reac-tion (immuno-PCR) offers the prospect of increasing the sensitivity of these approaches by 100,000 times or more.[9] Of course, increased sensitivity in this range again raises the issue of our ability to detect these adducts outstripping our ability to interpret their biologic significance. Furthermore, it is now clear that more than just the number of adducts is important; especially important is the formation of adducts that are not easily repaired and that are formed at a few key sites in the genome where they lead to fixed mutations in the genes that control the disease process. Hence, it is logical to examine biomarkers of response to the formation of these critical DNA adducts.

BIOMARKERS OF RESPONSE

The importance of the biologically effective dose is that it is presumed to produce some significant change in a critical cellular component, such as mutation in DNA, that alters the function of the cell in such a way as to lead to disease, such as cellular transformation in carcinogenesis. Thus, the detection of these significant cellular changes may be considered biomarkers of response to the biologically effective dose. Many such biomarkers of response are well established and widely used. The increased interest in biomarkers of response in recent years has derived from our ability to detect the cellular response to the effects of genotoxins.

Genotoxins have been known for some time to be able to produce gross chromosomal changes in cells, such as chromosome breaks and rearrangements. Researchers have been able to examine chromosomal aberrations, sister chromatid exchanges, and micronuclei formation in individuals exposed to genotoxins.[10] With the advent of DNA amplification technology (polymerase chain reaction) and DNA sequencing techniques it has become possible to identify particular acquired genetic changes (such as point mutations—single base changes in the DNA) in the specific genes that are directly related to the disease process.

In the case of cancer, for example, it now appears likely that tumors arise from the occurrence of such genetic alterations in a particular small subset of the human genome, the oncogenes (genes that have the potential to cause a normal cell to become cancerous) and the tumor suppressor genes. In some cases, it may be possible to link the particular type of mutation in these cancer-related genes to the type of carcinogen exposure (mutational spectrum), so that these gene mutations represent much more specific biomarkers of response.[11]

Although in certain instances it may be possible to detect such biomarkers in DNA isolated from biological fluids,[12] generally such analysis requires the extraction of DNA from target samples, which usually are not available for routine monitoring. However, the protein products of oncogenes and tumor suppressor genes can frequently be found in easily accessible biological fluids, such as blood and urine, and can be used as surrogate biomarkers of response.[13] These proteins can be detected using such immunochemical techniques as Western blotting (electrophoretic separation of a mixture of proteins on a gel transferred to a membrane for identifying protein bands with immunologic probes) or enzyme-linked immunosorbent assays based on monoclonal antibodies.[14]

BIOMARKERS OF SUSCEPTIBILITY

The area of susceptibility represents the nature versus nurture intersection between environmental exposure and how different individuals react to that exposure. The modulating influence of susceptibility can have a great impact on the linear progression from exposure to disease at many steps in the process. Probably the most important source of this variability lies in differences in the metabolism of toxins. Much of this variability is genetically determined through the inheritance of different alleles for the genes that encode metabolic enzymes. These different genotypes represent potential biomarkers of susceptibility. These potential biomarkers are no different from other inherited genetic variants that contribute to disease, such as those being sought through the

Human Genome Project, discussed elsewhere. In some cases, however, even though the inherited genotype is fixed, the phenotypic expression may be variable and related to the environmental exposure, since the expression of some of the metabolic enzymes is inducible by the exposure. Thus, both the genotype (measured, e.g., by DNA sequencing) and the phenotype (measured, e.g., by biochemical analysis of enzymatic activity) may be considered biomarkers of susceptibility.

Examples of phenotypic polymorphisms in enzymes that metabolize toxins and may affect disease outcome include N-acetyltransferase. Mutations in the N-acetyltransferase gene result in less functional enzymes such that slow acetylators cannot detoxify aromatic amines and other toxins as well as fast acetylators. Because occupational exposure to aromatic amines is associated with bladder cancer, it is not surprising to note that occupationally exposed fast acetylators are at decreased risk for bladder cancer compared to occupationally exposed slow acetylators.[15] Similarly, the extensive debrisoquine metabolizing phenotype and the high inducibility arylhydrocarbon hydroxylase phenotype have been associated with an increased risk of lung cancer in cigarette smokers.[16] Other examples include: glutathione-S-transferase μ genotype and phenotype (involved in phase II detoxification processes) associated with a decreased risk of lung cancer;[17] apolipoprotein B genotype (involved in cholesterol metabolism) associated with premature coronary artery disease;[18] and α-1-antitrypsin genotype and phenotype (involved in the prevention of proteolytic tissue destruction) associated with chronic obstructive pulmonary disease.[19]

Genetic susceptibility to the risk of developing cancer in some cases may also be related to inherited mutations in tumor suppressor genes, similar to the acquired mutation that can be produced by environmental exposures. For example, Li-Fraumeni syndrome—inherited mutations in the p53 gene—can dramatically increase the risk for cancer at many sites in susceptible individuals.[20] The same types of techniques used for DNA or protein analyses in acquired cases of p53 alteration can be used in these cases as biomarkers of susceptibility.

THE IMPLICATIONS OF BIOMARKERS

The application of molecular biomarkers to examine at-risk populations raises both hopes and concerns. In scientific terms, the use of such biomarkers provides the opportunity to validate disease mechanisms that have been postulated from model in vitro or animal systems in vivo in human populations. Mechanistic comparisons based on biomarkers—for example, between species used in the toxicologic testing of environmental agents and humans—can shed light on the validity of risk assessments of toxins. Biomarkers allow the potential to confirm or refute the protection afforded by permitted exposure levels, for example, if biomarkers of toxicologic significance are absent or can still be detected at such levels. Molecular biomarkers have also been touted for their potential to permit the refinement of epidemiologic analyses (molecular epidemiology), for example, in reducing the misclassification of exposure and disease variables and in accounting for variability and effect modification.

As techniques for the detection of molecular biomarkers become increasingly sophisticated and sensitive, there is a risk that the ability to detect biomarkers may outstrip the ability to interpret their significance. For the exposed or at-risk individual, the interpretation of most significance may be the predictive value of molecular biomarkers to determine the future occurrence of disease (diagnosis) or the outcome of disease (prognosis). Because many of the biomarkers discussed here are presumed to represent a point on a causal pathway to disease, their presence contributes to the development of disease, and they can occur before the disease is detected by other routine methods and so could have significant predictive value. This characteristic will be particularly relevant for cohorts with known high occupational or environmental exposures (hence already suspected to be at increased risk of disease), since predictive value depends on the prevalence of the disease in the population as well as on the sensitivity and specificity of the biomarker itself. Thus, populations already known to be at elevated risk of a disease due, for example, to their workplace or other environmental exposures, may yield high predictive values for biomarkers (or combinations of biomarkers) related to the process of their disease. Because not all individuals in such at-risk populations will develop the disease, biomarkers of high predictive value will allow those individuals at greatest risk for the disease to be identified.

For example, ingestion of foodstuffs contaminated with the fungal by-product aflatoxin and chronic infection with hepatitis B virus are considered risk factors for hepatocellular carcinoma, but the likelihood that a given individual with a history of exposure to aflatoxin or hepatitis B virus will develop hepatocellular carcinoma is still relatively small. Biomarkers may be able to better predict those individuals in such populations who will actually develop hepatocellular carcinoma. Thus, in a recent study in Shanghai (an endemic area for both aflatoxin and hepatitis B), middle-aged males were recruited between 1986 and 1989 and monitored for hepatocellular carcinoma to 1992. At the time of recruitment, blood and urine samples were obtained and subsequently analyzed for serum hepatitis B virus surface antigen positivity and urinary aflatoxin metabolites, including DNA-aflatoxin adducts, in the resultant cancer cases and matched controls. A highly significant association was found between the presence of the biomarkers (serum viral antigen and urinary aflatoxin metabolites) at the time of recruitment and the subsequent development of cancer.[21] In another study, serum mutant *ras* p21 and mutant p53 were determined in vinyl chloride–exposed workers at risk for the development of angiosarcoma of the liver, since mutations in these proteins are felt to be a likely consequence of this exposure and to contribute to the development of the disease. The estimated positive predictive value for having the presence of both biomarkers was 0.67 with a negative predictive value of 0.88 if both biomarkers are absent or only one biomarker is present.[22]

In the future, therefore, combinations of various biomarkers of exposure, response, and susceptibility may be brought to bear to predict with great certainty the disease outcome in occupationally and environmentally exposed populations. The useful applicability of such predictive biomarkers will depend on a balance of the certainty of the outcome against the risk of the intervention to prevent the outcome. For example, biomarkers of exposure, being farther removed in the disease continuum from the clinical outcome, may be of lower predictive value (due to the necessary occurrence of further steps in the causal pathway) and may thus warrant less risky interventions than biomarkers of response that, being closer to the clinical end point, may have higher predictive value.

This raises another important issue. The predictive value of biomarkers is of little clinical importance if there is no appropriate intervention available that can abort or ameliorate the disease process. Thus, to be meaningful, biomarker research should be coupled with research on intervention (e.g., the development of specific chemoprophylaxis that attempts to correct or negate the defect identified by the biomarker or to short-circuit subsequent steps in the disease pathway), if it is to prevent or ameliorate disease. Appropriate counseling of tested individuals will also be necessary. Some individuals may wish to know their presumed disease status as predicted by biomarkers with or without the existence of a suitable intervention, but this brings the potential for considerable psychological distress.

The predictive value of biomarkers may have additional significance. When, for example, is the detection of certain biomarkers (or an ensemble of biomarkers) of sufficient predictive value to be considered a stage of the disease itself and, therefore, potentially a compensable event? Indicators of disease risk are currently not usually viewed in this way. As biomarkers increase in robustness, however, a reasonable argument may be made that a worker who has suffered a toxic exposure and now manifests a biomarker of very high predictive value should be eligible for some form of workers' compensation, at the very least on the basis of the psychologic burden imposed on the worker. An analogy may be drawn to medical malpractice litigation, in which several jurisidictions have upheld the awarding of damages to individuals for enhanced risk of future harm incident to a current injury.[23] Plaintiffs in occupational and environmental torts also have been awarded damages for emotional distress from enhanced likelihood of future harm, but they often require some present harm.[24] Biomarkers may be important in these cases in establishing the subclinical or preclinical harms upon which damages for future harms may be based.

There are related issues. How, for example, should the presence of such biomarkers affect the individual's status under the Americans with Disabilities Act (ADA)? Suggested amendments to the act would include under the term *disability* "having a risk of a future physical or mental impairment that would substantially limit one or more of the major life activities."[25] Such future risk could be defined by biomarkers of high predictive value. Even without such an amendment, it could be argued that an individual who is subject to discrimination based on biomarkers is being regarded as an individual with a disability, for purposes of coverage under the ADA. It is unclear how these issues would be resolved.

The application of biomarkers, and particularly their use in industry, also raises serious issues of information control and transfer, including concerns of privacy and confidentiality. These issues are in many ways the same as those for inherited genetic markers of disease discussed in relation to the Human Genome Project, but when biomarker testing is performed in the workplace, they may assume additional urgency. For one thing, the employer, in whose workplace the exposure has occurred, may have a disincentive to share information about biomarkers with employees. Even if the testing is performed by an employer with the best intentions of early detection and prevention, the information typically becomes part of the employer-owned medical record of the employee and is therefore subject to potential misuse and abuse, particularly as more of such records are retained in electronic databases.

Ethical standards of occupational medicine practice mandate that employers are "entitled to counsel about an individual's medical work fitness, but not diagnoses or specific details,"[26] but examples abound of instances where this level of confidentiality has been breached.[27] As corporations continue to be increasingly concerned with containing costs, particularly with regard to health care and workers' compensation, the abuse of predictive information on individuals from biomarkers may be too tempting to ignore in the pursuit of profitability. Unfortunately, the disastrous outcome for the individual, already burdened with the psychological and clinical implications, may be that he or she becomes unemployable and uninsurable.

Laws relating to the confidentiality of medical information, especially medical information in the workplace, are varied and confusing. With advances in biomarkers as well as other changes in the nature of the workplace and the way information is handled, it will become increasingly important to develop a consensus on this important issue. The proposed Medical Records Confidentiality Act, introduced in 1995 in the Senate, would have added sanctions for the failure to protect medical information, which, broadly defined by the bill, would apparently include genetic information.[28] In addition, the American College of Occupational and Environmental Medicine (ACOEM) endorsed the statement of the National Conference on Uniform State Laws, which recommended "the development of uniform comprehensive legislation addressing the confidentiality of medical records . . . that encompass the treatment of employee medical information in the workplace."[29]

Regarding issues related to biomarkers more specifically, ACOEM has approved a position statement on genetic screening in the workplace that covers "tests for the detection of disease and for increased susceptibility for disease."[30] Among other things, the statement warns against the misuse of testing for discrimination in employability or insurability and endorses the notion that "the guiding ethical principles for such testing should be voluntary, informed consent and confidentiality with due respect for autonomy, equity and privacy considerations of those tested."[31] Adherence to such notions will help to ensure the fulfillment of the promise and the avoidance of the problems generated by the rapid scientific advances in biomarker research.

NOTES

1. National Research Council, "Biological Markers in Environmental Health Research," *Environmental Health Perspectives* 74 (1987): 1–191.
2. See Mortimer L. Mendelsohn, John P. Peeters, and Mary Jane Normandy, eds., *Biomarkers and Occupational Health—Progress and Perspectives* (Washington, D.C.: Joseph

Henry Press, 1995); Paul A. Schulte and Frederica P. Perera, *Molecular Epidemiology— Principles and Practices* (New York: Academic Press, 1993).

3. Nicholas E. Preece and John A. Timbrell, "The Use of NMR in Drug Metabolism Studies: Recent Advances," in G. Gordon Gibson, ed., *Progress in Drug Metabolism* (London: Taylor and Francis, 1990), 147–203.

4. Samy Abdel-Baky and Roger Giese, "Gas Chromatography Electron Capture Negative-Ion Mass Spectrometry at the Zeptomole Level," *Analytic Chemistry* 63 (1991): 2986–89.

5. Eric Eisenstadt, "Biological Assays for Mutagens in Human Samples," *Annual Review of Public Health* 4 (1983): 391–95.

6. Randal van Welie et al., "Mercapturic Acids, Protein Adducts, and DNA Adducts as Biomarkers of Electrophilic Chemicals," *Critical Review of Toxicology* 22 (1992): 271–306.

7. Preece and Timbrell, "Use of NMR in Drug Metabolism Studies."

8. Margareta Tornquist, "Tissue Doses of Ethylene Oxide in Cigarette Smokers Determined from Adduct Levels in Hemoglobin," *Carcinogenesis* 7 (1986): 1519–21; Frederica Perera et al., "Molecular and Genetic Damage in Humans from Environmental Pollution in Poland," *Nature* 360 (1992): 256–58; Nathaniel Rothman et al., "Formation of Polycyclic Aromatic Hydrocarbon-DNA Adducts in Peripheral White Blood Cells During Consumption of Charcoal-Broiled Beef," *Carcinogenesis* 11 (1990): 1241–43; Peter Farmer et al., "Monitoring Human Exposure to Ethylene Oxide by the Determination of Haemoglobin Adducts Using Gas Chromatography-Mass Spectrometry," *Carcinogenesis* 7 (1986): 637–40; Anne Marie Fichtinger-Schepman et al., "Kinetics of the Formation and Removal of Cisplatin—DNA Adducts in Blood Cells and Tumor Tissue of Cancer Patients Receiving Chemotherapy: Comparison with In Vitro Adduct Formation," *Cancer Research* 50 (1990): 7887–94; John Groopman et al., "Aflatoxin Metabolism and Nucleic Acid Adducts in Urine by Affinity Chromatography," *Proceedings of the National Academy of Sciences* 82 (1985): 6492–96; Byung Lee et al., "Immunologic Measurement of Polycyclic Aromatic Hydrocarbon-Albumin Adducts in Foundry Workers and Roofers," *Scandinavian Journal of Work and Environmental Health* 17 (1991): 190–94; Ainsley Weston et al., "Fluorescence and Mass Spectral Evidence for the Formation of Benzo(a)pyrene Anti-diol-epoxide-DNA and Hemoglobin Adducts in Humans," *Carcinogenesis* 10 (1989): 251–57.

9. Takeshi Sano, Cassandra Smith, and Charles Cantor, "Immuno-PCR: A Very Sensitive Antigen Detection System Using a DNA-Antibody Conjugate," *Science* 258 (1992): 120–22.

10. Hans Stich and Bruce Dunn, "DNA Adducts, Micronuclei, and Leukoplakias as Intermediate End Points in Intervention Trials," in Helmut Bartsch, Kari Hemminki, and I. K. O'Neill, eds., *Methods for Detecting DNA Damaging Agents in Humans: Applications in Cancer Epidemiology and Prevention* (Lyon: IARC, 1988), 1661–63; Henry Evans, "Cytogenic Studies on Industrial Populations Exposed to Mutagens," in Bryn Bridges et al., eds., *Indicators of Genotoxic Exposures* (Cold Spring Harbor, N.Y.: Cold Spring Harbor Laboratory, 1989), 325–40; Timothy Wilcosky and Susan Rynard, "Sister Chromatid Exchanges," in Barbara Hulka, Timothy Wilcosky, and Jack Griffith, eds., *Biological Markers in Epidemiology* (New York: Oxford University Press, 1990), 28–35.

11. Paul Brandt-Rauf, Marie-Jeanne Marion, and Immaculata DeVivo, "Mutant p21 as a Biomarker of Chemical Carcinogenesis in Humans," in Mendelsohn, Peeters, and Normandy, eds., *Biomarkers and Occupational Health*, 163–73; Douglas Brash et al., "A Role of Sunlight in Skin Cancer: UV-Induced p53 Mutations in Squamous Cell Carcinoma," *Proceedings of the National Academy of Sciences* 88 (1991): 10124–28; Ih-Chang Hsu et al., "Mutational Hot Spot in the p53 Gene in Human Hepatocellular Carcinoma," *Nature* 350 (1991): 427–28; Hiroko Suzuki et al., "p53 Mutations in Non-Cell Lung Cancer in Japan: Association Between Mutations and Smoking," *Cancer Research* 52 (1992): 734–36; Kirsi Vahakangas et al., "Mutations of p53 and Ras Genes in Radon-Associated Lung Cancer from Uranium Miners," *Lancet* 339 (1992): 567–80.

12. Gloria Sorenson et al., "Soluble Normal and Mutated DNA Sequences from Single-Copy Genes in Human Blood," *Cancer Epidemiology and Biomarkers Preview* 3 (1994): 67–71.

13. Paul Brandt-Rauf et al., "The Molecular Epidemiology of Growth Signal Transduction Proteins," *Journal of Occupational and Environmental Medicine* 37 (1995): 77–83.

14. Immaculata deVivo et al., "Mutant c-Ki-ras p21 Protein in Chemical Carcinogenesis in Humans Exposed to Vinyl Chloride," *Cancer Causes and Control* 5 (1994): 273–78.

15. Paolo Vineis and Benedetto Terracini, "Biochemical Epidemiology of Bladder Cancer," *Epidemiology* 1 (1990): 448–52.

16. Charles Crespi et al., "A Tobacco Smoke-Derived Nitrosamine, 4-(Methyl-nitrosamino)-1-3-(Pyridyl)-1-Butanone, Is Activated by Multiple Human Cytochrome p450s Including the Polymorphic Human Cytochrome p4502D6," *Carcinogenesis* 12 (1991): 1197–201.

17. Janeric Seidegard et al., "Isoenzyme(s) of Glutathione Transferase (class mu) as a Marker for the Susceptibility to Lung Cancer: A Follow Up Study," *Carcinogenesis* 11 (1990): 33–36; Shan Zhang et al., "Glutathione S-transferase Mu Locus: Use of Genotyping and Phenotyping Assays to Assess Association with Lung Cancer Susceptibility," *Carcinogenesis* 12 (1991): 1533–37.

18. Jacques Genest et al., "DNA Polymorphism of the Apolipoprotein B Gene in Patients with Premature Artery Disease," *Atherosclerosis* 82 (1990): 7–17.

19. Ronald Klayton, Robert Fallat, and Alan Cohen, "Determinants of Chronic Obstructive Pulmonary Disease in Patients with Intermediate Levels of Alpha 1-Antitrypsin," *American Review of Respiratory Disease* 112 (1975): 71–75.

20. Frederick Li, "Familial Cancer Syndromes and Clusters," *Current Problems in Cancer* 49 (1991): 75–113.

21. Geng-Sun Qian et al., "A Follow-up Study of Urinary Markers of Aflatoxin Exposure and Liver Cancer Risk in Shanghai, People's Republic of China," *Cancer Epidemiology and Biomarkers Preview* 3 (1994): 3–10.

22. Marie-Jeanne Marion et al., "The Molecular Epidemiology of Occupational Carcinogenesis in Vinyl Chloride Exposed Workers," *International Archives of Occupational and Environmental Health* 68 (1996): 394–98.

23. Petriello v. Kalman, 576 A.2d 474 (Conn. 1990).

24. Sterling v. Velsicol Chem. Corp., 855 F.2d 1188 (6th Cir. 1988).

25. Mark A. Rothstein, "Genetic Secrets: A Policy Framework," Chapter 23 in this volume.

25. American College of Occupational and Environmental Medicine, "Code of Ethical Conduct," *Journal of Occupational Medicine* 36 (1994): 28.

26. Paul Brandt-Rauf, "Ethical Conflict in the Practice of Occupational Medicine," *British Journal of Industrial Medicine* 46 (1989): 63–66.

27. U.S. Congress, Senate, Medical Records Confidentiality Act of 1995, S. 1360, 104th Cong., 1st Sess.

28. American College of Occupational and Environmental Medicine, "Position Statement on the Confidentiality of Medical Information in the Workplace," *Journal of Occupational and Environmental Medicine* 37 (1995): 594–99.

29. American College of Occupational and Environmental Medicine, "Position Statement on Genetic Screening in the Workplace," *Journal of Occupational and Environmental Medicine* (in press).

30. Ibid.

Chapter 11 Environmental Population Screening

Jonathan M. Samet and Linda A. Bailey

Epidemiology, a scientific method used to describe the occurrence of disease in populations and to identify the causes of disease, has long held a central role in providing the evidence needed to advance the public's health.[1] Routine tracking of vital statistics has identified new epidemics of acute and chronic disease and documented the success of interventions directed at the epidemics. For example, mortality from coronary artery disease rose progressively across the twentieth century, reflecting the aging of the population and the effects of new risk factors including cigarette smoking, changing dietary patterns, and an increasingly sedentary way of life. The well-known Framingham epidemiologic study on heart disease identified risk factors for coronary artery disease, and its findings became the basis for interventions intended to reduce the disease burden.[2] As a result, mortality from the disease began to fall in the 1960s, reflecting the initial decline of smoking in men and more aggressive management of hypertension as well as improving treatment. Epidemiologic investigation has proved equally informative concerning risk factors for infection with HIV and for progression to full-blown AIDS following infection with the virus.

Epidemiology's domain is the population, contrasting with the focus of the clinician on an individual or of the employer on those who have been employed. Epidemiologic research may involve entire populations, randomly sampled members of populations, or groups selected on the basis of some special characteristic, such as being employed in a certain industry or having a particular disease. Some epidemiologic studies may be conducted passively, without active contact with study participants, by record linkage techniques, or by routine collection of information on disease occurrence, such as cancer registries. Epidemiologic studies, though often involving direct contact with participants, collection of biologic specimens, and even application of clinical assessment tools, do not directly engage researchers in a clinical relationship with the study participants. Typically, any clinically relevant information is referred to the participants' physicians, but the research team does not offer treatment or make therapeutic interventions.

Access to data on factors determining health status and on health status itself is central to the success of epidemiologic research. The epidemiologist uses routinely collected data on births, deaths, disease incidence and prevalence, and risk factor distributions to develop and test hypotheses concerning disease etiology. Cross-sectional studies or surveys may be used to further characterize risk factors and disease in population groups. Hypotheses concerning disease etiology are tested using the analytic designs of case control and cohort studies.[3] The case control design involves the comparison of exposures of persons having the disease of interest with those of appropriate control individuals not having the disease. In the cohort design, persons having one or more exposures of interest are followed over time and the occurrence of disease is monitored; rates of disease are compared in the exposed cohort members to those in an unexposed group or rates of disease may be calculated across a range of exposures. Intervention studies may be conducted to assess the consequences of reducing exposures. In the controlled clinical trial, participants are randomly assigned to either a treatment group or a control group, not receiving the new intervention or either receiving the standard intervention or a placebo therapy. Intervention programs might also be implemented at the population level.

A variety of sources of information have been used in epidemiologic research. Routinely collected, anonymous data are available through national, state, and local repositories. Although these data are a rich resource for hypothesis generation and surveillance, the testing of hypotheses about disease etiology nearly always involves collecting data related to specific and identified

Table 11.1 Examples of information
collected in epidemiologic studies

1. Lifestyle information
         Smoking habits
         Diet
         Exercise
2. Environmental exposures
         Residence location
         Occupation
         Water source
3. Personal health history
         Past illness history
         Reproductive and sexual history
         Use of medications
4. Family history
         History of cancer
         History of cardiovascular disease
         History of asthma
5. Sociodemographic factors
         education
         income
         race and ethnicity

individuals (table 11.1). In collecting data, the epidemiologist gives assurance of confidentiality and implements a systematic approach to assuring confidentiality for all data collected from study participants. The elements of assuring confidentiality for a study typically include the following: (1) training staff members about the importance of confidentiality and their signing a pledge of confidentiality; (2) anonymous linkages between personal identifiers for an individual and the data about them; (3) storage of all data in protected repositories, whether the data exist as hard copies or in electronic form; and (4) eventual destruction of linkages between the individuals and their data or destruction of the data themselves. Participants actively enrolled in epidemiologic research sign an informed consent document that gives an assurance about the confidentiality of data and describes the approach for maintaining privacy.

The potential for breach of confidentiality has arisen largely from inappropriate disclosure, involving either leakage of confidential information or the negligent and improper use of information by members of the investigative

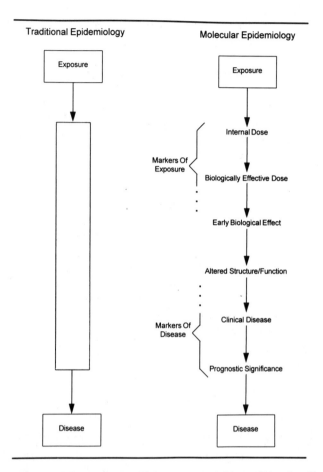

Figure 11.1 The progression of disease as viewed by traditional and molecular epidemiology

team. For example, an interviewer might indiscreetly reveal confidential information during a conversation with someone outside the investigative group. More deliberate disclosure might involve release of information to interested, outside parties. The consequences for the individual participants depend largely on the sensitivity of the information collected and the possibility of damage to individuals by its leakage. For a study, a breach of confidentiality carries the possibility of jeopardizing the research by compromising participation.

A changing paradigm of epidemiologic research has added a new overlay of concern to the confidentiality concerns that have long been familiar to epidemiologic researchers. Investigations of disease etiology increasingly follow a research approach known as "molecular epidemiology."[4] Central to this approach is the collection of biological specimens for characterization of biomarkers of exposure, dose, response, and susceptibility (fig. 11.1). This new paradigm reflects the emergence of new and informative markers that complement information that might be obtained directly from participants in epidemiologic studies, from environmental measurements, from historical records of exposures, or from other data resources.

Application of biomarkers of exposure and dose to a population provides information of presumed direct biologic relevance about the population as well as about specific individuals. Biomarkers of response, indicators of intermediate levels of outcome in the spectrum that begins with a healthy individual and ends with clinically evident disease, are also informative at the individual and population levels. A biomarker of susceptibility could be either an individual's genotype or some acquired characteristic of the individual, such as respiratory tract injury from cigarette smoking. In contemporary epidemiologic research, emphasis is largely on genotypic markers of susceptibility, reflecting the explosive pace of technologic development for investigating genetic markers and anticipation of the full sequencing of the human genome. Because an individual's constitutional genetic makeup is constant, genetic susceptibility can be readily studied by accessing appropriate biological samples, even samples taken before the start of the research project or samples taken for other purposes.

In this chapter, we consider the implications of using new technologies in epidemiologic investigation. Our context is set by the population level at which epidemiologic research takes place: a contextual level distinct from clinical contact between patient and health care provider and from the employer-employee relationship. In epidemiologic research, emphasis is on associations at the population level, although epidemiologic data may have substantial implications for individuals. We begin by defining privacy and confidentiality; next, we review present approaches to maintaining privacy and confidentiality in epidemiologic research; finally, we address the challenges raised by the new genetic technologies.

To date, there has been surprisingly little treatment of these issues in the epidemiologic literature; two of the first books on molecular epidemiology and biomarkers do not specifically address privacy and confidentiality.[5] However, privacy is a growing concern of the American public. According to a Louis Harris poll conducted in 1993, 79% of the public is very or somewhat worried about threats to personal privacy.[6] The survey also found that (1) 80% of respondents agreed that consumers have lost all control over how personal information about them is circulated and used by companies; (2) 68% agreed strongly or very strongly that computers are an actual threat to personal privacy; and (3) nearly 90% agreed that computers have made it much easier to obtain confidential personal information improperly. The increasing importance of privacy to the public and its concerns about confidentiality of data warrant a review of the adequacy of procedures to safeguard privacy and confidentiality for all epidemiologic studies as well as for studies involving new genetic technologies.

AN OVERVIEW OF PRIVACY AND CONFIDENTIALITY

In the context of epidemiology, privacy refers to an individual's right to control the conditions under which personal information is conveyed to others.[7] Privacy has been defined as "the capacity of the individual to determine which information is communicated to whom"[8] and, in a succinctly modern way, as "the protection of people from computers."[9] Although researchers have a stake in privacy to the extent that individuals are more likely to participate in research if privacy is protected, the concept of privacy refers specifically to the implicit rights of an individual research subject.[10]

Researchers have historically protected an individual's privacy through the process of informed consent. Through this process, an individual is apprised of the types of information that are sought in a research project, how the information will be used, and the potential harms and benefits of participating. Then the individual is given the choice whether to participate. A thorough informed consent procedure ensures that a subject is knowledgeable about the ramifications of participation, thereby protecting the autonomy of the individual. Properly obtained informed consent should minimize the liability of the researcher and the institution conducting the research.

The institutional review board (IRB) process is relevant to privacy in that it evaluates the benefit-risk ratio of proposed research, the distribution of risk to the population, and the adequacy of the consent process.[11] An IRB has the authority to determine which studies an institution will permit its staff to conduct; it functions as an important institutional mechanism for protecting the privacy of individuals.

Confidentiality refers to a researcher's duty to protect from disclosure private information about individuals.[12] Implicit in the issue of confidentiality is the knowledge that uncontrolled access to some types of personal information could result in harm to an individual. For example, if an individual conveys information about illegal drug use to a researcher and such information falls into the hands of an employer or police officials, the individual could be subject to loss of his or her job or to criminal sanctions. Epidemiologists generally safeguard confidentiality of data by implementing the internal study procedures.

THREATS TO PRIVACY AND CONFIDENTIALITY FROM NEW GENETIC TECHNOLOGIES

The new genetic technologies have brought unprecedented opportunities to investigate the genetic basis of disease, including the genetic basis of response to environmental agents. With new automated methodologies for using genetic markers, assays are now feasible on a scale compatible with large-scale epidemiologic research. Epidemiologists can grasp the potential of future developments for genetic research even though specifics remain to be developed. We make the following presumptions about future approaches to using genetic technologies in epidemiologic research:

- Population-based epidemiologic studies will continue to have a key role in investigating the genetic basis of disease;
- Genetic technologies will be further integrated into epidemiologic studies with increasing storage of biological specimens; and
- The current pace at which new technologies are emerging predicts future capabilities dramatically more informative than those now available; epidemiologists will design studies to maintain opportunities for application of the latest technologies.

Although maximizing the informativeness of epidemiologic investigations using the new genetic technologies will undoubtedly have benefits to society, epidemiologists need to respect the privacy of research participants and to assure the confidentiality of information about them. Epidemiologists need to be informed about how to consider and resolve conflicts that arise between investigative strategies intended to provide the most powerful tests of hypotheses and the safeguarding of privacy and confidentiality of individuals.

How can we assure the future informativeness of epidemiologic studies while protecting the privacy and confidentiality of information obtained from subjects and making certain that fully informed consent has been obtained? The epidemiologist may seek and need full permission for use of genetic materials, including for purposes not envisioned at the time of obtaining informed consent. We presume that privacy and confidentiality can be assured with the same confidence for the future as for the present. Informed consent, however, hardly seems possible if all future uses of materials cannot be anticipated. Is informed consent needed for each future use? Can specimens be shared with other investigators, having potentially informative methods, without requesting informed consent for this sharing?

Some research designs do not involve direct contact with participants. For example, population-based cancer registries, an extremely powerful research resource, passively follow large cohorts of people from entire regions for the development of incident cancer. Diagnoses of incident cancers are obtained through passive and active reporting systems and survival is tracked by many registries through record linkages. Tissues can be retrieved from hospital pathology laboratories for research purposes. Thus, studies can be readily conducted, for example, on genes determining cancer susceptibility or on genetic determinants of cancer prognosis. Cancer registries operate with legal authority given by a requirement to report cancer, usually implemented at the state level; one of their purposes is to facilitate research. Does this authority extend to genetic research? Is participant consent needed if the scope of the research involves individual-level data linkages and genetic analyses? Failure to address these issues will threaten privacy and confidentiality.

A second threat to privacy and confidentiality is posed by decisions about whether to maintain a link between personal identifiers and epidemiologic data sets. Privacy and confidentiality can be jeopardized by a third party, such as an employer, insurer, or other who has an interest in acquiring information about particular individuals or populations. Epidemiologic studies that include information about genetic susceptibility of individuals for diseases may be sought through court orders by third parties with a pecuniary interest in the information. If a court deems the information to be relevant to a dispute (i.e., a lawsuit), it has the authority to compel a researcher to disclose confidential information. Although the researcher and his or her institution can object to disclosure, the cost of engaging in legal battles and the likelihood of success need to be considered. What limits of privacy and confidentiality can epidemiologists maintain? Can the risks posed by third-party interference be reduced? Should personal identifiers be eliminated from data sets to prevent interference by third parties? What are the risks and benefits of eliminating personal identifiers from data sets?

In considering this issue, it is essential to balance the need for future contact with study participants to provide feedback about tests that were performed (e.g., the genotype, biomarker, etc., that will be available shortly after the test is conducted) and to provide interpretative information (i.e., the implications of the tests, which may not be available at the time of testing or for many years thereafter).

A third threat operates at the population level. Population-based studies will undoubtedly indicate genetically increased risks for some diseases in some populations. Population anonymity is typically not maintained in epidemiologic studies with populations being identified, for example, by location or race and ethnicity. Such information could be used in discriminatory ways by insurers, employers, and others.

The management of these threats is no different from that for the threats to privacy and confidentiality arising for the types of information long collected in the course of epidemiologic research. However, given the potential value of the information on genetic risk in large populations, the adequacy of current approaches to safeguarding privacy and confidentiality in epidemiologic studies merits reconsideration.

CONDUCTING INFORMATIVE STUDIES

An informative epidemiologic research study that incorporates genetic information on participants might typically involve data collection by questionnaire on demographics, relevant exposures, illness history, and family history and sampling of biologic materials for genetic analyses. The information about the participants may be maintained in hardcopy and electronic files; biologic specimens may be processed in one or more laboratories for various genetic analyses; and white cells, buccal swabs, or DNA may be stored for future analyses. Results from the laboratory analyses would be merged with the other kinds of information to create analytic files.

In this typical scenario are there opportunities for privacy and confidentiality to be breached? With appropriate procedures, the answer should be "no." For the laboratory analyses, there is no need to reveal information that could identify individuals, and analytic files that merge genetic with other types of information need not include identifying information. Anonymous identification numbers can be used to merge the information for individual participants. Further protection would be gained by appropriate protection of electronic files against access by unauthorized persons or by breach of security against incursions through networks.

MAINTAINING A LINK BETWEEN PERSONAL IDENTIFIERS AND DATA SETS

It is essential for future contact with research subjects that links be maintained between personal identifiers and data sets. Contact may be necessary to ask subjects for their "informed consent" to conduct additional studies on their stored samples, thereby advancing scientific knowledge. It is also necessary to notify subjects about findings from genetic tests conducted on their tissue samples and to interpret the test results (the interpretation may not be available at testing time).

The issue of informed consent is discussed in Part II of this volume. However, the issue of participant notification about test results and the interpretation of results merits discussion.

The provision of information on genotype has received extensive consideration in the context of patient care. The ethics of transmitting and of not transmitting information have been of concern, as has the impact of being informed about a genotype associated with disease risk. For the epidemiologist, who is not engaged in a therapeutic relationship at an individual level, providing the findings of genetic analyses to individual research participants may not be practicable. Participant numbers and lack of expertise may preclude the communication of results to participants. Nevertheless, participants may ask for findings or the implications of the findings may necessitate their communication.

The epidemiologic researcher has three alternatives in addressing this issue: (1) to implement the research with an announced intent of not providing individual genetic information to participants; (2) to assemble a research team with the capability for appropriately informing participants as to their individual findings; and (3) to provide the genetic information to the participants' physicians for interpretation to the individuals. Of these alternatives, the first can be readily implemented and would arguably be appropriate, assuming that the implications of the genetic information obtained in the research are of uncertain significance for individuals. However, some potential participants might ask for access to their information, and the findings of the research could shift the weight of the evidence and make feedback an ethical and legal imperative. The epidemiologic research team may not include a trained genetic counselor; in addition to this feasibility constraint, the second alternative would place the epidemiologic researcher in a potentially inappropriate therapeutic relationship with research subjects. The third alternative shifts responsibility to the participants' physicians. Few will be capable of interpreting the information. More important, genetic information could be included in clinical records and therefore potentially available to insurers and others who might use the information to assess disease risk and potential for liability.

None of these alternatives is satisfactory. The first, providing no information, assures privacy and confidentiality but may deprive research participants of information that is of potential benefit to their health. The second alternative is generally impracticable, particularly in the context of large-scale population-based studies, and places the researcher in an inappropriate, clinical relationship with research participants. The third alternative shifts responsibility without any assurance the genetic information will be properly interpreted and carries the potential for leakage of information in a way that could harm the research subject.

A separate issue for consideration is notification of participants, perhaps years in the future, when test results can be accurately interpreted. The concept of participant notification evolved in epidemiologic studies of the consequences of occupational exposures. The cohort study design was widely used to investigate worker populations. If conducted retrospectively, information became available about the risks of past exposures in the present, whereas if conducted prospectively, information about disease risks became available at some point in the future. Paul Schulte proposed that study participants should be notified as to the findings and offered criteria for determining whether notification was warranted.[13]

The same ethical bases might be extended to cohort studies of the genetic basis of disease. For example, a prospective cohort study might be undertaken to identify genetic determinants of cancer risk. Markers might be identified in the future as specimens are analyzed for the population, including those who have and have not developed cancer. If markers are identified, should those participants who are at increased risk be notified? Should a commitment to notify be made at the time of enrolling in the study? To our knowledge, the issue of notification has not yet been addressed by epidemiologists in the context of genetic research.

The need to maintain a link between personal identifiers and the data set is supported by the continuing interest in being able to contact research subjects regarding informed consent for additional testing of stored samples and notification about test results and their interpretation. However, keeping data linked poses a threat to privacy and confidentiality. If a link exists, an investigator can be compelled by a court to disclose confidential information to employers, insurers, or others with a pecuniary interest.

Under Rule 26 of the Federal Rules of Civil Procedure, courts can compel researchers to disclose their data if the information is relevant to a dispute before the court. In considering whether information should be compelled, courts often draw on the Supreme Court case of United States v. Nixon, which quoted the Court's earlier decision in Branzburg v. Hayes: "The public has a right to every man's evidence, except for those persons protected by a constitutional, common law, or statutory privilege."[14] Unless disclosure of information would violate a protection offered under the Constitution, statute, or common law, a court can compel researchers to disclose confidential information. Risk of compelled disclosure should be viewed as a limitation of confidentiality.

Court-compelled disclosure of confidential research information is not a common occurrence, but it is a reality. In 1983, a federal court ordered Dr. Arthur Herbst to disclose a data set of more than 500 medical research records that contained evidence of a link between the drug Diethylstilbestrol (DES) and cancer in the daughters of women who took the drug.[15] The pharmaceutical manufacturer sought access to the data set, including the names and addresses of women who participated in the study, to verify the research methodology and to cross-examine the opposing experts regarding the accuracy of the reported findings. Herbst was not a witness or expert in the case. His article, however, offered a scientific basis for the lawsuit. More recently, Dr. Irving Selikoff was compelled to provide data supporting his findings that smoking, combined with exposure to asbestos, heightens the risk of lung cancer. The parties seeking the data were tobacco companies.[16] Maintaining links between personal identifiers and data has benefits and liabilities. On the benefits side, links enable researchers to reach subjects to provide relevant information and make relevant inquiries. On the liability side, maintaining links raises questions vis-à-vis the researcher's duty to keep information confidential, given that a court can compel the information and an employer can misuse information.

Ethical guidelines provide a framework for thoughtful consideration of these issues. The International Guidelines for Ethical Review of Epidemiological Studies provides a useful starting place for such consideration.[17]

POPULATION ANONYMITY

To date, discussions of privacy and confidentiality have focused on protection of the individual. Should the same concern be extended to populations? What are the implications of labeling a population as having an increased frequency of a disease-causing mutation?

For example, breast cancer gene 1 (BRCA1), a major gene responsible for inherited breast cancer, has been found to have a specific mutation in a relatively high proportion of women of Ashkenazi Jewish descent, approximately 1%.[18] This observation was made in 895 DNA samples from three independent sets of samples of Ashkenazi Jewish women in the United States and Israel; the frequency of the mutation was much higher than in reference populations. In the general Caucasian population, the frequency of BRCA1 mutations is 1 in 833. Researchers have found that the BRCA1 mutation accounts for 16% of breast cancer and 39% of ovarian cancer diagnosed before age 50 in Ashkenazi Jewish women.

The report has now been verified and the role of the mutation in premenopausal breast cancer has been shown.[19] What are the implications of these reports for women of Ashkenazi descent? Will their insurance coverage be limited? Will their insurance costs be increased? Will employers and others use the information to discriminate against individuals who test positive? Will information about an increased "population" risk be used in a discriminatory way against the Ashkenazi Jewish population or the larger Jewish population?

Epidemiology carries the risk of labeling populations. It may not be possible to ensure confidentiality of information at the population level without severely compromising the epidemiologist's ability to conduct informative studies.

RECOMMENDATIONS

There has been surprisingly little discussion in the epidemiologic literature on the implications of the new genetic technologies for the conduct of epidemiologic research. We suggest a two-pronged approach in considering these complex issues: (1) What are the scope and limitations of privacy in research? How can we ensure that an individual research subject controls the uses of his or her biological samples by researchers to the fullest extent possible? (2) What are the scope and limitations of confidentiality? How can we ensure that researchers fulfill their duty to keep confidential the private information about research subjects?

To answer these questions, we propose the following steps:

First, as a long-term goal, a dialogue about the scope and limitations of privacy and confidentiality needs to occur within professional epidemiology organizations and between epidemiologists and the public. It will be essential to clarify the expectations of the public and epidemiologists and the implications of pressures and actions that are beyond the control of researchers and their institutions (i.e., the rule of law). Epidemiologists should consider ways to include consumer panels in planning and implementing these discussions.

Second, as a long-term goal, we recommend that professional associations of epidemiologists begin to address the very real threats posed by third-party interest in research information. Third parties may try to gain access to personal information by direct request, or they may ask a court to compel researchers to provide confidential information. This goal is relevant to epidemiology in general as well as to "molecular epidemiology."

A number of potential solutions exist. Researchers can develop guidelines for permanently removing identifiers after research has been concluded, if this is acceptable to professionals and the public. This may be an especially important concern for research in controversial areas. Researchers can also support the establishment of certificates of confidentiality for genetic research through the federal government. Such protection is provided by statute for research in the areas of substance abuse and sexuality. Certificates of confidentiality are a powerful tool for protecting confidential information from disclosure. The current statute for certificates of confidentiality could be used as a model for a certificate of confidentiality in genetics research.

Third, as a long-term goal, we also suggest that epidemiologists consider using the dialogue (described at item 1) as a basis for developing a professional code of ethics. The International Guidelines for Ethical Review of Epidemiological Studies provides a starting point for such work.[20]

Fourth, based on the dialogue, informed consent procedures can be improved for epidemiologic studies that use new genetic technologies by attempting to develop informed consent procedures that (1) allow for some reuse of biologic samples, if this is acceptable to the public; and (2) consider the issue of notification of subjects with test results as well as notification of others whose health may be affected by the test results (i.e., children and siblings at risk for the same condition). Both procedures should be guided by the expectations and concerns of the public and epidemiologists. In addition, thought should be given to providing subjects with information about whether the results of the research will be used in any for-profit ventures.

Last, as a short-term goal, we suggest that training about privacy and confidentiality issues be improved (in both quantity and quality) for professionals and students. Professionals and teachers should look to professional organizations of epidemiologists to circulate recommendations about curricula.

NOTES

1. C. W. Tyle, Jr., and John M. Last, "Epidemiology," in John M. Last and Robert B. Wallace, eds., *Public Health and Preventive Medicine*, 13th ed. (Norwalk, Conn.: Appelton and Lange, 1992).

2. Thomas R. Dawber, *The Framingham Study: The Epidemiology of Atherosclerotic Disease* (Cambridge: Harvard University Press, 1980).

3. Kenneth J. Rothman, *Modern Epidemiology* (Boston: Little, Brown, 1986).

4. Barbara S. Hulka, Timothy C. Wilcosky, and Jack D. Griffith, *Biological Markers in Epidemiology* (New York: Oxford University Press, 1990); Paul A. Schulte et al., eds., *Molecular Epidemiology: Principles and Practices* (New York: Academic Press, 1993).

5. Ibid.

6. National Academy of Sciences, Institute of Medicine, *Health Data in the Information Age* (Washington, D.C.: National Academy Press, 1994).

7. Ibid.

8. C. J. Lako, "Privacy Protection and Population-Based Health Research," *Social Science and Medicine* 23 (1996): 293–95.

9. Daniel M. Robinson, "Health Information Privacy: Without Confidentiality," *International Journal of Biomedical Computing* 5, supp. (1994): 97–194.

10. John M. Last, ed., *A Dictionary of Epidemiology*, 3d ed. (New York: Oxford University Press, 1995).

11. Alexander M. Capron, "Protection of Research Subjects: Do Special Rules Apply in Epidemiology?" *Journal of Clinical Epidemiology* 44, supp. 1 (1991): 81–89.

12. Robinson, "Health Information Privacy."

13. Paul A. Schulte, "The Epidemiologic Basis for the Notification of Subjects of Cohort Studies," *American Journal of Epidemiology* 121 (1985): 351–61.

14. United States v. Nixon, 418 U.S. 683, 709 (1973); Branzburg v. Hayes, 408 U.S. 665, 688 (1972).

15. Deitchman v. Squibb & Sons, 740 F.2d 556 (7th Cir. 1984); Andrews v. Eli Lilly Co., 97 F.R.D. 494 (N.D. Ill. 1983).

16. In re American Tobacco Co., 880 F.2d 1520, 1523 (2d Cir. 1989).

17. Council for International Organizations of Medical Sciences, "International Guidelines for Ethical Review of Epidemiologic Studies," in S. S. Coughlin, ed., *Ethics in Epidemiology and Clinical Research* (Newton, Mass.: Epidemiology Resources, 1995).

18. Jeffrey P. Struewing et al., "The Carrier Frequency of the BRCA1 185delAG Mutation Is Approximately 1 Percent of Ashkenazi Jewish Individuals," *Nature Genetics* 11 (1995): 198–200.

19. Michael G. FitzGerald et al., "Germ-Line BRCA1 Mutations in Jewish and Non-Jewish Women with Early-Onset Breast Cancer," *New England Journal of Medicine* 334 (1996): 143–49.

20. Council for International Organizations of Medical Sciences, "International Guidelines."

Chapter 12 Are Developments in Forensic

Applications of DNA Technology Consistent

with Privacy Protections?

Randall S. Murch and Bruce Budowle

Physical evidence from criminal investigations is subjected to inter-comparative examinations, between known and questioned sources, to determine whether relationships can be established between victims, suspected perpetrators, and locations where a criminal offense has been alleged to have taken place. Probative information can potentially be derived from forensic analyses in a number of scientific disciplines, which assists the police and legal parties involved in determining what happened, who was involved and how, and when and where the alleged crime may have taken place. Forensic science has increasingly become more important in assisting or resolving crime investigations and therefore has come under greater scientific and legal scrutiny.[1] As a result, even legal standards for the use of scientific methods are changing, with the most recent change on the admissibility of scientific evidence from the Frye standard (a 1923 case holding that scientific evidence is admissible if it is "generally accept-

The authors wish to thank Steven Niezgoda for his assistance in the preparation of this chapter. This document is publication number 96-7 of the Federal Bureau of Investigation.

able" in the scientific community) to the Daubert decision (a 1993 Supreme Court case holding that the Frye test was superseded by the Federal Rules of Evidence).[2]

The value and power of physical evidence analyzed in criminal investigations lie in the inherent informational content and the ability of scientists to recognize, extract, format, interpret, and explain the results. The goal of the forensic scientist is to determine, via scientific analysis of physical evidence, whether two samples (one known and one questioned) originate from the same source. The better one can determine the absolute source of evidentiary material, the greater is the confidence with which one can establish the relationship, or lack thereof, between the known and the questioned sources (victim, suspect, and scene). This permits the relation to the criminal event to be determined with some degree of confidence. Such comparative analyses of samples can result in a continuum of interpretations from "did not originate from the same source" to "could have originated from the same source" to "did absolutely originate from the same source."

The greatest advance in forensic science over the past decade, in approaching absolute individualization of the source of forensic biospecimens, has been in the application of DNA analysis. The inherent stability and high informational content of DNA, the access to a variety of genetic markers, and the development of techniques to process DNA from dried biological materials have resulted in widespread forensic application of molecular biological tools to characterize biological materials deposited during the commission of a crime, particularly a violent crime such as homicide, rape, assault, or kidnapping. In fact, the use of DNA typing analyses to characterize biological evidence is the best avenue for the forensic scientist to exclude individuals who have been falsely associated with that evidence. With the development of community standards for forensic DNA applications, a high degree of confidence is derived regarding the relationship of the parties thought to be involved in a criminal act and the residual biological materials from the event.[3]

Most existing and forthcoming technological advances in forensic DNA analysis evolved independently but can be advantageously used to better address the demands of investigators, attorneys, courts, and citizens for more and better information at a faster pace. What is evolving in the microcosm of forensic DNA technology is merely another variation of the information age.

When current digital imaging and computing technologies are combined with forensic DNA technology, faster and more standardized intercomparisons as well as more comprehensive and readily accessible DNA data archiving emerge. Add in high-speed telecommunications, and the boundaries for inter-comparing DNA profiles transcend the confines of an individual laboratory to those in other states or throughout the nation.

In a highly mobile society, where violent crime is a substantial concern, advanced technologies such as DNA typing must be integrated and fully applied by law enforcement for the public good, and appropriate scientific and legal guidelines must be implemented, also for the public good. Forensic DNA technology will be more effectively used toward the crime problem when DNA profiles from questioned specimens can be efficiently compared by automated means against forensic DNA databases composed of, for example, those individuals who have committed (i.e., been convicted of) certain violent crimes. In forensic DNA parlance, this is commonly contrasted in the ability to perform unbiased "cold searches" (when the suspect is unknown or when probable cause does not necessarily exist) versus being limited to only "warm searches" (when there is probable cause). The former substantially extends the technology's investigative usefulness. Forensic DNA technology has simply evolved to the same point one uses when performing a computerized library search to find the most useful information possible in the shortest time.

In concert with scientific and legal concerns over the quality assurance and quality control employed with forensic DNA technology, the rapid development and application of such genetic and information management technologies have triggered concerns on the use of and access to information derived from DNA typing data.[4] In this chapter, we address forensic DNA technology; what information is and is not provided; how that information is used; the necessity for forensic databases; the construction and intended mechanism for the use of databases; the proposed architecture of a national database; and privacy issues regarding various analytical and information management aspects.

CURRENT FORENSIC DNA TECHNOLOGY

Most of the DNA in human cells is packaged and organized into 46 chromosomes in the nucleus. Only a portion of the chromosomal DNA codes for proteins; the remainder either serves in a regulatory capacity or does not serve any known function. Most of the DNA-based genetic markers that have been used for forensic analyses serve no known function. Arlene Wyman and Ray White have demonstrated that multiple repeats of particular nucleotide sequences exist within noncoding regions of genomic DNA.[5] The number of the repeated sequences has been demonstrated to be highly variable within the human population. These repetitive sequence sites are called variable number of tandem repeat (VNTR) regions. A DNA profile composed of several of these VNTR sites can be uniquely identifying (excluding identical twins).

The molecular biology approach most often used for genetic characterization by VNTR markers is restriction fragment length polymorphism (RFLP) analysis via Southern blotting.[6] This procedure is well defined, robust, and highly informative. The concept of RFLP analysis is simple. After DNA is extracted from a biological specimen, it is cut into small fragments by specific restriction endonuclease (bacterial enzyme) digestion. The DNA fragments are sorted by size using agarose gel electrophoresis. While residing in the agarose gel, the fractionated double-stranded DNA fragments are denatured into single-strand fragments by exposure to an alkali environment. The denatured fragments are then transferred out of the gel by capillary action onto a membrane support, where they are immobilized. Subsequently, specific VNTR markers are detected through hybridization (complementary binding) with labeled DNA probes. The resultant profiles are band patterns; the bands vary in their position based on their respective size (which ultimately is related to the number of repeat sequences contained within the fragments).

Because the genetic polymorphism of VNTR markers is based on differences in size, data on fragment lengths are desirable. The size or length of a VNTR band in a DNA profile can be determined by the distance traveled through the agarose gel relative to some standard(s) of known length. An interactive system of image analysis is used to determine the length of fragments rapidly and objectively.[7] The fragment lengths are expressed as numerical values resulting from specific VNTR markers. These values can be used to refute or confirm a putative match of an evidentiary sample with a suspect profile or to construct a profile that may be compared with those in a database of convicted felons or in open case files.

An alternative molecular biological approach for typing DNA is based on the sample amplification technique—the polymerase chain reaction (PCR).[8] PCR is nothing more than a sample preparation technique. It enables the scientist to increase the number of DNA target molecules in a sample from subanalytical to analytical levels in a relatively short time. Although there are many approaches for PCR analysis, it is basically an in vitro enzymatic synthesis of millions of copies of a target DNA sequence. PCR amplifies specific DNA sequences by repetitively denaturing template DNA, hybridizing specific DNA primers flanking the region of the template DNA to be amplified, and extending the primers. In this way, multiple copies of the target region can be generated.

In principle, PCR analysis is easy to accomplish. One needs only a DNA template sample, primers, a mixture of four phosphorylated nucleotide bases, buffer, and a thermostable DNA polymerase. All ingredients can then be placed in a small tube and inserted into a programmable thermal cycler, which permits the temperature to change in the tubes. At high temperatures (e.g., 94°C), DNA will denature; at lower temperatures (37–72°C), primers can anneal, and at 72°C Taq polymerase, a thermostable DNA polymerase, will then extend the primers. PCR can be performed in about an hour once the tube has been placed in the thermal cycler.

PCR-based technology offers several advantages over RFLP typing; augmented sensitivity and specificity, the ability to detect DNA types in highly degraded samples, decreased assay time and labor, and less consumption of evidentiary material. In addition, PCR analysis takes only a few days for an assay, compared with weeks for RFLP analysis, and PCR systems are generally amenable to automation. Further, small amounts of evidentiary DNA and several distinct markers can be simultaneously amplified in one PCR mixture, a technique known as multiplexing, which saves both time and reagents.[9] These qualities make PCR an extremely useful tool for analyzing small or degraded biological materials found in criminal investigations.

Once a sample has been amplified by PCR, the product can be analyzed through three general approaches, each dictated by the genetic marker and its type of polymorphism. The PCR-based markers can be either noncoding regions such as repetitive DNA markers (i.e., VNTR sites) or coding regions (or genes). The analytical methods that have been and are being evaluated for the characterization of forensic materials are (1) dot-blot assays using allele-specific oligonucleotide (ASO) probes to detect sequence polymorphisms, (2) electrophoretic separations to resolve size variants (similar to RFLP typing of VNTR markers), and (3) sequencing.

The first PCR-related approach used for forensic purposes was the detection of sequence polymorphisms by the use of ASO hybridization probes in a dot-blot format. Under appropriate conditions, ASO probes hybridize only to DNA sequences that contain their exact complement. Thus, a different ASO probe is required for each genetic variant that will be detected for a DNA marker system. The reverse dot-blot format has become the method of choice.[10] In this situation, the ASO probes that detect each variant of a particular marker are immobilized on a nylon membrane strip, and the variants of the amplified DNA of the sample are identified through hybridization with the immobilized probes. If the particular variant is carried by the DNA sample, a colored reaction in the form of a dot will result.

HLA-DQA1 is the most characterized PCR-based system using the reverse dot-blot format for the analysis of forensic specimens.[11] The HLA-DQ molecule is expressed in B-lymphocytes, macrophages, thymic epithelium, and activated T-cells.[12] Eight variants can be identified via a commercially available kit, and they are designated 1.1, 1.2, 1.3, 2, 4, 4.1, 4.2, and 4.3.

It now is possible to amplify six loci simultaneously: HLA-DQA1, low-density lipoprotein receptor, glycophorin A, hemoglobin G gammaglobin, D7S8, and group-specific component.[13] All these markers except D7S8 are coding genes. After amplification, the markers are typed simultaneously in a manner similar to that of HLA-DQA1, using a reverse dot-blot approach in which the ASO probes are also immobilized on a nylon membrane strip. Thus, more information can be obtained in one analysis to assist in characterizing evidentiary samples.

Regardless of the ease of typing sequence polymorphisms afforded by ASO typing, VNTR markers remain the most informative genetic markers for attempting to individualize biological material. As described above, the size of the amplified fragment is dictated by the number and size of the repeat sequences contained within it. With appropriate VNTR loci and high-resolution electrophoretic systems, amplification by PCR and typing of specific VNTR sequences have proven useful for the purposes of testing identity.[14] These markers have been termed AMP-FLPs (amplified fragment length polymorphisms).[15]

A subgroup of these AMP-FLPs is the short tandem repeat (STR) markers. These markers are highly polymorphic and are abundant in the human genome.[16] The STR markers, which contain shorter repeat sequences than the RFLP/VNTR markers, are composed of tandemly repeated sequences of 2–5 base pairs in length. Several STR markers have been evaluated for forensic applications, including HUMTHO1, CSF1PO, TPOX, and VWA.[17]

The PCR technique is also an effective means for producing a template for DNA sequencing. Basically, sequencing is reading the genetic code along a specified DNA fragment. Sequencing was not considered practical for revealing genetic variation for forensic purposes until the recent development of instruments that provide automated analysis of fluorescently labeled sequence reaction products. Automation simplified a cumbersome assay, enabled more effective interpretation of sequences, and eliminated the need for radioactivity.

Markers that are carried on the nuclear chromosomes are generally not practical candidates for a sequencing approach in forensic analyses, because the presence of two copies of each gene in the nucleus makes interpretation more complicated. This is further confounded when the evidence contains fluids from multiple individuals, a frequent occurrence during acts of violent crime. However, mitochondrial DNA (mtDNA) can serve as a useful genetic marker(s) for the characterization of evidentiary material. The mtDNA is an extrachromosomal, circular piece of DNA that has been completely sequenced, resulting in the mapping and identification of all mt genes. The features that make mtDNA desirable for forensic analyses are: (1) mtDNA can occur in more than 5,000 copies per cell, which, in essence, is an amplification process in itself; (2) mtDNA is maternally inherited and therefore monoclonal; (3) mtDNA generally appears to be homogeneous within different tissues of an individual, which facilitates comparisons of DNA derived from different body tissues; and (4) portions of mtDNA's noncoding region (called the D-loop) are highly polymorphic. In fact, amplified mtDNA has been successfully sequenced on such items as 7,000-year-old brain tissue, 5,500-year-old bone, and 4,000-year-old mummified tissue.[18]

Besides bones, an important tissue for potential application of mtDNA sequencing in forensics is hair. Since individual hairs contain very small quantities of DNA, mtDNA sequencing may be the only viable technique for analysis. Forensic researchers have applied mtDNA sequencing to the characterization of human hairs.[19]

Criminal investigators collect biological evidence left at a crime scene to identify the perpetrator (and to exclude those falsely associated with an evidentiary sample). DNA typing is a powerful tool for assisting in the inculpation or exculpation of an individual as the source of biological evidence left at a crime scene. There are three interpretations of DNA profile comparisons between a known sample (e.g., a suspect) and an evidentiary sample (e.g., a vaginal swab containing semen). These are: (1) inconclusive—there is insufficient information to render a conclusion; (2) exclusive—the two DNA profiles are sufficiently different such that the samples did not originate from the same source; and (3) inclusive (or match)—the two DNA profiles are similar operationally and potentially could have originated from the same source. An estimation of the frequency of occurrence of a DNA profile in a general population group or groups does not arise with the first two interpretations. However, with an inclusion, it is desirable to convey a valid estimate as a guideline of how common or rare the DNA profile is in the general population of potential perpetrators.

To assess the rarity of a DNA profile (which ultimately assists the trier of fact in a case), general population databases are generated. DNA samples from anonymous individuals from major population groups (such as African Americans and Caucasians) or geopolitical groups (such as Hispanics) are typed for various genetic markers. The number of the various forms of each marker, whether they are fragment sizes, the presence or absence of dots, or specific DNA sequences, are tallied, and these tallies provide a basis for estimating the rarity of DNA profiles in the various population groups.

All profile data (whether population or casework data) can be archived numerically in a computer. The profile data in a database can be retrieved readily and compared with evidentiary profiles. Although comparisons of DNA profiles can be made within a case or among profiles in a database, the quality issues are slightly different. In a particular case, when comparing, for example, a suspect's profile with that of an evidence sample, one is more concerned with the false-positive scenario (i.e., that one or both of the samples have been typed incorrectly and a match has resulted when the samples are genetically different at those markers). Laboratories practice standard protocols to minimize the occurrence of a false positive; if there are serious concerns about the occurrence of a false positive, samples can usually be reanalyzed. A false negative scenario is more tolerated in a particular case because it would not result in wrongly inculpating an individual. In contrast, for a database search for a potential matching profile to be effective, a false negative result is less tolerated. If matches cannot be made in a database, where matches exist, then there would be no need to generate databases for identifying repeat offenders or serial perpetrators. A false positive can be eliminated in a database search by requiring a reanalysis of the known sample by the querying laboratory. A false negative can be minimized by establishing validated and robust protocols and establishing proper guidelines for quality assurance and control.

TECHNOLOGICAL AND INFORMATION MANAGEMENT BASES FOR FORENSIC DNA DATABASES

In 1989, the forensic community, through the body known as the Technical Working Group on DNA Analysis Methods (TWGDAM), began to address the need for comprehensive standards in applying DNA to forensic specimens.[20] TWGDAM has since addressed such issues as laboratory organization, personnel qualifications, documentation, materials and equipment, validation of analytical procedures, generation and validation of genetic marker frequency databases, evidence-handling procedures, internal controls and standards, data analysis and reporting, proficiency testing, quality audits, and safety. A natural evolution for establishing DNA typing standards was the creation by Congress of the DNA Advisory Board (DAB) via the DNA Identification Act of 1994.[21] The DAB is responsible for promulgating national standards of forensic DNA analysis.

Since the inception of forensic DNA profiling (and certainly since the beginning of TWGDAM), considerable benefit has been gained from integrating information management and communication technologies with the data derived from forensic DNA analyses. The establishment of various forensically useful databases, for both population and forensic data, was also recognized as pivotal to the process of resolving crimes where there is no suspect or multiple crimes that may be committed by the same individual. The result was the birth in 1989 of the Federal Bureau of Investigation's Combined DNA Index System (CODIS). CODIS is a powerful tool for the use of forensic DNA technology in generating investigative leads.[22] With the evolution of CODIS, the scientific (including forensic) and legal communities are addressing forensic genetic information management in the establishment of standards.[23] Most forensic DNA laboratories have built their respective DNA analysis programs in four areas: (1) casework, (2) research and development of technology, (3) technology and data sharing, and (4) a computerized indexing system.

As noted above, forensic science is founded on comparisons of specimens from known and questioned sources toward the derivation of probative information, not simply the independent analysis of physical evidence, which by itself would be of little value. DNA data comparisons generally entail a stringent, systematic comparison of a set of digitized DNA typing results from one or more questioned specimens against a library of known specimens. With CODIS, large amounts of information can be sifted, permitting an examiner to perform an efficient side-by-side comparison of the putative specimens of interest. This side-by-side comparison by the analyst is desirable because the scientist, not a computer, renders the opinion.

At the user level, CODIS is configured physically into workstations from off-the-shelf, commercially available personal computer hardware, commercially available and customized software, and an image capturing device. This setup can be configured as either a standalone or local area network, depending on laboratory requirements. CODIS is currently actively employed in 46 laboratories in 22 states and in the District of Columbia, and the number of laboratories seeking and acquiring CODIS is rapidly increasing.

CODIS is a distributed database with three distinct levels: local, state, and national. At the local level, CODIS is operated by forensic laboratories that support police departments, sheriff's offices, or other state police agencies. These laboratories use CODIS to search their own DNA databases. Local laboratories can share their data by forwarding it to the state level. At the state level, CODIS is typically operated by the agency responsible for implementing the state's convicted offender statutes. At this level, interlaboratory searching takes place—that is, the DNA profiles submitted by different laboratories within the state are compared. A state can share this data by forwarding it to the national level. The National DNA Index System (NDIS) is operated by the FBI as authorized by the DNA Identification Act. NDIS permits forensic crime laboratories throughout the country to compare DNA profiles automatically.

NDIS will *not* be connected to other repositories of genetic information, such as those containing comprehensive or medical genetic information at the Department of Defense, universities, insurance companies, research institutes, or hospitals, *nor* will it be connected to criminal history databases.

A number of layers of control over access to forensic DNA information exist in CODIS or any of its component parts. At the workstation, user access can be limited (user name, password protection) and the system administration can detect and archive logon and logoff activity. Workstations can be placed in restricted areas of the laboratory. In considering broader networks of participating CODIS laboratories, security of the information over telecommunication pipelines is realized against unauthorized third-party access through use of the Secure Telephone Unit III (STU III, with inherent resident DES [Data Encryption Standard] and connectivity authentication); software-based encryption may be used in the future.[24]

Automated searches are conducted systematically using a set of forensic typing criteria (e.g., specifying protocols and DNA probes) from DNA types identified on the questioned specimen, without "benefit" of personal identifying information. If a putative match is obtained (i.e., the two samples cannot be excluded as potentially originating from the same source) from an automated query, only the laboratory, sample-identifying information, and DNA typing data are provided. The laboratory making the query must then contact the laboratory that has the sample of interest, properly identify itself, and appropriately explain why it needs access to a particular specimen profile. Only when a match is verified by the laboratory that has the sample of interest should further identifying information be released under controlled circumstances (i.e., "need-to-know" demonstrated and documented).

FORENSIC DNA DATABASES

Like all databases, forensic DNA databases are simply organized bodies of information that can be accessed based on certain criteria. Forensic DNA databases consist of (1) a convicted offender database, (2) an unsolved cases (or no available suspect cases) database, (3) population frequency databases, and (4) a missing persons database. Contained in the forensic databases are the DNA profile, identifiers for the laboratory, examiner, case, sample, and population statistics.

A convicted offender database consists of DNA profiles from known individuals convicted of crimes for which the deposition of biological materials by a suspect is likely (e.g., homicide, attempted homicide, sexual assault, kidnapping, assault). A biological sample, which may be a liquid blood or buccal sample, is collected at the time of incarceration or before the convicted felon is released. Dried replicate specimens are prepared and frozen in a restricted access facility in case future analysis is required. A portion of each donor's sample is subjected to analyses against genetic loci known to be forensically informative. Typing information (e.g., band size, numerical type designations) is then determined and entered into the database with the appropriate identifying information (e.g., sample numbers) to permit only sample identification and retrieval.

The forensic database consists of DNA typing results from biological materials from crime scenes or victims for which the donor (i.e., the suspect) has not been or cannot be determined by other investigative means. Examples of DNA profiles that can be contained in a forensic database may include those from semen left behind at an unsolved rape, blood typed on a knife found at the scene of a homicide that did not come from the victim, or hair not originating from a victim or other known person who had access to the scene.

Population databases contain population statistics information on how frequently forensically important genetic markers occur among various geographic areas or racial and ethnic groups. Population databases are required to convey an estimate of how rare a DNA profile is. The identity of donors of individual samples is not carried within population databases; generally, the source of each sample is anonymous.

Other potential forensic database applications might include profiles derived from body parts whose origin is unknown and profiles from the parents of missing children.

Forty states have enacted legislation permitting the acquisition of biological samples from known convicted offenders for the purpose of including DNA profiles into forensic databases. A sampling of statutes in this regard is contained in a 1994 report of the Ohio DNA Advisory Council to the governor.[25] Common elements of these statutes include: the authority to establish database(s); the declared purpose of the use of the database(s); who can and cannot be subjected to sample collection; what offenses are covered; the type of sample to be collected and by whom; the assignment of responsibility for the construction, maintenance, and administration of the database records; unauthorized uses of DNA databases and penalties for that unauthorized use; provisions for the expungement of DNA data from such an archive; and specifications for the unauthorized disclosure of DNA records.

More than 250,000 convicted offender forensic database samples have been collected nationwide, with Virginia, Florida, and California having collected the largest number.

In 1996, the FBI drafted legislation requiring individuals convicted of violent offenses under federal law to provide DNA samples for databasing purposes. Also in 1996, the FBI began operating NDIS, the upper tier of CODIS. Because NDIS contains information about individuals, it falls under the federal Privacy Act of 1974. To comply with this act, in 1996 the FBI published a description of NDIS in the *Federal Register* for a 30-day period of public comment. This description includes: a statement of purpose for the system; the authority for the maintenance of NDIS; probable or potential effects on the privacy of individuals; system security; authority for uses for and access to information contained in the system; categories of records stored in NDIS; policies and practices for storing, retrieving, accessing, retaining, disposing, and contesting the accuracy of records; and various exemptions that apply.

Like the local and state levels in the CODIS hierarchy, NDIS does not contain such sensitive information as name, date of birth, Social Security number, driver's license number, FBI number, or criminal history. When NDIS matches two or more DNA profiles, it provides the following information to all parties to the match: laboratory identifier, sample identifier, the associated DNA profile, and details of the search parameters.

PRIVACY CONCERNS AND THE EVOLUTION OF FORENSIC DNA DATABASES

Concerns exist over the privacy and confidentiality of forensic and medical genetic data banking. In articles on this issue, George Annas and Andrea DeGorgey have recognized the considerable power and accuracy of DNA typing and commented on the natural evolution and usefulness of databasing DNA profiles for more efficient scientific investigative purposes. Both have expressed the need to balance the benefits of genetic information to society, particularly in the medical and forensic realms, with the right of individuals to control information about themselves and prevent its use for purposes other than those for which it was created.[26] Because of the information and specificity of genetic typing, the potential sensitivity of DNA information, and the ability to store and retrieve genetic information via electronic means, a call has been sounded for safeguards to be developed and implemented.

Forensic applications of DNA technology are evolving with stringent privacy considerations and controls in mind, and the forensic community has addressed a number of potential privacy issues. Unlike medically oriented DNA analyses, forensic DNA typing does not derive the donor's predisposition to genetic diseases or the expression of genetic disease conditions. The genetic loci used in forensic DNA typing are selected for certain attributes, which include genetic variability among individuals, stability, and ease of assay. The majority of genetic markers used in DNA typing are noncoding segments in the human genome. No known function encoded in these repetitive DNA sequences might predispose an individual to a particular disease or attribute. Furthermore, there has been little evidence for any association of the forensically used noncoding DNA markers with particular diseases. However, some genetic markers employed in forensic analyses encode certain proteins (e.g., HLA-DQA1). There have been reports of associations with these coding markers and particular diseases. But the relative risk of the association is so low as to provide little or no information regarding an individual's health status or future well-being; the DNA types from coding marker data do not provide the level of information as, for example, the disease-causing gene itself.

The predisposition of a donor to one or more genetically induced conditions is generally not retrievable from forensic genetic data; only the potential for the individualization of a donor to the exclusion of all others (or an exclusion as the source of the evidence sample) by the genetic information can be obtained. Medically sensitive information cannot be derived from forensic DNA analyses. The genetic loci used in forensic DNA typing are well established and known by the scientific, forensic, and legal communities. The limited dissemination of forensic DNA information to authorized recipients during court proceedings or pretrial activities has no medical or other value.

Other than the name and type of investigation, the laboratory performing the analysis usually has little, if any, sensitive identifying information about the donor that may or could be included in a database. Investigative information as to the nature of the crime is often provided to the forensic scientist so that the proper analyses can be performed and information or conclusions about leads can be derived, but the information is not directly associated with the samples themselves and therefore would not be part of a database. Sensitive identifying information about a donor (e.g., Social Security number) has no bearing on or value to the forensic analytical process. Submissions of evidence are usually identified by a unique sequential number (e.g., year, month, day, and order received) or alphanumeric generated by the laboratory and, perhaps, the contributing agency. Sample designators (often alphanumeric) are assigned to individual specimens and used for efficiency during the analyses.

As a result of the intensity of judicial and scientific scrutiny since its inception, forensic DNA analyses must be conducted under TWGDAM guidelines, using established protocols, by qualified personnel. Obviously, the quality of the information produced as a result of the analyses and proper evidence handling are of prime concern. TWGDAM has produced guidelines to which the DNA forensic and legal communities subscribe. The DNA Advisory Board is reviewing these guidelines and refining them from a number of perspectives, including information management. Further, a CODIS Subcommittee has been generated under the TWGDAM umbrella to address issues concerning system design, function, acceptable loci, data quality, and information management. TWGDAM participants also have benefit of legal counsel regarding forensic issues through their respective organizations.

Forensic laboratories and police agencies are subject to strict legal and procedural requirements as to the chain of custody of the physical evidence (i.e., source of genetic information) and the release of information to unauthorized personnel. Forensic laboratories are restricted access facilities or are contained in such facilities, making unauthorized access difficult. Usually, access to physical evidence and forensic information is even further restricted inside a facility by either physical or electronic security measures.

Direct random access by the public to forensic genetic information and its potential sources is minimal. However, regardless of how many controls and barriers are constructed, it is difficult to defend absolutely against unlawful access by "authorized" persons from within an organization.

Jean McEwen has raised the issue of privacy and access to stored DNA samples.[27] Most laboratories will store data bank samples for retesting purposes or for typing additional genetic markers that become desirable for human identity-typing purposes. Although safeguards and penalties are in place for the unauthorized dissemination and obtaining of DNA data, there appear to be no protections against the dissemination of DNA samples. If samples are disseminated, then it is possible for someone to type the samples for genetic markers or genes that may compromise an individual's privacy concerns. The FBI recommends that similar confidentiality safeguards for the acquisition and distribution of DNA data be considered regarding the potential abuse of samples. The DNA samples should be analyzed only for the purposes that they were collected for, forensic identity markers. Safeguards can include numerical coding of samples (i.e., no personal information associated with the DNA samples), locked storage facilities, and substantial penalties for the unauthorized release or use of the samples.

Consider the scenario of the forensic DNA data bank as described earlier. The authorization to collect, preserve, and analyze samples to be contained within such a database, and the restrictions and limitations of such uses, including privacy and confidentiality issues and penalties for violation, are created by a legislative body with associated legal review, scientific comment, and recommendations. This becomes part of the public record. With NDIS, for example, the FBI has submitted a privacy impact statement (including assigning responsibility for privacy guidelines and enforcement) for publication in the *Federal Register* to provide for public comment. The purposes for the new system of records are clearly stated in the notice. From the FBI's point of view, uses for purposes other than those stated should result in expulsion from NDIS, in addition to whatever other penalties are levied.

The federal statute that establishes NDIS also requires that the FBI and other criminal justice agencies participating in NDIS disclose an identification match only: (1) to criminal justice agencies for purposes of law enforcement identification; (2) in judicial proceedings, if otherwise admissible pursuant to applicable statutes and rules; (3) for criminal defense purposes to a defendant, who shall have access to samples and analyses performed in connection with the case in which the defendant is charged; or (4) if personally identifiable information is removed, for a population statistics database, for identification research and protocol development, or for quality control purposes.

The samples themselves are collected and transported to the analytical facility (governmental or commercial) by specified personnel under strict chain-of-custody rules. Samples are prepared within the confines of a restricted access facility under established quality assurance and control procedures. Donor reference specimens are stored in locked containers within these facilities and are labeled only with identifying or archival numbers, which cannot be directly linked to the source without proper access to the local database. Even with physical access to a terminal, access in turn would provide only minimal identifying information for the source, administrative housekeeping information, and forensic DNA typing data. The extraction of specific information from a particular sample must be performed by someone with specific expertise in a laboratory. DNA profiles developed by outside contractors can be submitted to NDIS only by a criminal justice agency with authorized access to NDIS. This agency is wholly responsible for the integrity of the submitted DNA records.

To acquire information from the database itself would require logon privileges (subject to legitimate system surveillance) for output via an authorized user designation, knowledge of a password, and, perhaps, the ability to manipulate the software effectively. To access other forensic DNA databases (within the state, in other states, or nationally), a query would have to be made from an authorized system and electronic authentication would be required. The only information that can be accessed is the "matched" DNA profile (no other profiles can be accessed) and other system-assigned numerical identifiers, not the identity of the sample source. Last, to acquire associated source information requires direct contact with the original submitting agency. From the perspective of external system security, data and communication encryptions of the forensic data bank network in all or any of its parts are isolated from other electronic archives to minimize unwanted access.

CONCLUSION

Within the span of control of the forensic scientist, a considerable array of scientific, legal, administrative, physical, electronic, practical, procedural, and technological safeguards have been or are being considered as forensic DNA data banking evolves toward comprehensive deployment. The misuse of or unauthorized access to forensic genetic information is made extremely difficult through a variety of safeguards and restrictions. Every reasonable attempt has been or will be made to protect the privacy of individuals while providing for the needs of the investigative and legal processes.

We conclude with a case that illustrates the considerable value of a forensic DNA database, even at the state level. In Virginia in March 1989, a woman whose husband is a police officer was abducted from her home by a man she had never seen before. Her assailant forced her from her kitchen to the woods behind her home and raped her. Before leaving the scene of the crime, the rapist threatened the victim, saying he knew where she lived and would kill her if she told anyone what had happened.

The local police department developed a suspect in the case and sent a sample of his blood and the evidence to their forensic laboratory. Conventional serology examinations excluded the suspect. However, the examiner instructed the investigating officer to preserve the evidence because there was a new examination based on DNA that could possibly solve this crime sometime in the future.

Five years later, in 1994, the county where the victim resides experienced an outbreak of sexual assaults and rapes. The police developed a suspect in these cases and sent a sample of his blood to the laboratory. They also resubmitted the evidence from the original victim's case, thinking this individual might be responsible. This time, DNA analysis was available and performed. The suspect of immediate interest was excluded from the original sexual assault. At this time, however, a DNA profile was developed for the unknown rapist in the original matter.

In the years since the original assault, the state had also undertaken the development of a forensic DNA data bank containing profiles of convicted felons. As examiners developed offender profiles, they periodically searched them against unsolved cases. During the summer of 1995, the rapist in the case described at the outset was identified from a match against the data bank.

This rapist was already serving a 161-year sentence for abduction and robbery. The commonwealth attorney has decided to prosecute this case. Because the subject is a two-time felon, a successful prosecution will produce the "third strike" (i.e., no chance of parole). When told that the man who raped her had been identified, the woman said, "I feel as if a weight has been lifted from my shoulders."

NOTES

1. Committee on DNA Technology in Forensic Science, National Research Council, *DNA Technology in Forensic Science* (Washington, D.C.: National Academy Press, 1992); George J. Annas, "Setting Standards for DNA-Typing Results in the Courtroom," *New England Journal of Medicine* 326 (1992): 1641–44; Paul R. Billings, ed., *DNA on Trial: Genetic Identification and Criminal Justice* (Plainview, N.Y.: Cold Spring Harbor Laboratory Press, 1992).

2. Frye v. United States, 293 F. 1013 (D.C. Cir. 1923); Daubert v. Merrell Dow Pharmaceuticals, Inc., 509 U.S. 579 (1993).

3. DNA Advisory Board, "Forensic DNA Technology Standards" (in preparation); Technical Working Group on DNA Analysis Methods (TWGDAM), "Guidelines for a Quality Assurance Program in DNA Analysis," *Crime Laboratory Digest* 22 (1995): 33–37.

4. George J. Annas, "Privacy Rules for DNA Data Banks: Protecting Coded 'Future Diaries,'" *Journal of the American Medical Association* 270 (1993): 2346; Andrea DeGorgey, "The Advent of DNA Databanks: Implications for Information Privacy," *American Journal of Law and Medicine* 16 (1990): 381–98; Nachama L. Wikler et al., "DNA Data Banking in the Public Interest," in Billings, ed., *DNA on Trial,* 141–49.

5. Arlene R. Wyman and Ray White, "A High Polymorphic Locus in Human DNA," *Proceedings of the National Academy of Sciences* 77 (1980): 6754–58.

6. Edwin M. Southern, "Detection of Specific Sequences Among DNA Fragments Separated by Gel Electrophoresis," *Journal of Molecular Biology* 98 (1975): 503–17; Bruce Budowle and F. S. Baechtel, "Modifications to Improve the Effectiveness of Restriction Fragment Length Polymorphism Typing," *Applied Theoretical Electrophoresis* 1 (1990): 181–87.

7. Keith L. Monson and Bruce Budowle, "A System for Semi-Automated Analysis of DNA Autoradiograms," in *Proceedings of the International Symposium on the Forensic Aspects of DNA Analysis* (Washington, D.C.: Government Printing Office, 127–32).

8. Randall K. Saiki et al., "Enzymatic Amplification of Beta-globin Genomic Sequences and Restriction Analysis for Diagnosis of Sickle Cell Anemia," *Science* 230 (1985): 1350–54.

9. Jeffrey S. Chamberlain et al., "Deletion Screening of Duchenne Muscular Dystrophy Locus via Multiplex DNA Amplification," *Nucleic Acids Research* 16 (1988): 11141–56.

10. Randall R. Saiki et al., "Genetic Analysis of Amplified DNA with Immobilized Sequence-specific Oligonucleotide Probes," *Proceedings of the National Academy of Sciences* 86 (1989): 6230–34.

11. Ibid.

12. Ibid.

13. Bruce Budowle et al., "Validation and Population Studies of the Loci LDLR, GYPA, HBGG, D7S8, and Gc (PM loci), and HLA-DQ Using a Multiplex Amplification and Typing Procedure," *Journal of Forensic Science* 40 (1995): 45–54.

14. Bruce Budowle et al., "Analysis of the VNTR Locus D1S80 by the PCR Followed by High-Resolution PAGE," *American Journal of Human Genetics* 48 (1991): 137–44; Al

Edwards et al., "DNA Typing and Genetic Mapping with Trimeric and Tetrameric Tandem Repeats," ibid., 746–56; Al Edwards et al., "Genetic Variation at Five Trimeric and Tetrameric Repeat Loci in Four Human Population Groups," *Genomics* 12 (1992): 241–53.

15. Budowle et al., "Analysis of VNTR Locus D1S80."

16. Edwards et al., "Genetic Variation."

17. Ibid.; Nu En Huang, James M. Schumm, and Bruce Budowle, "Chinese Population Data on Three Tetrameric Short Tandem Repeat Loci—HUMTHO1, TPOX, and CSF1PO—Derived Using Multiplex PCR and Manual Typing," *Forensic Science International* 71 (1995): 131–36; Roberto Anker, T. Steinbreuck, and Helen Donnis-Keller, "Tetranucleotide Repeat Polymorphism at the Human Thyroid Peroxidase (hTPO) Locus," *Human Molecular Genetics* 1 (1992): 137; Colin Kimpton, A. Walton, and P. Gill, "A Further Tetranucleotide Repeat Polymorphism in the VWF Gene," ibid., 287.

18. Svante Paabo, J. A. Gifford, and A. C. Wilson, "Mitochondrial DNA Sequences from a 7000-Year-Old Brain," *Nucleic Acids Research* 16 (1988): 9775–8; Svante Paabo, R. Higuchi, and A. C. Wilson, "Ancient DNA and the Polymerase Chain Reaction: The Emerging Field of Molecular Archaeology," *Journal of Biologic Chemistry* 264 (1989): 9707–12; Svante Paabo, "Ancient DNA: Extraction, Characterization, Molecular Cloning, and Enzymatic Amplification," *Proceedings of the National Academy of Sciences* 86 (1989): 6196–200.

19. Linda Vigilant et al., "Mitochondrial DNA Sequences in Single Hairs from a Southern African Population," *Proceedings of the National Academy of Sciences* 86 (1989): 9350–54; Keun M. Sullivan, R. Hopgood, and P. Gill, "Identification of Human Remains by Amplification and Automated Sequencing of Mitochondrial DNA," *International Journal of Legal Medicine* 105 (1992): 83–86; Mark R. Wilson et al., "Guidelines for the Use of Mitochondrial DNA Sequencing in Forensic Science," *Crime Laboratory Digest* 20, no. 4 (1994): 68–77; Mark R. Wilson et al., "Extraction, PCR Amplification, and Sequencing of Mitochondrial DNA from Human Hair Shafts," *Biotechniques* 18 (1995): 662–69.

20. TWGDAM, "Guidelines for Quality Assurance Program."

21. DNA Identification Act, 42 U.S.C. § 14132(b)(3) (1994).

22. Jay V. Miller, "The FBI's DNA Analysis Program," *Law Enforcement Bulletin* (July 1991): 11–15.

23. DNA Advisory Board, "Forensic DNA Technology Standards"; TWGDAM, CODIS Subcommittee, "Standards for CODIS Acceptance of Data" (in preparation).

24. Peter Wayner, "DragNET—G-Men Launch Distributed Database: Criminals Baffled," *Byte* 20, no. 12 (1995): 106–12.

25. Ohio DNA Advisory Council, Offices of the Ohio Attorney General and Lieutenant Governor, *Using DNA Analysis to Fight Crime in Ohio* (Columbus: Ohio Attorney General, 1994).

26. Annas, "Privacy Rules for DNA Data Banks"; DeGorgey, "Advent of DNA Databanks."

27. Jean E. McEwen, "Forensic DNA Databanking by State Crime Laboratories," *American Journal of Human Genetics* 56 (1995): 1487–92.

Chapter 13 DNA Data Banks

Jean E. McEwen

Rapid and continuing developments in our understanding of human genetics, coupled with ongoing advances in information science, are leading us into a new era of DNA data banks. These data banks—repositories of genetic information about individuals obtained from the analysis of DNA samples—take many forms. Typically, however, they involve the routine storage of genetic information about large numbers of people; the information is generally maintained with individual identifiers and in computerized form, making it easy to access and (potentially) to share. Frequently housed with DNA data banks are DNA banks—that is, collections of the tissue samples from which the banked DNA data has been derived (or may be derived in the future).

DNA data banks and DNA banks can be used for a variety of purposes and are emerging in a range of settings. Although DNA tissue and data banking had their inception in the context of clinical medicine and medical research, today the main use of the technology is occurring in the forensics context, where government agencies are setting up DNA data banks to assist in establishing individual identification. For example, many states, pursuant to statutory mandate, have begun to collect DNA samples from certain convicted criminals and to analyze them for their unique identification characteristics. These DNA identification "profiles" are then stored (along with the samples themselves) for future law enforcement use—to help identify suspects in violent crime cases where biological evidence for comparison is available. The United States military is also establishing an enormous repository of DNA samples that will be tested as necessary in order to help identify soldiers missing in action in war.

DNA banks and DNA data banks are also being created outside the context of forensics for use in genetic research and clinical medicine. University- and hospital-based research labs are developing banks of DNA samples drawn from members of families affected with particular genetic disorders so that the DNA can be used in gene mapping and related studies. As the samples in these banks are tested and the test results recorded, DNA data banks are simultaneously being created. Some biotechnology companies have set up commercial DNA banks (and associated data banks) that for a fee will store DNA as a service to researchers, physicians, or genetic counselors. Some people are even banking their own DNA so that it can be made available to family members who in the future may need it for predictive testing, diagnosis, or treatment. In a few cases, parents have begun to bank their children's DNA so that it can be used to help locate the child and verify identity in the (however unlikely) event of a future abduction.

Whether established for the purpose of finding genes, predicting, diagnosing, or treating genetic disease, or identifying criminal suspects, soldiers missing in action, or other missing persons, DNA banks and DNA data banks hold tremendous promise. But DNA banking and DNA data banking also raise novel legal, ethical, and public policy challenges.

STATE FORENSIC DATA BANKS

Although DNA banking and data banking take place in a variety of contexts, nowhere have these activities proliferated more rapidly than in the area of law enforcement. By September 1996, 40 states had enacted statutes to establish forensic DNA data banks: collections of DNA samples (and the unique DNA identification profiles derived from their analysis) taken from various categories of criminals.[1] These laws generally require specified convicted offenders (especially violent sex offenders or other violent felons) to provide blood (and in some cases saliva) samples for DNA identification testing, either at the time of sentencing or before release from prison. State crime labs then extract DNA from the samples and, using what is becoming a standardized set of enzymes and probes, create for each offender a DNA profile.[2] These profiles—arguably unique to each individual, with the exception of identical twins—are then digitized and entered onto computer.[3] If in the future biological material of unknown origin (such as semen or blood) is found at a crime scene, investigators will be able to profile that sample and compare it with the reference profiles of known offenders that are already in the data bank—much in the same way as has long been done with conventional fingerprints.[4] A proposal is also being developed to set up a federal DNA data bank; this would include DNA profiles from persons convicted in federal or military courts of offenses similar to those covered under most states' data banking laws.

By September 1996, 32 of the states that had enacted forensic DNA data banking laws had begun to collect samples for their data banks. Cumulatively, samples from almost 380,000 offenders nationwide had been amassed, with most of those in Virginia and California. In those states that had already begun to analyze the samples, about 116,000 samples, or 30%, had been tested. The rate at which crime labs will be able to process samples for their data banks (and the evidence samples against which to compare them) should increase significantly over the next few years as the technology becomes cheaper and better automated and as more resources for DNA testing become available. The DNA Identification Act, a federal law passed in 1994, will make $40 million in federal matching grants available to states for DNA analysis activities over a five-year period in exchange for the states' adherence to specified uniform standards.[5] This law also formally authorized the Federal Bureau of Investigation to establish a national computer network called CODIS (an acronym for the Combined DNA Identification System) to facilitate the exchange of DNA information between data banks in different states.[6]

The CODIS network, when fully operational, should enable law enforcement officials to identify many suspects who in an earlier day might never have been identified—including those who move across state lines. By September 1996, data banks had already achieved "cold hits" in at least 58 cases (mostly sexual assault and murder cases)—where DNA extracted from biological evidence of unknown origin found at a crime scene was found to match that of a known offender whose DNA profile was in the data bank. In addition, in at least 80 instances, DNA data banks had been used to establish associations between two or more as-yet unresolved cases, where DNA data derived from unknown evidence samples and entered into the data bank were linked to the same (as-yet unidentified) individual. Minnesota's DNA data bank, for example, was used to tie one individual to 18 separate sexual assaults.

Forensic DNA data banks hold particular promise for rape and sexual assault cases—where biological evidence is often available, the victim often cannot identify the perpetrator, and rates of recidivism are extraordinarily high.[7] DNA data banks may also be useful in homicide investigations where biological evidence from the assailant is left at the scene and other leads are limited. They may be significantly less useful in the investigation of nonviolent crimes, but even in such cases they may have some utility (e.g., should a white collar criminal leave saliva on an envelope flap from which DNA can be extracted for comparative analysis).

WHO SHOULD BE IN A FORENSIC DNA DATA BANK?

Accompanying the dramatic recent growth in the number of forensic DNA data banks has been a marked expansion in the scope of the population the laws target.[8] Originally drafted to cover primarily persons convicted of violent sex offenses, a number of statutes now require samples from nonviolent felons, including, for example, those convicted only of drug or white collar offenses.[9] In some states, samples are collected from those convicted only of certain misdemeanors, despite legislative guidelines issued by the FBI that recommend against taking samples from misdemeanants.[10] One state requires samples from persons who have merely been arrested (not convicted) of a covered offense,[11] and several other states are considering bills that would extend their data banking laws to arrestees. States are also moving increasingly to cover juvenile offenders under the ambit of their data banking laws.

The historical trend toward broadening the scope of coverage under forensic DNA data banking laws raises the question of how far such a law may extend before it would be invalidated on Fourth Amendment grounds as an unreasonable search and seizure. The case for requiring samples from violent convicted sex offenders seems compelling: Bureau of Justice Statistics data regarding the recidivism of convicted criminals shows that rapists released from prison are 10.5 times more likely than other released prisoners to subsequently be arrested for rape and that released prisoners who have served time for other sexual assaults are 7.5 times more likely to be arrested later for a like offense.[12] Other violent offenders also have high recidivism rates, and it is not uncommon for persons initially convicted of such offenses as burglary, robbery, and assault to later be arrested for such "crossover crimes" as sex crimes (the type of crime most likely to be solved with a DNA data bank).[13] However, in relative terms, it is less likely that a person convicted of a nonviolent offense that is not sex related will later commit an offense involving biological evidence suitable for comparison through a DNA data bank.

So far, courts that have entertained Fourth Amendment or other constitutional challenges to forensic DNA data banking laws have consistently rejected them.[14] Even Virginia's data banking law, which encompasses all convicted felons, has been upheld as bearing a rational relationship to the state's legitimate interest in facilitating the investigation of future crimes without suspects.[15] Courts have also uniformly upheld laws that require samples from persons already incarcerated on the law's effective date (rather than just from those convicted thereafter), rejecting the argument that such retroactive application violates the Constitution's ex post facto clause.[16] The collection of samples from juveniles convicted of offenses otherwise covered by a state's data banking law has also been upheld,[17] although one court, ruling on another state's data banking statute, found that a juvenile court lacked statutory authority to require samples for the data bank from juveniles who had merely been adjudicated delinquent.[18]

The opinions upholding state DNA data banking laws have not always been unanimous, and some judges have cautioned against unrestrained expansion in the scope of the statutes, emphasizing the need for a rational relationship between the categories of offenders covered and the data bank's stated purpose.[19] The National Academy of Sciences has also recommended against launching massive data banks too hastily lest crime labs find themselves prematurely locked into a "dinosaur" technology.[20] Nevertheless, the historical experience in the United States with conventional fingerprinting suggests that the range of persons required to provide samples for DNA data banks will probably continue to broaden—especially as the technology becomes better automated.

Popular support for high-tech approaches to fighting crime is also likely to fuel the continued growth of forensic DNA data banks. But critics of data banking fear that DNA data banks—initially aimed at a narrow "pariah" group of violent repeat sex offenders but already expanding in scope—will inexorably lead to the taking of samples from other unpopular segments of the population regardless of criminal history—such as new immigrants, welfare recipients, and people in drug and alcohol treatment programs.[21]

Great Britain has already taken a major step toward establishing a forensic DNA data bank that will, over time, include a substantial portion of the country's population. Since 1995, British police have been authorized to take "nonintimate samples" (such as hair or saliva) for data banking without consent from anyone convicted of or charged with a recordable offense.[22] About 135,000 samples are expected to be taken in the first year alone, and as many as 5 million records will eventually be entered into the data bank. Britain has also been the site of several mass "bloodings" in which, following the commission of several brutal, highly publicized crimes, large numbers of men in the surrounding neighborhoods have been asked to provide samples "voluntarily" for DNA profiling in order to "rule themselves out" as suspects and place pressure on the perpetrator to come forward. The first case of this (which was a major impetus for the initial concept of a DNA data bank) was chronicled in 1989 in Joseph Wambaugh's best-seller *The Blooding*.

Some civil libertarians worry that even in the United States, DNA data banks, despite their currently limited objectives, are promoting a kind of "surveillance creep" in which eventually everybody in the population, perhaps at birth, will be required to provide a DNA sample to the state.[23] In fact, some have suggested that our unique DNA identification profiles will, over time, become our national identifiers, effectively replacing today's Social Security number.[24]

On one hand, having a reference DNA profile on file for everyone in the population could dramatically increase crime resolution rates—especially in serial sex crime cases. It could also be argued that only the guilty should have reason to fear having their DNA data in a forensic DNA data bank. On the other hand, a population-wide DNA data bank could fundamentally alter the relationship between individuals and the state, essentially turning us into a nation of suspects.[25] In addition, large-scale DNA data banks, even if intended solely for identification purposes, raise significant policy challenges for society at large. Ultimately, determining who should be in a forensic DNA data bank will require balancing the quantifiable law enforcement benefits that large data banks can confer against the less quantifiable, but nonetheless real, risks to civil liberties that they may implicate.

PRIVACY IMPLICATIONS OF FORENSIC DNA DATA BANKS

Understanding the privacy concerns that forensic DNA data banks raise requires differentiating between the DNA data stored in the data banks and the samples from which those data are derived. The DNA identification profiles that most forensic DNA data banks are creating for their data banks are based on restriction fragment length polymorphism (RFLP) analysis techniques, which focus only on segments of the DNA that do not code for structural proteins and thus (apart from their ability to identify individuals uniquely) are genetically uninformative.[26] Even this limited information, however, could be of some interest outside the law enforcement community, such as to child support or immigration authorities seeking to track people's whereabouts or familial relationships for reasons unrelated to criminal investigations.[27]

In addition, most crime labs are moving toward polymerase chain reaction-based technologies to analyze samples for their data banks.[28] Because these techniques focus directly on genes and not just on "spacer" material, they may at least indirectly generate information about matters such as one's predisposition to genetic disease[29]—although the amount of such information that could be gleaned through examining a PCR-based DNA identification profile would likely be quite limited. In addition, whether created with RFLP or PCR methods, a DNA identification profile, when run through a data bank, has the unique capability to implicate biological relatives of the perpetrator (whose profiles, though not identical to the perpetrator's, may be similar).[30] Thus, the genetic data held in a DNA data bank, even if intended solely for identification purposes, raises unique privacy concerns that go beyond those associated with conventional fingerprints.

However, the major privacy issues in DNA data banking arise not from the maintenance of the DNA data but from the retention of the samples themselves.[31] This is because DNA samples, unlike identification profiles, contain a potential wealth of genetic and other medical information. As new genes are found and tests are developed to determine who has them, it will become increasingly possible to discern from examining an individual's DNA predispositions and traits that may be highly personal, sensitive, or stigmatizing. Critics of forensic DNA data banks worry that the samples collected for data banking will be retested, perhaps many years in the future, for reasons unrelated to those for which they were originally collected—and for the resulting information to be misused.[32] For example, insurance companies, employers, school systems, adoption agencies, and other state and federal agencies could all be expected to have an interest in accessing genetic information of a type that could be derived from testing banked DNA samples. Research investigators—particularly behavioral geneticists—may also be keenly interested in the captive repository of samples from convicted criminals stored along with forensic

DNA data banks.[33] Indeed, one state's data banking law specifically authorizes the use of samples collected for its data bank for "educational research or medical research or development"—an authorization that would presumably encompass behavioral research into, for example, genetic predispositions to violence.[34]

The National Academy of Sciences, recognizing the risks to privacy and individual autonomy that stored DNA samples can present, has recommended that samples taken from convicted offenders for data banks be destroyed "promptly" after being analyzed.[35] However, crime labs that maintain data banks currently plan to retain their samples indefinitely (except in situations warranting expungement, such as where the conviction that supplied the basis for drawing the sample is reversed on appeal).[36] Crime labs cite a need to save samples so that they can be reanalyzed at a later date as testing technologies improve, so that they can be made available to defense counsel in a future case should a person in the data bank be targeted through a data bank search, or so that they can be accessed for routine quality control checks.[37]

So far there have been no reported instances of unauthorized dissemination of either DNA samples or DNA data by crime labs with DNA data banks. In addition, the FBI has made computer security a major priority for the CODIS network by incorporating, for example, data encryption capabilities.[38] The DNA Identification Act also provides some protection for the privacy interests of those required to provide samples for data banking.[39] Specifically, it requires crime labs, as a condition of participating in the CODIS network, to limit the disclosure of stored individually identifiable DNA samples and data to criminal justice agencies for "law enforcement identification purposes" (and for use in judicial proceedings if otherwise admissible and to criminal defendants in connection with the cases in which they are charged).[40] The law also provides criminal fines of up to $100,000 for the knowing, unauthorized obtaining of DNA samples and for the knowing, unauthorized obtaining or disclosure of individually identifiable DNA data.[41] These provisions may ameliorate some of the informational privacy concerns raised by DNA data banks—risks to which state data banking statutes have sometimes tended to give short shrift.[42] However, whether they will prove to have real "teeth" or remain primarily symbolic remains to be seen. The statute essentially entrusts its enforcement to the FBI and other law enforcement agencies, in spite of an earlier National Academy of Sciences recommendation that primary oversight over forensic DNA activities be placed with an independent agency such as the Department of Health and Human Services.[43]

THE DEPARTMENT OF DEFENSE DNA REPOSITORY

Law enforcement is not alone in banking DNA for identification. In fact, the world's largest DNA bank is operated by the United States military. Since June 1992, the Department of Defense has required all military inductees and all active duty and reserve personnel to provide blood and saliva samples for its DNA Specimen Repository at the time of enlistment, reenlistment, or preparation for operational deployment. Almost 1.5 million samples had already been collected by September 1996; more than 3 million are expected to have been amassed by 2001, when the repository will be complete. The Armed Forces Institute of Pathology plans to use this DNA bank for humanitarian purposes: to identify the remains of missing soldiers so they can be returned to their families, making the Tomb of the Unknown Soldier a relic of the past.

Before the era of DNA technology, missing soldiers typically could be identified, if at all, only through dog tags, fingerprints, or dental X-rays. Each of these methods, however, had significant limitations—especially given the destructiveness of modern weaponry. The advent of DNA testing technology, used for the first time in Operation Desert Storm, made identifying missing soldiers much less onerous—but even in that conflict (which predated the establishment of the DNA repository), identifications typically required comparing DNA from the unknown remains with samples provided by surviving relatives of the missing soldier. The DNA repository will now permit the direct comparison of DNA from remains with banked DNA known to have come from the missing service member. This will permit identifications to be made even in cases where paternity is uncertain or where no biological relatives of the service member are available for testing.

The military plans to extract DNA from the samples warehoused in its repository only as needed. However, it plans to keep the samples themselves for 50 years, although pursuant to a revised policy announced in 1996, service members will be permitted to request that their samples be destroyed when they leave the military.[44] But as with the DNA samples being housed in state crime labs, the samples in the military's repository are inherently subject to being used for purposes other than those for which they were collected. For example, in 1994, following the murder of the young daughter of a U.S. Army sergeant stationed in Germany, military authorities, in the largest "Dragnet"-style DNA investigation ever undertaken, made a sweeping request for blood samples from all soldiers living in the area.[45] The operation resulted in the taking of some 1,900 samples and was ultimately successful in identifying the perpetrator. However, the operation's success raises the question of whether the role of the military's DNA repository will eventually be expanded, with samples no longer used solely for identifying remains but also for the routine investigation of crime.

Other, more futuristic uses of the repository can be envisioned. For example, some research suggests that genes influence sexual orientation. Should a so-called gay gene someday be found and a test developed to determine who has it, the question may arise whether anything would prevent the Department of Defense from screening the samples in its repository to identify those thought to be predisposed to engage in homosexual behavior. In an effort to alleviate such concerns, the military in 1996 clarified its policy regarding the range of permissible uses of samples. Under the revised policy, samples cannot be used without consent for any purpose other than the identification of human remains (and routine quality assurance), except where subpoenaed for the investigation or prosecution of a felony.[46]

The requirement that all service members provide samples for the military's DNA repository was challenged in a 1995 lawsuit filed by two marines who refused to submit to having their blood drawn for this purpose and who as a result were subjected to court martial proceedings.[47] A federal district court upheld the program, rejecting the service members' claims that it violated the First, Fourth, Fifth, or Ninth Amendments, violated the terms of their enlistment contracts, or was inconsistent with military regulations regarding the protection of human subjects in research. The lawsuit did, however, provide an impetus for the military to clarify and revise certain of its policies.[48]

RESEARCH AND CLINICAL SERVICE DNA BANKS

Although identification-related DNA banks and DNA data banks are the largest and fastest-growing repositories of DNA, DNA banking and DNA data banking had their inception in clinical service and research contexts. Today a considerable number of DNA samples are still stored in these settings, and DNA banking in academic institutions and commercial labs, though still a relatively novel activity, is on the increase. A 1992 poll of 11 biotechnology companies that examined the extent of commercial DNA banking going on at the time suggested that fewer than 10,000 samples were being banked in the United States and that many of those were being stored at the request of researchers rather than for individual patients.[49] However, a 1995 survey of 148 DNA diagnostic labs—both commercial and academic—showed that 90%

had begun to bank DNA in at least some form or forms and that more than half of those already had 500 or more samples in storage.[50] In addition, almost one-third of the labs indicated that they planned to develop DNA banking services further over the next two years.

Biotechnology companies and university- or hospital-based laboratories that store DNA generally do so for one of two purposes.[51] Some labs, especially in the commercial arena, bank DNA as a service to individuals or families who are at risk for particular genetic conditions and who thus are interested in making their samples available for family-based linkage testing in the future; these samples are frequently stored at the request of an intermediary such as a physician or genetic counselor. Other labs bank DNA for research purposes, such as for gene mapping studies, which frequently require samples from numerous family members over several generations. The line that separates these two types of DNA banking is not always clear; for example, a sample provided for linkage testing might later (in the absence of any agreement to the contrary) be used for genetic research—perhaps on an unrelated condition. A very small number of samples banked in commercial DNA labs are stored for identification purposes; these are typically reference samples from children stored by parents who believe it may be beneficial to have their child's DNA on hand for identification profiling should the child someday be abducted.

Most DNA samples housed in commercial and academic facilities, however, are stored for medical rather than identification purposes. Thus, when samples in these banks are tested and the results entered into DNA data banks, the information will tend to be much more personal and sensitive than that which can be gleaned from the DNA identification profiles in forensic data banks—particularly when the data are correlated with information about familial relationships. But the samples themselves also raise particular privacy concerns; indeed, even information regarding the mere existence in a disease-related DNA bank of a sample from an individual may be highly stigmatizing—independent of any associated test results.[52]

In assessing the privacy implications of DNA banking secondary to research and clinical service activities, one must thus again distinguish between the storage of the samples and the storage of the data derived from testing them; one must also differentiate between DNA storage in the clinical service and research contexts. DNA storage raises more potential privacy problems in the clinical service context than in the research context because in the clinical context, such information as the depositor's name, address, birth date, diagnosis, family history, and physician's or genetic counselor's name and address will often be stored along with the sample. In the research context, by contrast, samples are generally stored without individual identifiers, although they may sometimes be traceable to their source through code numbers or other means.[53]

Research- and clinical service–oriented DNA banks, unlike those in the forensics context, are essentially unregulated.[54] In addition, although several sets of guidelines have been proposed for drafting consent forms and other relevant documentation for DNA banking,[55] few facilities that store DNA have developed comprehensive written internal protocols, depositor's agreements, or other documents governing important aspects of this activity.[56] This has led some to call for strict laws to govern DNA banks; one proposal, for example, has advocated requiring all DNA banks to file a "privacy impact" statement with a national licensing agency. Under this approach, the burden of proof would be on the DNA bank to demonstrate that DNA storage is necessary to achieve an "important medical or societal goal."[57] The American Society of Human Genetics and the American College of Medical Genetics have also issued policy recommendations for DNA banking;[58] both sets of guidelines are based on the principle that those who provide samples for banking have the right to control the samples' future disposition.

ETHICAL AND LEGAL ISSUES

DNA banking in academic institutions and commercial settings raises complex ethical and legal issues, especially relating to informed consent.[59] For example, for research or testing on many genetic disorders to proceed, samples must be obtained from multiple family members. But this may create situations in which some family members are pressured by others to provide samples for banking, raising questions about voluntariness and informed consent. Some people may be reluctant to bank their DNA because they do not wish to learn (or have others learn) their genetic status or because they are concerned that undisclosed evidence of nonpaternity, incest, or adoption in the family may surface.

The characteristically long storage period can also create problems.[60] Genetic research typically proceeds in stages, and the course of most such research is impossible to predict. For example, research involving a banked DNA sample may begin with efforts to localize a gene through linkage analysis and continue through the isolation of the gene to the study of mutations and the development of a direct DNA test. Implications may thus arise for the use of a banked sample in the future that could not have been anticipated when the sample was provided. Requiring the bank to obtain informed consent from the depositor before each new phase of the study may be extremely burdensome. And yet, basic principles of informed consent and individual autonomy suggest that those who bank their DNA, whether for linkage testing or for research, should retain some control over what happens to their samples over time. This is particularly true where it is anticipated that transformed cell lines will be created from a sample and made available (anonymously) for research on unrelated genetic conditions—perhaps to investigators at other institutions.[61]

The often murky line between research and testing can compound the difficulties in obtaining informed consent—especially where the activities of the DNA bank and the affiliated research lab are closely intertwined, making absolute anonymity of the banked samples hard to preserve.[62] For example, a sample from a person who is a member of an at-risk family but is presumed to be unaffected may be analyzed in the course of a research study and found to have the mutant gene that was expected to be found only in the affected family members. Or a sample initially banked in connection with research on one genetic condition may later be used for research on an unrelated condition, unexpectedly revealing the presence of the mutant gene. In such cases, if the samples have not been irrevocably stripped of identifiers, the researcher may find himself or herself in an ethical bind, having acquired information about a person that, if known to that person or his or her physicians, might lead to closer medical surveillance or other preventive measures. Does the researcher then have an ethical obligation to recontact that person with the incidental, potentially clinically relevant finding? What if the person would prefer not to know? These questions have no easy answers, but they point to areas in which agreement should be sought at the time samples are collected.

Occasionally, research conducted using transformed cell lines created from banked DNA samples will lead to the development of a drug, therapy, or other commercially valuable product, resulting in substantial economic benefit to the researcher or the bank. The question may then arise as to whether those who provided the samples are entitled to share in the profits thus derived. Although the law regarding the property status of extracorporeal DNA is unsettled, the court in Moore v. University of California, a pathbreaking case involving the unauthorized commercial use of a patient's cell lines by a physician and various researchers, held that the patient had no property right in the cell lines and thus could not state a claim for conversion.[63] However, the Moore court held that the patient could state a claim for breach of fiduciary duty or lack of informed consent, reasoning that a physician must disclose personal interests, including economic interests, unrelated to the patient's health that may affect his or her professional judgment.[64] This decision highlights the importance of communicating, at the time a sample is being banked, the possibility (however remote) that some commercial benefit may inure to others based on the sample's use and of clarifying the depositor's rights (if any) with respect to any such profits.

Misunderstandings between persons who bank their DNA and facilities that store it may also occur in other areas.[65] For example, who "owns" the sample and is entitled to control its disposition—the "depositor" of the sample, a designated representative from the depositor's family, or the DNA bank? How long will the sample be kept, and in what form or forms? What will be the bank's liability (if any) for accidentally destroying a sample, for keeping a sample beyond the agreed upon storage period, or for mixing up samples? What fee (if any) will be charged for storing the sample, and what are the consequences of non-payment? Might the sample be made available in the future for related or unrelated research, and if so, can the depositor's anonymity be guaranteed? Under what (if any) circumstances will the bank re-contact the depositor with new information derived from the sample? What will happen to the sample should the bank suspend operations or significantly change its identity (for example, should the company in which the bank is housed dissolve or change ownership)?

WHO MAY HAVE ACCESS TO BANKED DNA SAMPLES?

One of the most difficult questions in academic or commercial DNA banking is who may have access to banked DNA samples and to the data derived from their analysis?[66] This issue is especially important where samples are being kept in an individually identifiable form and where the banking is being done by someone other than the depositor's physician (such as by a biotechnology company or a researcher in an academic institution) who has no direct relationship with the depositor.

Issues may arise with respect to both access within families and access to third parties. Regarding access within families, the approach of requiring the depositor's consent before the sample can be made available to other family members would accord to the depositor the greatest confidentiality protection. Some banks, however, take the position that depositors, by entering the bank, agree to allow automatic access to the sample by any family members who may need it. This approach works well where family members' views about genetic privacy are not in conflict, but can create problems where relatives disagree. Access by third parties to individually identifiable DNA samples (or data) can be controlled through depositor's agreements that specifically prohibit their release (for example, to an insurance company) without the depositor's express written consent. However, compelled disclosure to third parties pursuant to subpoena or court order may be impossible to prevent.

In Britain, a proposal has been made to establish centralized registries that would collaborate to maintain a directory of all DNA banks in the country and of all individuals and families who have banked samples.[67] This proposal is designed to ensure that persons who might be able to benefit from knowing about a relative's banked sample (such as one provided by a now-deceased relative or a relative in a distant location) can learn about the sample's availability. However, this approach would pose privacy risks that to many people in the United States would seem unacceptably high.

INCHOATE DNA BANKS AND DNA DATA BANKS

Although this discussion has focused on organized DNA banks and DNA data banks (facilities that store DNA as a matter of routine, for the specific purpose of performing some type of DNA analysis, either now or in the future), any facility where blood or other tissue is stored, whatever the stated purpose of the storage, has the potential to become, in the future, a kind of DNA bank.[68]

Thus, for example, the archives of newborn screening cards, or "Guthrie cards," that many state public health labs have retained (after testing the blood spots on the cards for PKU and other inborn errors of metabolism) collectively constitute an enormous inchoate DNA bank.[69] The trend in most states is toward saving these cards for a longer time, and given the stability of DNA in dried blood and the increasing ability to screen such samples for particular DNA sequences, interest in using Guthrie cards as a resource for population-wide genetic epidemiological studies is likely to grow.[70]

Other collections of tissue samples kept for reasons unrelated to DNA analysis, such as stored pathological specimens in paraffin blocks and even samples in ordinary blood banks, can also be seen as "inchoate" DNA banks, providing a major potential resource for large-scale retrospective genetic research studies. In fact, because DNA may be found wherever biological materials are present, even such places as post offices (where DNA may be found on millions of licked stamps), barbershop floors (where DNA may be found in hair roots), and manicure salons (where DNA may be found in clipped fingernails) can be viewed as at least potential DNA "banks." The fact that DNA can often be extracted from biological materials found even in places like these makes the very notion of a "DNA bank" difficult to define, and helps to explain why comprehensive attempts to regulate DNA banks as distinct entities tend to be difficult.

Just as inchoate DNA banks exist wherever biological materials are being stored, inchoate DNA data banks exist wherever genetic information is recorded and stored—even if the information is not being kept in a very systematic fashion. Thus, for example, even ordinary medical records that contain genetic information are potential DNA data banks. As these medical records are computerized (which is becoming the norm in most health maintenance organizations), it will become increasingly difficult to control the flow of this information.[71] DNA test results recorded in medical records may begin to make their way on to wider electronic networks and be linked to information in other data banks. This, in turn, may raise the potential for genetic discrimination.

The insurance context provides an example of how this could occur. Insurance applicants must routinely consent to the release of their medical records as a condition of obtaining coverage. To an insurance underwriter, even a reference in a medical record to the fact that a person has banked his or her DNA in a particular disease-related bank could trigger suspicion that a genetic disorder runs in the family. This, in turn, could be used as a basis to deny coverage or at least to require DNA testing before issuing a policy.

The uniquely familial nature of genetic information exacerbates the potential for discrimination. Insurers already use traditional family histories to make decisions about their applicants' insurability. In the future, it will become possible to correlate family relationships and DNA test results at the click of a button, to make decisions about the insurability not only of individuals but of entire families. In addition, insurance companies routinely share information—for example, through the Medical Information Bureau (MIB), a massive data bank that serves more than 650 major insurance companies by providing information about the health of their applicants. As computer matching techniques become increasingly sophisticated, other data banks like the MIB can be expected to evolve in other contexts, and to be used in determining the eligibility of individuals for a range of important societal benefits.

CONCLUSION

Whether intended for identification, research, or clinical medicine, most DNA banks and DNA data banks serve important and socially beneficial purposes. In the criminal justice arena, state forensic DNA data banks are helping police apprehend violent repeat criminals who in an earlier day might never have been brought to justice. In the military, stored DNA samples will help to ensure that no American soldier need ever again be buried in the Tomb of the Unknown Soldier. In the context of genetic research, DNA banking is leading to some of the most exciting progress in medicine today. And in the clinical service context, DNA banks are helping individuals and families to make important decisions regarding their health.

But DNA banking and DNA data banking—whether done for purposes of identification or for medical testing or research—raise complex questions of law, ethics, and public policy. Although DNA data banks in the forensics contexts are subject to some degree of state and federal regulation, it remains to be seen whether current laws will adequately protect the privacy and related interests of those required to provide samples. The military's DNA repository is subject only to internal Department of Defense control, and most research and clinical service banks housed in academic and commercial labs remain completely unregulated. In this new age of genetic discovery and electronic data interchange, controlling the flow of banked DNA information will become increasingly difficult. Continued vigilance is essential if DNA banks and DNA data banks are to perform their important functions without impinging on the rights and interests of individuals who—whether by state mandate or by choice—have their DNA in a bank.

NOTES

1. Ala. Code §§ 36–18–20, et seq. (1994); Alaska Stat. § 44.41.035 (1996); Ariz. Rev. Stat. Ann. § 31–281 (1993); Ark. Code Ann. § 12–12–1101 (West 1994); Cal. Penal Code §§ 290.2, 3060.5, Cal. Gov't Code § 76104.5 (West 1994); Colo. Rev. Stat. Ann. § 17–2–201(5)(g)(1) (West 1995); Conn. Gen. Stat. Ann. § 54–102g (West 1994); Del. Code Ann. tit. 29, § 4713 (1994); Fla. Stat. Ann. § 943.325 (West 1994); Ga. Code Ann. § 24–4–60 (1992); Haw. Rev. Stat. § 706–603 (1992); Ill. Ann. Stat. ch. 730, ¶5/5–4–3 (Smith-Hurd 1992); Iowa Code Ann. § 13.10 (West 1991), Iowa Admin. Code r. 61–8.1(13), et seq. (1991); Kan. Stat. Ann. § 21–2511 (1991); Ky. Rev. Stat. Ann. §§ 17.170, 17.175 (Baldwin 1992); Me. Rev. Stat. Ann. tit. 25, § 1571 (West 1996); Md. Code Ann., art. 88B, § 12A (1994), Md. Code Ann., Cts. & Jud. Proc. § 10–915 (1994); Mich. Comp. Laws Ann. § 750.520m (West 1994); Minn. Stat. Ann. §§ 299C.155, 609.3461 (West 1993); Miss. Code

Ann. § 45–33–15 (1995); Mo. Ann. Stat. §§ 650.050, 650.055 (Vernon 1991); Mont. Code Ann. § 44–6-101 (1995); Nev. Rev. Stat. Ann. § 176.111 (Michie 1989); N.J. Stat. Ann. §§ 53:1–20.17, et seq. (West 1994); N.Y. Exec. Law §§ 995, et seq. (McKinney 1994); N.C. Gen. Stat. §§ 15A-266, et seq. (1993); N.D. Cent. Code §§ 31–13–02, et seq. (1995); Ohio Rev. Code Ann. §§ 109.573, 2151.315, 2901.07 (Baldwin 1995); Okla. Stat. Ann. tit. 22, §§ 751.1, 991a (West 1996), Okla. Stat. Ann. tit. 57, § 584 (West 1996), Okla. Stat. Ann. tit. 74, §§ 150.27, et seq. (West 1996); Or. Rev. Stat. §§ 137.076, 181.085 (1991); Pa. Cons. Stat. tit. 35, §§ 7651.101, et seq. (1996); S.C. Code Ann. §§ 23–3-600, et seq. (Law. Co-op. 1995); S.D. Codified Laws Ann. §§ 23–5-14, et seq. (1990); Tenn. Code Ann. §§ 38–6-113, 40–35–321 (1991); Tex. Gov't Code Ann. §§ 411.141, et seq. (Vernon 1995); Utah Code Ann. §§ 53–5–212.1, et seq. (1994); Va. Code Ann. § 19.2–310.2 (1993); Wash. Rev. Code §§ 43.43.752, 43.43.754 (1990); W. Va. Code §§ 15–2B–1, et seq. (1995); Wis. Stat. Ann. §§ 165.76, 165.77, 973.047 (West 1993).

2. National Academy of Sciences, National Research Council, Commission on Life Sciences, Board of Biology, *DNA Technology in Forensic Science* (Washington, D.C.: National Academy Press, 1992); U.S. Congress, Office of Technology Assessment, *Genetic Witness: Forensic Uses of DNA Tests* (Washington, D.C.: Government Printing Office, 1990); Jack Ballantyne, George Sensabaugh, and Jan Witkowski, eds., *DNA Technology and Forensic Science,* Banbury Report 32 (Cold Spring Harbor, N.Y.: Cold Spring Harbor Laboratory Press, 1989).

3. National Academy of Sciences, *DNA Technology in Forensic Science.*

4. Ibid.

5. DNA Identification Act of 1994, Pub. L. No. 103–322, 108 Stat. 1796, § 210304 (1994).

6. 42 U.S.C. § 14132 (1994).

7. National Academy of Sciences, *DNA Technology in Forensic Science.*

8. Jean E. McEwen and Philip R. Reilly, "A Review of State Legislation on DNA Forensic Data Banking," *American Journal of Human Genetics* 54 (1994): 941–58.

9. See, e.g., Va. Code Ann. § 19.2–310.2 (Michie 1993).

10. U.S. Department of Justice, Federal Bureau of Investigation, *Legislative Guidelines for DNA Databases* (Quantico, Va.: Federal Bureau of Investigation, 1991).

11. See S.D. Codified Laws Ann. §§ 23–5–14, et seq. (1990).

12. U.S. Department of Justice, Bureau of Justice Statistics, *Recidivism of Prisoners Released in 1983* (Washington, D.C.: Government Printing Office, 1989).

13. Ibid.

14. See, e.g., Gilbert v. Peters, 55 F.3d 237 (7th Cir. 1995) (ex-post facto challenge); Jones v. Murray, 962 F.2d 302 (4th Cir. 1992) (Fourth Amendment), *cert. denied,* 506 U.S. 977 (1992); Rise v. Oregon, 59 F.3d 1556 (9th Cir. 1995) (Fourth Amendment); Ryncarz v. Eikenberry, 824 F. Supp. 1493 (E.D. Wash. 1993)(Fourth Amendment); Sanders v. Coman, 864 F. Supp. 496 (E.D.N.C. 1994) (Fourth Amendment); People v. Calahan, 649 N.E.2d 588 (Ill. App. 1995) (state constitutional right to privacy); People v. Wealer, 636 N.E.2d 1129 (Ill. App. 1994) (search and seizure), *appeal denied,* 642 N.E.2d 1299 (Ill. 1994); and State ex rel. Juvenile Dep't v. Orozco, 878 P.2d 432 (Or. App. 1994) (Fourth Amendment).

15. Jones v. Murray, 962 F.2d 302 (4th Cir.), *cert. denied,* 506 U.S. 977 (1992).

16. Ewell v. Murray, 11 F.3d 482 (4th Cir. 1993), *cert. denied,* 511 U.S. 1111 (1994); Gilbert v. Peters, 55 F.3d 237 (7th Cir. 1995); Jones v. Murray, 962 F.2d 302 (4th Cir. 1992), cert. denied, 506 U.S. 977 (1992); Rise v. Oregon, 59 F.3d 1556 (9th Cir. 1995); Sanders v. Coman, 864 F. Supp. 496 (E.D.N.C. 1994); Vanderlinden v. Kansas, 874 F. Supp. 1210 (D. Kan. 1995); Doe v. Gainer, 642 N.E.2d 114 (Ill. 1994), *cert. denied,* 115 S. Ct. 1139 (1995).

17. Matter of Welfare of ZPB, 474 N.W.2d 651 (Minn. Ct. App. 1991).

18. Matter of Appeal in Maricopa County, 901 P.2d 1205 (Ariz. Ct. App. 1995).

19. See, e.g., Rise v. Oregon, 59 F.3d 1556, 1564 (9th Cir. 1995) (dissenting opinion); Jones v. Murray, 962 F.2d 302 (4th Cir. 1992) (dissenting opinion), *cert. denied,* 506 U.S. 977 (1992); and Washington v. Olivas, 856 P.2d 1076 (Wash. 1993) (concurring opinion).

20. National Academy of Sciences, *DNA Technology in Forensic Science.*

21. Philip L. Bereano, "DNA Identification Systems: Social Policy and Civil Liberties Concerns," *International Journal of Bioethics* 1 (1990): 146–55; E. Donald Shapiro and Michelle L. Weinberg, "DNA Data Banking: The Dangerous Erosion of Privacy," *Cleveland State Law Review* 38 (1990): 455–86.

22. Criminal Justice and Public Order Act of 1994, Part IV, § 55 (amending Police and Criminal Evidence Act of 1984, § 63).

23. Philip L. Bereano, "The Impact of DNA-Based Identification Systems on Civil Liberties," in Paul R. Billings, ed., *DNA on Trial: Genetic Identification and Criminal Justice* (Plainview, N.Y.: Cold Spring Harbor Laboratory Press, 1992), 119–28; Shapiro and Weinberg, "DNA Data Banking."

24. Shapiro and Weinberg, "DNA Data Banking."

25. Andrea DeGorgey, "The Advent of DNA Databanks: Implications for Information Privacy," *American Journal of Law and Medicine* 16 (1990): 381–98.

26. National Academy of Sciences, *DNA Technology in Forensic Science.*

27. McEwen and Reilly, "Review of State Legislation."

28. Jean E. McEwen, "Forensic DNA Data Banking by State Crime Laboratories," *American Journal of Human Genetics* 56 (1995): 1487–92.

29. National Academy of Sciences, *DNA Technology in Forensic Science.*

30. McEwen, "Forensic DNA Data Banking."

31. American Society of Human Genetics (ASHG), Ad Hoc Committee on Individual Identification by DNA Analysis, "Individual Identification by DNA Analysis: Points to Consider," *American Journal of Human Genetics* 46 (1990): 631–34; Philip R. Reilly, "Reflections on the Use of DNA Forensic Science and Privacy Issues," in Ballantyne, Sensabaugh, and Witkowski, eds., *DNA Technology and Forensic Science,* 43–54.

32. DeGorgey, "Advent of DNA Databanks"; Shapiro and Weinberg, "DNA Data Banking."

33. Barry Scheck, "DNA Data Banking: A Cautionary Tale," *American Journal of Human Genetics* 54 (1994): 931–33; Nachama L. Wikler et al., "DNA Data Banking and the Public Interest," in Ballantyne, Sensabaugh, and Witkowski, eds., *DNA Technology and Forensic Science,* 141–49.

34. See Ala. Code §§ 36–18–31(b)(3) (1994).

35. National Academy of Sciences, *DNA Technology in Forensic Science.*

36. McEwen, "Forensic DNA Data Banking."

37. Ibid.

38. Technical Working Group on DNA Analysis Methods (TWGDAM), "The Combined DNA Index System (CODIS): A Theoretical Model," in Lorne T. Kirby, ed., *DNA Fingerprinting: An Introduction* (New York: Stockton Press, 1989), 279–317.

39. DNA Identification Act of 1994.

40. Ibid.

41. Ibid.

42. McEwen and Reilly, "Review of State Legislation."

43. National Academy of Sciences, *DNA Technology in Forensic Science.*

44. Assistant Secretary of Defense (Health Affairs) Memorandum and Policy Statement, "Establishment of a Repository of Specimen Samples to Aid in Remains Identification Using Genetic Deoxyribonucleic Acid (DNA) Analysis," Jan. 5, 1993.

45. Rick Atkinson, "DNA Samples Catch American Killer of Toddler in Germany," *Washington Post,* Jan. 1, 1995, A27.

46. Assistant Secretary of Defense (Health Affairs) Memorandum and Policy Statement, "Establishment of Repository of Specimen Samples."

47. Mayfield v. Dalton, 901 F. Supp. 300 (D. Haw. 1995).

48. Assistant Secretary of Defense (Health Affairs) Memorandum and Policy Statement, "Establishment of Repository of Specimen Samples."

49. Philip R. Reilly, "DNA Banking," *American Journal of Human Genetics* 51 (1992): 1169–70.

50. Jean E. McEwen and Philip R. Reilly, "A Survey of DNA Diagnostic Laboratories Regarding DNA Banking," *American Journal of Human Genetics* 56 (1995): 1477–86.

51. Ibid.

52. Lori B. Andrews, "DNA Testing, Banking and Individual Rights," in Bartha M. Knoppers and Claude M. Laberge, eds., *Genetic Screening: From Newborns to DNA Typing* (Amsterdam: Excerpt Medica, 1990), 217–42.

53. Ellen Wright Clayton et al., "Informed Consent for Genetic Research on Stored Tissue Samples," *Journal of the American Medical Association* 274 (1995): 1786.

54. George J. Annas, "Privacy Rules for DNA Databanks: Protecting Coded 'Future Diaries,'" *Journal of the American Medical Association* 270 (1993): 2346–50.

55. R. L. Gold et al., "Model Consent Forms for DNA Linkage Analysis and Storage," *American Journal of Medical Genetics* 47 (1993): 1223–24; Bartha M. Knoppers and Claude Laberge, "DNA Sampling and Informed Consent," *Canadian Medical Association Journal* 140 (1989): 1023–28.

56. McEwen and Reilly, "Survey of DNA Diagnostic Laboratories."

57. Annas, "Privacy Rules for DNA Databanks."

58. American Society of Human Genetics (ASHG), Ad Hoc Committee on DNA Technology, "DNA Banking and DNA Analysis: Points to Consider," *American Journal of Human Genetics* 42 (1988): 781–83; American College of Medical Genetics (ACMG), Storage of Genetic Materials Committee, "Statement on Storage and Use Of Genetic Materials," ibid. 57 (1995): 1499–1500.

59. Annas, "Privacy Rules for DNA Databanks."

60. Peter S. Harper, "Research Samples from Families with Genetic Diseases: A Proposed Code of Conduct," *British Medical Journal* 306 (1993): 1391–94.

61. Ibid.

62. Ibid.

63. Moore v. Regents of Univ. of Cal., 793 P.2d 479 (Cal. 1989), *cert. denied*, 499 U.S. 936 (1991).

64. Ibid.

65. McEwen and Reilly, "Survey of DNA Diagnostic Laboratories."

66. Andrews, "DNA Testing, Banking and Individual Rights."

67. John R. W. Yates, Sue Malcolm, and Andrew P. Read, "Guidelines for DNA Banking," *Journal of Medical Genetics* 26 (1989): 245–50.

68. Clayton et al., "Informed Consent for Genetic Research."

69. Jean E. McEwen and Philip R. Reilly, "Stored Guthrie Cards as DNA 'Banks.'" *American Journal of Human Genetics* 55 (1994): 196–200.

70. Ibid.

71. See Marc Rotenberg, "Institute of Medicine; Health Data in the Information Age: Use, Disclosure, and Privacy," *Journal of Health Politics, Policy and Law* 20 (1995): 235 (book review); Harriet S. Meyer, "Protecting Privacy in Computerized Medical Information," *Journal of the American Medical Association* 271 (1994): 1549 (book review).

Part Four **Nonmedical Uses of**

Genetic Information

Chapter 14 Gen-Etiquette: Genetic Information, Family Relationships, and Adoption

Lori B. Andrews

Genetic information shares many features with other types of medical information, but it has several characteristics that raise heightened concerns about its protection. First, genetic information often affects central aspects of our lives. Because genes are usually viewed as immutable and central to the determination of who a person is, information about genetic mutations may cause a person to change his or her self-image and may alter the way others treat that person. Second, there is a chance that people will get genetic information without sufficient advance consideration of its potential effects. In most instances, people seek medical services because they are already ill. But with predictive genetic testing, there may be an incentive for biomedical companies and physicians to aggressively market such tests and asymptomatic people may not consider the psychological, social, and financial impact of learning genetic information about themselves before they agree to genetic testing. In addition, because most genetic treatment and prevention strategies for asymptomatic individuals have not yet been proven, positive results on a genetic test may lead to interventions that are costly, ineffective, or even harmful.

Genetic information has another unique feature. Information about a particular individual also reveals genetic risk information about his or her relatives. A parent and a child have half their genes in common, as do siblings. Cousins share one-quarter of their genes, as do grandparents and grandchildren. Family bonds raise new and profound questions of gen-etiquette, questions of the moral obligations to relatives that may be raised by the acquisition and disclosure of genetic information.

Genetic technologies place new stresses on family relationships. Some forms of genetic testing require linkage studies in which all blood relatives must provide tissue samples to determine whether a mutant gene (such as a form of one of the breast cancer genes) runs in the family. Only by learning about that family's form of the mutation can a diagnosis in an individual be made. With breast cancer, for example, one of the two genes thus far identified can be defective in hundreds of ways, and clinicians must narrow down the particular defects for which to test.

Even short of situations in which a family member might be asked to undergo genetic testing, questions arise as to whether and when relatives have a duty to share genetic information. If a woman learns that she has a mutation of a breast cancer gene, does she have a responsibility to tell her sister that she, too, might be at risk? If she decides not to disclose, may her physician breach confidentiality and warn her sister?

The web of relationships around genetic information runs in many directions. Children may want genetic information about their parents in order to be able to make reproductive plans. Parents may want genetic information about their young children to make medical and financial decisions about their children's futures. In every instance, the acquisition of genetic information has familial and social implications. A child may be denied health insurance later in life due to a genetic test on the child requested by the parents. A woman at risk for Huntington disease (HD) who has refused testing may learn that she has the HD gene when her adult son chooses testing and finds out he has the gene mutation.

Biological bonds are given great weight in our society and can serve as the basis for the assignment of rights and responsibilities. This chapter analyzes the precedents for finding moral and legal responsibilities within families based on genetic information. It assesses the rights and responsibilities of parents, children, and other relatives. It analyzes whether an obligation exists to undergo genetic testing to benefit a relative and whether an obligation exists to share genetic information with a relative. Last, it addresses whether physicians may breach confidentiality to warn a relative about genetic risks.

THE ANTHROPOLOGICAL AND PHILOSOPHICAL CONTEXT

The family, as Charles Fried describes it, is a "complex moral object at the intersection of a number of negative rights (personal, political, and legal), a number of primary and secondary positive rights, and a congruence of simply adventitious circumstances."[1] The adage "You can choose your friends, but you can't choose your relatives" is not quite true. Anthropological kinship studies indicate that, although blood ties may identify who one's relatives are, individual social decisions allow one to choose which relatives are considered "family." In most industrialized countries, people readily acknowledge the biological links between parents and children, as well as among more distant relatives. Yet, write Marilyn Strathern and Sarah Franklin, "What people do with these natural facts in terms of kin obligation, family formation, and so forth, is held to be a matter of *social* (pertaining to relationships) or *cultural* (pertaining to ideas and values) fact." Strathern and Franklin note that "the definition and recognition of kin is *selective*" and that in northern Europe, the nuclear family, rather than the extended family, "is more often encountered as the dominant kinship ethos."[2] In a study focusing on cystic fibrosis, Joanna Fanos detected a similar trend in the United States. Fanos found that families of patients with cystic fibrosis viewed information about genetic disorders as relevant to the nuclear family rather than to the extended family.[3]

As with the anthropological literature, philosophical writing about duties within families does not support the imposition of a broad set of duties merely because of biological connectedness. Rather, familial duties focus primarily on rights and responsibilities between parents and children.

Many philosophers have measured parents' duties by assessing children's needs.[4] Some have suggested that people should not bring a child into the world unless they are willing to meet the child's needs. Onora O'Neill has even argued that people have no independent right to procreate, if that is understood as an unrestricted right to beget and bear children whenever one desires. As O'Neill sees it, the right to procreate is contingent on having or making some feasible plan for rearing children adequately, either by the begetters and bearers themselves or by willing others.[5]

Similarly, Charles Fried has recognized that children have positive rights to what they need to develop into moral persons and that parents have a corresponding duty to meet these needs.[6] This emphasis on parents' duties to meet children's needs is echoed in legal requirements. Parents have a duty to support children and to provide them with certain necessities of life, including medical care. In the realm of genetics, the philosophical literature and legal precedents would argue in favor of parents sharing their genetic information with their children to the extent that it is needed to meet their children's health requirements.[7]

The philosophical literature does not provide guidance about an individual's duty to other relatives, however. It could be argued that there is no duty to other relatives as relatives;[8] that is certainly the standpoint of the legal precedents. Laws that require children to support their parents, people to support their cousins or great aunts, and so forth are rarely encountered. As a result, it could be argued that responsibilities assigned in the family sphere are designated on the basis of assumed obligations. Parents must provide support and appropriate care for their child because, if they did not, they would be seen to have caused the child's harm, since they brought him or her into the world.[9] Under such an analysis, a parent would have a duty to share genetic information with children but not with other relatives since they have not assumed responsibility for the other relatives.

PARENTS' RESPONSIBILITIES TOWARD CHILDREN

Parents have a clear moral responsibility to provide their children with the necessities of life. Statutes also mandate legal responsibilities, requiring parents to provide their children with appropriate food, clothing, shelter, and medical care. These precedents, however, would probably not be interpreted to substantiate a *legal* requirement that parents undergo genetic testing (for example, as part of a family linkage study) for the benefit of their children.

The strong protection that the law accords bodily integrity allows a parent to refuse medical interventions, even when such interventions would benefit that person's child. Recent cases have held that a pregnant woman can refuse a cesarean section even when such a refusal might cause significant morbidity or mortality to the fetus.[10] In situations when the medical intervention proposed for the parent is less intrusive, courts still may not be willing to order interventions over parents' refusals. This seems appropriate in the case of genetic testing. Forcing parents to undergo genetic testing for the benefit of their children is inappropriate. A variety of advisory and regulatory bodies have recognized that a genetic test is not a simple blood test. For example, the Office for the Protection from Research Risks of the Department of Health and Human Services warns of a variety of potential hazards from receiving genetic information, including psychological risks, changes in family relationships, and social risks of "stigmatization, discrimination, labeling and potential loss of or difficulty in obtaining employment or insurance."[11] The psychological, social, and financial ramifications of genetic information are sufficiently serious that parents should not be required to undergo genetic testing over their refusal and obtain genetic information they did not want.

A different situation exists when the parent has already undergone genetic testing or has otherwise obtained genetic information (for example, through a family history or through the manifestation of a genetic disease). There would be a moral obligation to share that information with one's child if the child would benefit from that disclosure. A legal obligation to share such information would arguably also exist.

In intact families, children obtain genetic information in the normal course of family affairs when their grandparents and parents become ill. When a child is separated from one or both biological parents (through adoption, egg donation, sperm donation, or embryo donation), however, courts and legislatures face questions about how much genetic information the child should receive about his or her parents.

An individual's genetic family history is increasingly being viewed as an important tool in medical diagnosis and treatment. The collection of genetic information is becoming easier, and technology has increased the number of genetic conditions identifiable through testing. These trends have led state legislatures over the past decade to pass statutes to require the collection of genetic information in the context of adoption, which can occur without revealing the identity of the adoptee's biological parents.

Thirty-six states require compilation of a medical history in the context of adoption,[12] 25 a genetic history or history of hereditary conditions,[13] and 21 a health history.[14] Of the 36 state statutes requiring compilation of medical history, 28 require information about both the adoptee and the biological parent(s),[15] six specify compilation of the biological parent(s) medical history,[16] one (Colorado) requires the adoptee's history, and one (Montana) does not specify whose information is compiled. Of the 25 statutes requiring compilation of a genetic history or history of hereditary diseases, 10 require the information about both the adoptee and the biological parent(s);[17] 13, about the biological parent(s);[18] and two are not specific.[19] And, of the 21 statutes requiring compilation of a health history, 12 require the information about the biological parent(s);[20] four, about both the adoptee and the biological parent(s);[21] three, about the adoptee,[22] and one (New Mexico) is not specific. Not only is this information compiled, but many states require its disclosure early on in the adoption process. Twenty-three states require disclosure by the state or county department of social services or licensed child placing agency or the court of the known medical history[23] of the adoptee and the biological parents to adoptive parents before or soon after finalization of the adoption.[24] Nine states have statutes which require disclosure of the biological parents' medical histories.[25] No current statutes require that biological parents actually undergo genetic testing. Instead, the statutes refer to collection of information that is "known," "available," or "reasonably known."[26]

These laws are in keeping with the recommendations of a number of professional organizations. The American Society of Human Genetics (ASHG) has taken the position that genetic history should be included in an adoptee's record, asserting that "every person should have the right to gain access to his or her medical record, including genetic data." The ASHG recommends that "when medically appropriate, genetic data may be shared among the adoptive parents, biological parents and adoptees."[27] The Child Welfare League of America similarly recommends disclosing known hereditary conditions of the biological parents and the child to the adoptive parents.[28]

Information collected at the time of the child's adoption may be limited in value. Parents who surrender children for adoption are often young, therefore there is only a limited amount of information known about the biological parents' own health; many diseases will not have manifested by that time. Requiring information about *other* family members, such as grandparents (as is done in 10 states),[29] will provide further clues, but the lack of a mechanism for updating the information will limit the potential benefits to the child of having genetic information. Currently, no state except Texas mandates updating health information. The Texas law states that "the department, authorized agency, parent, guardian, person, or entity who prepares and files the regional report is required to furnish supplemental medical, psychological, and psychiatric information to the adoptive parents should it become available, and to file such supplemental information where the original report is filed."[30] Although the statute imposes no penalties for failure to supplement the record, it places great emphasis on updating medical information. A Delaware statute, though it does not require affirmative steps to amass updated information, does require that "if the Family Court receives a report stating that a birth parent or the adoptee has a genetically transmitted disorder or family pattern of a disease, Family Court shall instruct the agency that was involved with the adoption . . . to conduct a diligent search for the adult adoptee, adoptive parents of a minor adoptee or birth parent(s) to inform them of the report."[31]

There is also a growing interest in genetic information in the context of such reproductive technologies as egg donation, sperm donation, and embryo donation. Several state statutes require the collection of genetic information about sperm donors[32] and, in one case, egg donors,[33] but the purpose of such information is generally not to inform the recipient or resulting child but rather to exclude as donors those men or women who have particular genetic mutations (such as Tay-Sachs carrier status). For similar reasons, Florida, Virginia, and New Hampshire have statutes requiring medical screening of surrogates.[34] Beyond the few statutes on point, a medical standard of care has been created by the practice of genetic screening of donors and the standards embodied in the American Fertility Society's Ethical Guidelines on the New Reproductive Technologies. The guidelines require the taking of a genetic history and the provision of certain genetic tests for the purpose of excluding potential sperm donors, egg donors, embryo donors, or surrogates who are thought to present high risks (for example, men or women with the Tay-Sachs disease allele). In addition, the guidelines provide that the genetic information collected without identifying information should be available on request to the infertile couple and the resulting child.[35] Generally, the statutes and recommendations regarding reproductive technologies contain no provision for updating the information. The only exception is with respect to surrogate motherhood, which, ironically, is handled by lawyers, not physicians. In that case, the lawyers require surrogate mothers to keep them informed of any medical changes and of any address changes for the next 18 years in case the child needs additional information.[36]

In states that do not provide adoptees or the children born of reproductive technologies with a statutory right to genetic information, and in all states in which the offspring later desires additional genetic information (such as when the individual reaches reproductive age and wants to know about genetic risks to select prenatal tests), questions arise regarding whether the individual can sue to obtain that information. When such additional information is sought, most states permit disclosure only if good cause is shown,[37] the court determines the information is necessary,[38] or the interested parties have mutually consented to such disclosure.[39] Under the "good cause" standard, adoptees have been able to get certain nonidentifying information (such as health history), but not identifying information.

In 18 states, artificial insemination laws, like adoption laws, permit access to records under the good cause standard or a similar proof of compelling reasons.[40] Thus, court cases from the adoption realm could be applied by analogy to children conceived through donated sperm. Children of artificial insemination, however, would receive information of a lesser scope. Because state agencies are not involved in artificial insemination, it may be difficult to determine where the record is, and because physicians attempt to protect the anonymity of donors, the record is unlikely to contain any identifying information that would allow the resulting child (or even the physician providing the insemination) to contact the donor for information.

Adoptees and the children born of reproductive technologies might ultimately wish to obtain the identities of their biological parents in order to ask them to provide genetic information or to participate in linkage analysis. The case law indicates that "good cause" is a stringent requirement to satisfy when the adoptee is attempting to obtain *identifying* information.

Mere curiosity is obviously not enough.[41] Some adoptees have tried to show that their need to know has had a disturbing effect on their lives that can be relieved only by receiving identifying information, but courts have not readily granted such requests. In one case, the court did not find an adoptee's need to know to be sufficiently strong because even though he argued that he had "a deep personal need to know the truth" and was distressed by not knowing, he had not received medical or psychological assistance nor had his distress adversely affected his professional life.[42]

Even when an adoptee shows good cause for contacting a biological parent, courts are reluctant to provide identifying information. In Application of George, the applicant, an adult adoptee, suffered from leukemia. He was in remission produced by drug therapy, but once the drug treatment ceased to be effective, the only other therapy to induce remission would have been a bone marrow transplant, a procedure that is most effective when the donor is a blood-related sibling. To try to locate his closest genetic match, he sought the identities of his biological parents. The trial court denied his request for disclosure of the biological parents' identities, and the court of appeals affirmed. The trial judge himself, however, contacted the biological mother and half-sister, who turned out not to be a match, and the biological father, who refused to be tested.[43]

Nor have adoptees been successful in trying to create constitutional claims to access to identifying genetic information. Courts have rejected the arguments that "refusing automatic access to birth records that nonadopted persons have, is abridging a constitutionally protected right to privacy and to receive important information,"[44] as well as their First Amendment right to receive information,[45] their right to equal protection under the law (which they argued would entitle them to the same information that nonadopted persons can receive about their natural parents),[46] and their fundamental liberty interest in learning the identity of their biological family.[47] Courts have found sealed record statutes and their attendant requirement of a showing of good cause before allowing access to the information in the adoption record to be constitutional. According to the Supreme Court of Illinois, in In re Roger B., there does not seem to be any "case holding that the right of an adoptee to determine his genealogical origin is explicitly or implicitly guaranteed by the Constitution,"[48] and even if such a right were to be recognized, it would be not absolute but subject to limitations based on a compelling state need.[49]

PARENTS' INFORMATION ABOUT CHILDREN

Although the moral right of children to useful information about their parents is fairly well established, the moral basis of parents' right to genetic information about their children is less clear. Under common law, parents have great discretion in making medical decisions on behalf of their minor children. When parents refuse to consent to treatment for their child, pursuant to their constitutional rights of privacy to make child-rearing decisions or to religious freedom, the courts must determine how much state law may legitimately limit parents' constitutional rights. That determination has straddled a delicate balance, with a strong presumption in favor of parental rights. The general rule has been to mandate treatment over parental objection only when the child's life is in imminent danger and if the treatment poses little risk of danger.[50] Where the minor does not have a life-threatening condition, courts may compel treatment if some permanent affliction will result.[51]

Parents might similarly be seen to have broad discretion in requesting diagnostic services for their children.[52] However, the genetic testing of children raises profound dilemmas that have led some commentators to recommend that parents' rights be circumscribed in some instances. A few years ago, a mother entered a Huntington disease testing facility with her two young sons. "I'd like you to test my sons for the HD gene," she said. "I only have enough money to send one to college." That request and similar ones to test young girls for the breast cancer gene or other young children for carrier status for recessive genetic disorders raise enormous questions about whether parents' genetic knowledge about a child will cause them to treat him or her differently. A variety of studies have indicated risks to giving parents such information.

The possibility that genetic testing of children can lead to a dangerous self-fulfilling prophecy led to the demise of one study involving testing children. Harvard researchers proposed to test children to see if they had the XYY chromosomal complement, which had been linked (by flimsy evidence) to criminality. They proposed to study the children for decades to see if those with that genetic makeup were more likely to engage in a crime than those without it. They intended to tell the mothers which children had XYY. Imagine the effect of that information—on the mother, and on the child. Each time the child took his little brother's toy or lashed out in anger at a playmate, the mother might freeze in horror as the idea that her child's genetic predisposition was surfacing. She might intervene when other mothers would normally not and thus distort the rearing of her child.

Dorothy Wertz, Joanna Fanos, and Philip Reilly have noted that there is no widely accepted standard among physicians for making decisions about genetic testing of children.[53] Even though the International Huntington Association and the World Federation of Neurology have issued guidelines recommending that minors not be tested for HD, 53% of British pediatricians say they would test for the disorder upon parental request.[54] The literature on the subject is also divided. Some commentators suggest that parents should be able to obtain genetic information about children even if there is no potential medical benefit.[55] Others would restrict or prohibit such testing unless there is a medical benefit.[56]

Test results, once obtained, follow the child throughout life. "'Planning for the future,' perhaps the most frequently given reason for testing, may become 'restricting the future' (and also the present) by shifting family resources away from a child with a positive diagnosis," write Wertz, Fanos, and Reilly. Such a child, they continue, "can grow up in a world of limited horizons and may be psychologically harmed even if treatment is subsequently found for the disorder."[57] A joint statement by the American Society of Human Genetics and the American College of Medical Genetics notes, "Presymptomatic diagnosis may preclude insurance coverage or may thwart long-term goals such as advanced education or home ownership."[58]

Because of this potential for psychological and financial harm, a growing number of commentators and advisory bodies are recommending that genetic testing not be undertaken on minor children unless there is an immediate medical benefit. For example, the Institute of Medicine Committee on Assessing Genetic Risks recommended that "in the clinical setting, children generally be tested only for disorders for which a curative or preventive treatment exists and should be instituted at that early stage. Childhood screening is not appropriate for carrier status, untreatable childhood diseases, and late-onset diseases that cannot be prevented or forestalled by early treatment."[59]

SHARING GENETIC INFORMATION WITH OTHER RELATIVES

Genetic information affects people's relationships with siblings, cousins, and other relatives. In one case, identical twin brothers, both air traffic controllers, have a parent with Huntington disease and thus each are at 50% risk of getting the gene and, hence, the disease. The first twin wants to learn if he has the gene. His brother does not. But even if the first brother vows he will keep his test results secret (since if he has the gene, his twin does as well), will he actually be able to? If he doesn't have the gene, won't he want to tell his brother the joyous news? And if he doesn't relay good news to his sibling, won't his brother then know that they both have inherited the gene? If the first brother's medical record indicates that he has the HD gene, the second, untested brother could be denied health and life insurance based on those results—and both may lose their jobs as air traffic controllers.

The fact that we are inextricably bound to our kin by shared genes reaches far beyond the case of identical twins since we share genes with a variety of close and distant relatives. Consequently, questions arise regarding whether there are moral or legal obligations to share genetic information with, for example, siblings or cousins (and whether physicians may breach a patient's confidentiality and disclose information to these third parties). In some instances, such disclosure may help the relative avoid harm. If a person has the genetic condition of malignant hyperthermia (fatal if the individual is exposed to certain anesthetics), a sibling may also have the condition and will need to avoid those anesthetics. In other cases, however, the benefit of the genetic information is less clear. If a woman has the gene for breast cancer, her sister may or may not want to know that she, too, is at risk. Thus far, there have been no randomized clinical trials indicating that either greater monitoring of women with the mutation or prophylactic mastectomy improves the quality of life, psychological well-being, or medical outcome of the women who have a mutation in the breast cancer gene. And although arguably some individuals at risk for Huntington disease may wish to change their financial planning as a result of that information, other people may not wish to know that they have a 50% risk of having an untreatable disease.

An analysis of the philosophical literature indicates that responsibilities to other relatives are not owed on the basis of a biological bond per se. But if that is the case, what other grounds might be a basis for a duty to warn relatives? The law provides little basis for such a duty. In fact, geneticists may be surprised at how little regard the law has for the plight of a third party absent a contractual duty or an action on the part of the person that actually causes harm to the third party. It is a well-known legal adage that there is no "duty to rescue."[60] A person who walks past someone else's child drowning in a wading pool has no legal responsibility to save that child, even if it could easily be accomplished without risk to the rescuer. The only exception would be if the person's actions put the child at risk in the first place. Because genetic disease is not contagious, an individual with a genetic mutation would appear to be under no legal obligation to warn relatives. The patient is not *causing* a potential risk to the relatives. The relatives either have or do not have the gene, no matter what the patient does.

HEALTH CARE PROVIDERS' RIGHTS AND DUTIES WITH RESPECT TO RELATIVES

The fact that patients may not be required to disclose genetic information to their relatives does not set well with some health care providers, who would like to see the relatives tested to see if they, too, share the genetic mutations. Various arguments could be used to support a wide array of differing approaches to health care providers' disclosure to relatives—from a position of never disclosing to one of always disclosing. Some commentators would find a duty to warn relatives.[61] For example, some geneticists speak of "the family" as the patient rather than the individual. Dorothy Wertz and John Fletcher suggest that it is "vital to recognize that hereditary information is a family possession rather than simply a personal one." Other commentators question, "Why should a mere biological link justify an encroachment on an individual's sphere, in which most relatives are not socially or psychologically involved . . . ?"[62]

Among health care providers, there is equal representation of both viewpoints—the desire to disclose and the desire to protect confidentiality. In response to a survey by Wertz and Fletcher, 58% of geneticists said they would disclose the risk of hemophilia A to a relative without the patient's permission, and 60% said they would disclose the risk of Huntington disease.[63] These results not only reveal the split in opinion about disclosure (with about half of geneticists favoring it) but also indicate that the decision to disclose does not depend on whether the disorder at issue is treatable. A definitive standard of care among health care providers appears to be lacking on this issue.

In legal cases dealing with confidentiality of medical information, if a physician does not have a relationship with the relative (or other third party), the physician may breach a patient's confidentiality only if the patient, by his or her action, will potentially present a risk of serious, imminent harm to the relative or other third party.[64] A duty to breach confidentiality has been found in psychiatric cases in which the patient disclosed to a mental health professional that he or she was going to commit violence against an identifiable individual.[65] Not every potential risk triggers a duty to disclose, just those that present serious, imminent harm.[66] Courts have also ruled that physicians are privileged to breach a patient's confidentiality, if they wish, to warn family members or other individuals who are likely to be exposed to a patient's serious infectious disease.[67] In a few cases, the courts have gone further and actually found that the physician had a duty to warn and that the relatives or other third parties could sue physicians for not warning them.[68] In some instances, the court indicated that the duty could be met, not by actually warning the relative or third party, but by warning the patient of the risks to the relative or other third party.[69]

Few cases deal directly with the issue of whether health care providers have a duty to breach confidentiality and warn relatives of a genetic risk. In a Florida case of 1995, Pate v. Threkel, a daughter whose mother was diagnosed as having a genetic disease, medullary thyroid cancer, sued the mother's physician for not warning her that she, too, might be at risk. The court held that even if the prevailing standard of care required disclosure of the genetic nature of a condition, the physician had no duty to warn the daughter, but should have told the mother that the condition was genetic. The court held that a state law protected patients' confidentiality, that patients could be expected to pass on the warning, and that "requir[ing] the physician to seek out and warn various members of the patient's family would often be difficult or impractical and would place to heavy a burden upon the physician."[70]

A 1996 New Jersey case, Safer v. Estate of Pack, took a different approach, however. In that case, a doctor had treated a man for retroperitoneal cancer, ulcerative adenocarcinoma of the colon, and adenomatous polyps. Twenty-six years after the man died, his daughter learned she had cancer of the colon and multiple polyposis. She sued, claiming that her father's doctor had breached a duty to warn of the hereditary risk to her health and thus deprived her of the chance for monitoring, early detection, and early treatment. The trial court judge dismissed the case because there was no physician-patient relationship between the doctor and the daughter and because genetic disease was distinguishable from infectious disease since " 'the harm is already present within the non-patient child as opposed to being introduced, by a patient who was not warned to stay away.' "[71]

The appellate court, however, eschewed the need for a doctor-patient relationship. Because of the procedural posture of the case on appeal, the court was required to accept as true the daughter's expert's assertions that it was the prevailing standard of care at the time of the father's treatment to "warn of the known genetic threat."[72] The appellate court pointed out that genetic risks are as foreseeable as infectious ones and "the individual or group at risk is easily identified, and substantial future harm is easily identified or minimized by a timely and effective warning."[73] Applying an infectious disease precedent, the court held that there can be a duty to warn relatives and remanded the case for a determination of whether that duty was breached in this case. The court noted that the trial court would need to take a number of things into account, such as the extent of the daughter's risk, what the costs of monitoring would have been as compared to the expenses associated with the breach of duty, and whether— if the father had instructed the doctor *not* to disclose to his daughter—that request should have been honored.

The case of genetic disease, however, differs from that of violence and infectious disease. Those cases have already established social policies aimed at preventing violence or the spread of infectious diseases. There are criminal laws against violence and public health laws about reporting infectious diseases and preventing their spread. Breach of confidentiality thus furthers an established social policy. In contrast, society's position on genetic disease is less clear-cut. For example, no laws have been adopted to prevent the birth of children with genetic disorders.

The cases involving infectious disease and violence could be interpreted as offering no precedent for a privilege or duty for health care providers to breach confidentiality to warn relatives of a genetic risk. As the trial court in Safer noted, in the context of genetics, the patient is not *causing* the relative to have the gene at issue.[74] Warning siblings or cousins about genetic risks will not prevent them from having the gene (that has already been programmed in at birth), although it might prevent a particularly risky gene and environment interaction. Warning them about their genetic risk may prevent them from conceiving a child with the gene (but such a future risk is not the type of serious, imminent harm about which the cases have generally required disclosure).

A close analysis of case law precedents and other materials suggests that, if health care providers are found to have a privilege or duty to disclose to relatives, it should be in limited circumstances, in which there is a high probability of imminent, avoidable risk to a close family member, there are no alternative means of protecting the relative, and the benefits of disclosure outweigh the risks of disclosure to the patient, the relative, and society. Health care providers could make a strong argument that they have no duty to breach confidentiality and disclose genetic information.[75] The existing genetics precedents—Pate and Safer—were in unusual procedural postures on appeal, where the courts were forced to assume that the standard of care was to disclose genetic information, but it certainly could be asserted that the standard of care was to disclose the genetic nature of the condition to the patient but not to relatives.

Health care providers who feel strongly that a situation permits a breach of confidentiality should analyze a variety of factors. They should assess how likely it is the relative has the genetic mutation at issue. The cases themselves do not provide guidance for what degree of consanguinity creates sufficient risk to warrant disclosure. The anthropological literature provides an argument for limiting disclosure to the nuclear family (children, siblings) because this comports with people's intuitive notions about family and because first-degree relatives are most likely to have the same genes as the patient.

The health care provider should also assess the severity of the risk. The philosophical literature generally acknowledges that parents owe their children certain necessities. Similarly, the law requires that parents provide their children with certain essentials—food, clothing, shelter, medical care to prevent against serious harm. The lack of these items or services would certainly harm the children. Similarly, the cases of breach of confidentiality generally deal with serious, potentially life-threatening risks. Early in the twentieth century such a risk was presented by untreatable infectious diseases like scarlet fever, bubonic plague, and syphilis. More recently, the cases have dealt with such serious and potentially fatal diseases as tuberculosis, hepatitis, Rocky Mountain spotted fever, and AIDS.

The foregoing suggests that, in the context of genetics, disclosure over the patient's refusal should only be made in situations in which the potential harm at issue presents a serious threat to life or health.[76] This approach was taken by three national committees that addressed the issue of contacting relatives to warn of genetic risks. The National Research Council's Committee for the Study of Inborn Errors of Metabolism suggested that unauthorized disclosures be made only in cases of a life-threatening or massively disabling condition.[77] Similarly, the President's Commission on Ethical Issues in Medicine and Biomedical and Behavioral Research and the Institute of Medicine's Committee on Assessing Genetic Risks would allow disclosure only when the condition was serious; the Institute of Medicine committee used as examples conditions that are irreversible or fatal.

Cases of infectious disease deal with imminent risks—risks that have a high probability of occurring once contact between the patient and another individual is made. These precedents support warning a relative if possible harm was imminent, as in the case of the person about to undergo surgery who might have the gene for hyperthermia. It would caution against a breach of confidentiality to warn relatives of carrier status, even of a serious disorder, because the probability is low that they would have a child with another carrier and because such an occurrence would not be imminent.

If privacy of medical information were to be viewed as protected by the federal or state constitution, then the imminence requirement would be underscored. With respect to other constitutionally protected spheres (such as that of free speech), the right may not be infringed unless the harm is "extremely serious and the degree of imminence extremely high."[78]

The cases and statutes dealing with infectious diseases make clear that breach of confidentiality is a measure of last resort. It is thought more appropriate to use other measures to attempt to protect a third party, even if those measures might be more risky to the third party or more costly to society. This is evinced in several ways in the cases and statutes. Some cases talk of a duty to disclose risks to the patient as a means of protecting the third party. One such case, for example, found that a physician has a duty to describe safe sex practices to a patient with hepatitis (rather than a duty to warn a sex partner).[79] In addition, some statutes provide for universal precautions against infectious diseases such as AIDS or hepatitis, so protection would be possible without breaching confidentiality. For example, a majority of states have statutes covering those who respond to emergencies (e.g., emergency medical technicians, fire fighters, police officers), who may come in contact with people who have an infectious disease. In such a situation, a policy choice has been made to adopt universal precautions rather than to permit disclosure. When such precautions are in place, the emergency responder does not have a right to know the patient's infectious disease status. However, when universal precautions fail (such as when there is a needle prick or the responder performs cardiopulmonary resuscitation without a mask), the responder has a limited right to be notified of the person's infectious disease status.[80]

The cases highlight the requirement that the disclosed information be "necessary" to prevent harm. Disclosure would not be necessary if the information could be learned in some other way. Thus, if a gene is common to a particular ethnic or racial group and the existence of the gene is well publicized and people of that group are routinely offered testing, there is less need to breach a patient's confidentiality to warn of the risk. Such an approach is similar to that which has been taken in certain AIDS statutes under which physicians are privileged to report a patient's HIV status to a spouse.[81] The logic behind such reporting requirements seems to be that while a gay sexual partner might realize that he was in a high risk group, a wife may not realize that her husband was engaging in high-risk sex outside their marriage, and thus disclosure by the physician is likely to give her information she would not get in another way.

The health care provider should also have proof that the information would prevent or ameliorate the serious risk. In all of the infectious disease cases where disclosure was permitted or required, there was something that the relative or other third person could have done to prevent infection or to prevent the physical harm from occurring. These precedents suggest that, with respect to genetic diseases, there would not be a privilege or a duty to warn of an untreatable or unpreventable disorder. Thus, there would not be a duty to warn relatives that they were at risk of Huntington disease or that they might have a genetic or chromosomal abnormality that could lead them to bear a child with a mild disorder.

Because the purpose of disclosure would be to protect the relative from harm, the health care provider should also consider the potential harms of disclosure to the relative. If the relative is given new risk information, he or she would have to disclose that on insurance applications. He or she would also have to adjust psychologically to that information. The potential psychological harms might vary depending on whether there is a definitive test the individual could take to learn of the actual risk. For example, it could be problematic to inform someone that he or she is at risk for a particular type of cancer when there is no definitive test for that disease. Although the individual might undergo more frequent monitoring, he or she might not actually need it and might be subject to increased worry and unnecessary procedures without sufficient benefit.

The health care provider should also assess the likely effect of the disclosure on the patient whose confidentiality would otherwise be protected. In the cases dealing with infectious diseases, consideration is given to how the patient might be harmed by the breach of confidentiality. This is particularly true with respect to disorders associated with great stigma—such as AIDS[82] (or, perhaps, in the genetics context, certain psychiatric disorders). In some cases, the potential for stigma may be so great that disclosure is prohibited altogether.[83]

Even if a particular case seems to provide compelling reasons to breach confidentiality, the health care provider should consider the systemic effects of such a breach, particularly the effect of a breach in confidentiality on people's willingness to seek genetic testing. In the legal cases, privacy of medical information is protected so that people will seek medical diagnosis and treatment. The logic of this approach is that "a patient should be entitled to freely disclose his symptoms and condition to his doctor in order to receive proper treatment without fear that those facts may become public property. Only thus can the purpose of the relationship be fulfilled."[84]

Because the rationale for confidentiality is to prevent people from being deterred from using medical services, attention should be given to whether the possibility of informing relatives will deter people from undergoing genetic testing. In a cystic fibrosis carrier study directed by Wayne Grody at the University of California, Los Angeles, people making testing decisions were concerned about how third parties would react to the resulting genetic information. Eleven percent of the subjects experienced concern over what others would think if the test were positive, and 30% said they would refuse testing if they knew that the results would be available to insurers.

Similarly, consideration should also be given to the eugenic symbolism of breaching confidentiality to warn relatives. The National Research Council's Committee for the Study of Inborn Errors of Metabolism cautioned that allowing a breach of confidentiality to warn relatives without consent implies "a medical-social judgment that genetic 'normality' is a prime childbearing goal for society to follow."[85]

A breach of confidentiality does not occur in isolation. Its effects are felt in myriad ways. The patient may suffer stigmatization by family members, the relatives may obtain information that they did not want and that may cause them to suffer stigma or discrimination, and people's willingness to seek genetic testing may be diminished. Just as the adoption cases sometimes refuse to authorize breaches of confidentiality even when circumstances seem compelling (because of the other factors that outweigh the benefits of disclosure), it is likely that courts reviewing physicians' requests to breach confidentiality will also find that the overall context of family relationships and the provision of health care services weighs against a breach.

CONCLUSION

What are the responsibilities to share genetic information within families? Under current law, no one can be required to undergo genetic testing (for example, by being compelled to be involved in a family linkage study) for the benefit of another individual. With respect to the sharing of existing genetic information, parents would probably be found to have a legal duty to share medically relevant genetic information with their children. Parents should not be seen as having a legal right to order genetic testing of their children unless such testing is necessary for prevention or treatment during the child's minority. With respect to an individual's duties toward other relatives (such as siblings or cousins), there might be a moral duty to disclose medically relevant information, but there probably would not be a legal one. Similarly, a health care provider should not be allowed to disclose a person's genetic information to a relative unless, at a minimum, the patient will not disclose to the relative voluntarily, there is a high probability that the relative has the gene mutation, the mutation presents a serious and imminent health risk, disclosure would prevent or ameliorate that serious risk, and there are no alternative means of protecting the relative. Even when these stringent standards are met in an individual case, the overall effects of disclosure should be considered. Consideration should be given to the potential psychological, financial, and other harms of disclosure to the individual whose confidentiality would be breached and the relative to whom the information would be disclosed. Consideration should also be given to the effect of the breach on people's willingness to seek genetic testing and the potential eugenic symbolism of breaching confidentiality.

Claude Lévi-Strauss observed, "The rules of kinship and marriage are not made necessary by the social state. They are the social state itself."[86] Whether one agrees with the way Lévi-Strauss privileges kinship and marriage, society cannot be considered in isolation from how it defines family and the responsibilities it sets forth for family members. Through legal cases and professional guidelines regarding duties to disclose genetic information to family members, the institutions of law and medicine will be defining certain rights and responsibilities thought to be inherent in family relations. In doing so, attention must be paid to the social context. At a practical level, this requires a concern for the influence of the rule on whether people will be discouraged from seeking medical care. At a larger conceptual level, attention should be paid to how the rule will influence, distort, enliven, or otherwise challenge the conception of family within which people currently operate.

NOTES

Author's note: I thank Nanette Elster for her help in preparing this chapter.

1. Charles Fried, *Right and Wrong* (Cambridge: Harvard University Press, 1978), 151–52.
2. Marilyn Strathern and Sarah Franklin, "Kinship and the New Genetic Technologies: An Assessment of Existing Anthropological Research," in University of Manchester, Department of Social Anthropology, *A Report Compiled for the Commission of the European Communities Medical Research Division (DG-XII) Human Genome Analysis Program under Ethically Social and Legal Aspects of Human Genome Analysis,* no. PL 9101041 (Jan. 1, 1993), 1.3, 2.4.7, 2.4.4.
3. Joanna Fanos, "Response to NCHGR Questions."
4. Jean-Jacques Rousseau, for example, saw the natural bond between children and father as based on need and as lasting only as long as the need lasts. After the need ends, a family remains united only through the choice of its members; Rousseau, *The Social Contract,* trans. Maurice Cranston (New York: St. Martin's Press, 1968), 50–51.
5. Onora O'Neill, "Begetting, Bearing, and Rearing," in Onora O'Neill and William Rudick, eds., *Having Children: Philosophical and Legal Reflections on Parenthood* (New York: Oxford University Press, 1979), 25–38, 25–26.
6. Fried, *Right and Wrong,* 121, 131.
7. This might require new efforts to provide genetic information in the contexts of the practices of adoption, artificial insemination, egg donation, embryo donation, and surrogate motherhood. It has not been common for children in these situations to have access to the genetic information about the biological parents who are not rearing them. In recent years, however, there have been some attempts to provide such information; see, e.g., National Center for Maternal and Child Health, *Genetic Family History: An Aid to Better Health in Adoptive Children* (Rockville, Md.: Department of Health and Human Services, 1984). A Wisconsin pilot project trained adoption workers to take a genetic history of birth parents; Lori B. Andrews, *Medical Genetics: A Legal Frontier* (Chicago: American Bar Foundation, 1987), 201. The American Fertility Society's *Ethical Guidelines* suggest providing the children with nonidentifying genetic information; Ethics Committee of the American Fertility Society, "Ethical Considerations of the New Reproductive Technologies," *Fertility and Sterility* 46, supp. 1 (1986): 37S, 44S.
8. Although there might not be a duty to a family member just because of a biological bond, there might be a duty owed to a family member (just as to any other member of society) based on some other theory of obligation.
9. Adopting parents assume similar obligations by agreeing to step into the biological parents' shoes. This can be viewed as almost a contractual assumption of obligation.
10. In re A.C., 573 A.2d 1235 (D.C. App. 1990); Baby Boy Doe v. Doe, 632 N.E.2d 326 (Ill. App. 1994).

11. U.S. Department of Health and Human Services, Public Health Service, National Institutes of Health, Office of Extramural Research, Office for Protection from Research Risks, *Protecting Human Research Subjects: Institutional Review Board Guidebook* (Washington, D.C.: Government Printing Office, 1993), 5–45.

12. Ala. Code § 26.10A–31 (1993); Alaska Stat. § 18.50.510 (1993); Cal. Fam. Code § 8706 (West Supp. 1994); Colo. Rev. Stat. § 19–5–401 (1993); Fla. Stat. Ann. § 63.022 (1993); Haw. Code Ann. § 578–14.5 (1993); Idaho Code § 16.1506 (Michie Supp. 1994); Ill. Rev. Stat. Ann. ch. 50, para. 18.4a (1992); Ind. Code Ann. § 31-3-1–2 (West Supp. 1994); Iowa Code Ann. § 600.8 (West Supp. 1994); Kan. Stat. Ann. § 59–2130 (West Supp. 1993); La. Child. Code art. 1125 (1994); Me. Rev. Stat. Ann. tit. 22, § 4008 (West Supp. 1993); Md. Code Ann. § 5–328 (Michie Supp. 1993); Mass. Gen. Laws Ann. ch. 15A, § 5D (West 1994); Mich. Comp. Laws Ann. § 710.68 (West 1992); Miss. Code Ann. § 93–17–205 (1994); Mo. Ann. Stat. § 453.121 (Vernon's Supp. 1994); Mont. Code Ann. § 40–8-122 (1993); Neb. Rev. Stat. § 43–107 (1993); N.H. Rev. Stat. Ann. § 170-B:15 (1994); N.J. Stat. Ann. § 9:3–41.1 (Michie 1994); N.M. Stat. Ann. § 32A-5–40 (Michie 1994); N.Y. Dom. Rel. Law § 114 (McKinney's Supp. 1994), N.Y. Soc. Serv. Law § 373–a (1990); Ohio Rev. Code Ann. § 3107.12 (Baldwin Supp. 1994); Okla. Stat. Ann. tit 10, § 57 (West Supp. 1994); Or. Rev. Stat. § 109.342 (1993); Pa. Comp. Stat. Dom. Rel. ch. 25, § 2533 (1994); R.I. Gen. Laws § 15–7.2–1 (1993); S.C. Code Ann. § 20–7–1740 (1993); Tex. Code Ann. § 16.032 (West Supp. 1994); Utah Code Ann. § 78–30–16 (1994); Wash. Rev. Code Ann. § 26.33.350 (West Supp. 1994); W. Va. Code § 48–4–7 (1994); Wis. Stat. § 48.425 (1993); Wyo. Stat. § 1–22–116 (1994).

13. Ariz. Rev. Stat. Ann. § 8–129 (1993); Ark. Code Ann. § 9–9–505 (Michie 1993); Cal. Fam. Code § 8606 (Deering Supp. 1994); Colo. Rev. Stat. §§ 19–5–302 (West Supp. 1993); Ga. Code Ann. § 19–8–23 (Michie Supp. 1994); Haw. Rev. Stat. § 578–14.5 (Michie Supp. 1993); Idaho Code § 16–1506 (Michie Supp. 1994); Ill. Rev. Stat. ch. 50, para. 18.4a (1992); Iowa Code Ann. § 600.8 (West Supp. 1994); Kan. Stat. Ann. § 59–2130 (West Supp. 1993); La. Child. Code art. 1125 (1994); Me. Rev. Stat. Ann. tit. 22, § 4008 (West Supp. 1993); Minn. Stat. § 259.46 (West 1993); Miss. Code Ann. § 93–17–205 (1994); N.J. Stat. Ann. § 9:3–41.1 (Michie 1994); N.M. Stat. Ann. §§ 32A–5–3, 32A–5–14 (Michie 1994); N.Y. Dom. Rels. Law § 114 (McKinney Supp. 1994); N.Y. Soc. Serv. Law § 373–a (1992); Ohio Rev. Code Ann. § 3107.12 (Baldwin Supp. 1994); Or. Rev. Stat. § 109.342 (1993); R.I. Gen. Laws § 15–7.2–1 (Michie Supp. 1993); S.C. Code Ann. § 20–7–1740 (1993); Tex. Code Ann. Civ. Prac. & Rem. § 16.032 (West Supp. 1994); Utah Code Ann. § 78–30–16, 17 (Michie Supp. 1994); Wis. Stat. § 48.425 (1993); Wyo. Stat. § 1–22–116 (West Supp. 1994).

14. Ala. Code § 26–10A–31 (1993); Ariz. Rev. Stat. Ann. § 8–129 (Michie 1993); Ark. Code Ann. § 9–9–505 (Michie 1993); Conn. Gen. Stat. § 45a–746 (1992); Ga. Code Ann. § 19–8–23 (Michie Supp. 1994); Ky. Rev. Stat. Ann. § 199.520 (Baldwin 1993); Minn. Stat. § 257.01 (West 1993); N.H. Rev. Stat. Ann. §§ 32A–5–3, 32A–5–14 (West Supp. 1994); N.J. Rev. Stat. Ann. § 170–B:19 (1993); N.M. Stat. Ann. §§ 257.01 (Michie 1993); N.Y. Dom. Rel. Law § 114 (McKinney Supp. 1994); N.C. Gen. Stat. § 48–25 (1993); N.D. Cent. Code § 14–15–01 (Michie Supp. 1993); R.I. Gen. Law § 15–17.2–1 (Michie Supp. 1993); S.C. Code Ann. § 20–17–1780 (1993); S.D. Codified Laws Ann. § 25–6–15.2

(1992); Tenn. Code Ann. § 36–1–141 (1993); Tex. Code Ann. Civ. Prac. & Rem. § 16.032 (West Supp. 1994); Utah Code Ann. § 78–30–16 (Michie Supp. 1994); Vt. Stat. Ann. tit. 4, § 436 (1993); Wash. Rev. Code Ann. § 26.33.350 (West Supp. 1994).

15. Alabama, California, Florida, Hawaii, Illinois, Indiana, Iowa, Kansas, Maine, Massachusetts, Michigan, Mississippi, Nebraska, New Hampshire, New Jersey, New Mexico, New York, Oklahoma, Oregon, Pennsylvania, Rhode Island, South Carolina, Texas, Utah, Washington, West Virginia, Wisconsin, and Wyoming.

16. Alaska, Idaho, Louisiana, Maryland, Missouri, and Ohio.

17. California, Hawaii, Illinois, Kansas, Maine, Minnesota, Mississippi, Texas, Wisconsin, and Wyoming.

18. Arizona, Arkansas, Colorado, Georgia, Idaho, Louisiana, New Jersey, New York, Ohio, Oregon, Rhode Island, South Carolina, and Utah.

19. Iowa and New Mexico.

20. Arizona, Connecticut, Georgia, Kentucky, New Hampshire, New York, North Carolina, North Dakota, South Dakota, Tennessee, Vermont, and Washington.

21. Alabama, Minnesota, South Carolina, and Texas.

22. Arkansas, Rhode Island, and Utah.

23. As used here, this term includes all health and genetic information.

24. See Ala. Code § 26–10A–19 (1992); Ark. Code Ann. §§ 9–9–501, 9–9–505 (Michie 1993); Cal. Fam. Code § 8706 (West Supp. 1994); Fla. Stat. Ann. § 63.082 (1993); Ill. Rev. Stat. Ann. ch. 50, para. 18.4a (1992); Ind. Code Ann. § 31–3–7–2 (West Supp. 1994); Iowa Code Ann. § 600.8 (West Supp. 1994); Me. Rev. Stat. Ann. tit. 9–B, § 533 (West Supp. 1993); Mont. Code Ann. § 40–8–122 (1993); Neb. Rev. Stat. § 43–107, § 43–128 (1993); N.J. Stat. Ann. § 9:3–41.1 (West Supp. 1994); N.M. Stat. Ann. §§ 32A–5–3, 32A–5–14 (Michie Supp. 1994); N.Y. Dom. Rel. Law § 114 (McKinney's Supp. 1994), N.Y. Soc. Serv. Law § 373–G (McKinney's 1992); Ohio Rev. Code Ann. § 3107.12 (Baldwin 1994); Or. Rev. Stat. § 109.342 (1993); Pa. Comp. Stat. ch. 25, §§ 2102, 2909 (1994); Tex. Code Ann. § 16.032 (West Supp. 1994); Utah Code Ann. §§ 78–30–16, 78–30–17 (1994); Va. Code Ann. § 63.1–223 (Michie Supp. 1994); Wash. Rev. Code Ann. §§ 26.33.350, 26.33.380 (West Supp. 1994); W. Va. Code §§ 48–4–6, 48–4A–6 (1994); Wis. Stat. §§ 48.93, 48.425 (1993); Wyo. Stat. § 1–22–116 (1994).

25. Ariz. Rev. Stat. Ann. § 8–129 (1993); Conn. Gen. Stat. § 45a-746 (1992); Idaho Code § 16–1506 (Michie Supp. 1994); Ky. Rev. Stat. Ann. § 199.520 (Baldwin 1991); La. Ch. Code Arts. 1124, 1125, 1126 (1994); Mo. Ann. Stat. § 453.121 (Vernon's Supp. 1994); N.H. Rev. Stat. Ann. § 170–B:19 (1993); N.C. Gen Stat. § 48–25 (1993); N.D. Cent. Code §§ 14–15–01, 14–15–16 (1993).

26. See, e.g., Ariz. Rev. Stat. Ann. § 8–129 (1993) (reasonably available); Ark. Code Ann. § 9–9–501 (Michie 1993) (when obtainable); Cal. Fam. Code § 8706 (Deering Supp. 1994) (if available; . . . so far as ascertainable); Colo. Rev. Stat. § 19–5–207 (West Supp. 1993) (if obtainable); Conn. Gen. Stat. § 45a–746 (1992) (to the extent reasonably available); Fla. Stat. Ann. § 63.022 (1993) (furnished by birth parent when available); Haw. Code Ann. § 578–14.5 (1993) (if known); Idaho Code § 16–1506 (Michie Supp. 1994) (reasonably known or available); Ill. Rev. Stat. ch. 50, para. 18.4 § 50/18.4 (1992) (if known); Iowa Code Ann. § 600.08 (West Supp. 1994) (known); Kan. Stat. Ann. § 59–2130 (West

Supp. 1993) (if available); Ky. Rev. Stat. Ann. § 199.529 (Baldwin 1993) (if known); La. Child. Code art. 1125 (1994) (if known), 1126 (good faith effort to obtain); Me. Rev. Stat. Ann. tit. 22, § 4008 (West Supp. 1993); Md. Code Ann. Cts. & Jud. Proc. § 5–328 (Michie Supp. 1993) (whenever possible); Mich. Comp. Law Ann. § 710.27 (West 1992) (if obtainable); Mo. Ann. Stat. § 453.121 (Vernon's Supp. 1994) (if known); Neb. Rev. Stat. § 43–146.02 (1993) (available); N.H. Rev. Stat. Ann. § 170–B:15 (1993) (reasonably available); N.J. Stat. Ann. § 9:3–41.1 (West Supp. 1994) (available); N.M Stat. Ann. § 32A–5–14 (Michie 1994) (in as much detail as available); N.Y. Dom. Rel. Law 114 (Michie Supp. 1994) (available); N.C. Gen. Stat. § 48–25 (1993) (if known); Ohio Rev. Code § 3107 (Baldwin 1989) (to the extent possible); Okla. Stat. Ann. tit. 10, § 60.5A (West Supp. 1994) (as far as ascertainable); Or. Rev. Stat. § 109.342 (1993) ("When possible, the medical history shall include . . . "); S.C. Code Ann. § 20–17–1740 (1993) (known); S.D. Codified Laws Ann. § 25–6-15.2 (1992) (if known); Tenn. Code Ann. § 36–1–141 (1993) (available, "any known information"); Tex. Code Ann. Civ. Prac. & Rem. § 16.032 (West Supp. 1994) ("to the extent such information is available"); Utah Code Ann. § 78–30–16 (Michie Supp. 1994) (when obtainable); Va. Code Ann. § 63.1–223 (Michie Supp. 1994) (known); Wash. Rev. Code Ann. § 26.33.350 (West Supp. 1994) (if available); Wyo. Stat. § 1–22–116 (West Supp. 1994) (to the extent available). Several states do not qualify the information: Ala. Code § 26–10A–19 (1993); Ind. Code Ann. § 31–3–1–2 (Burns Supp. 1994); Kan. Stat. Ann. § 59–2130 (1993) (in a personal communication with the Kansas Department of Social and Rehabilitative Service, I learned that no request is made for the medical records of the birth parents); Md. Code Ann. Cts. & Jud. Proc. § 5–328 (Michie Supp. 1993); Vt. Stat. Ann. tit. 4, § 436 (West Supp. 1993); W. Va. Code § 48–4–7 (1994); Wis. Stat. § 48.425 (1993).
27. American Society of Human Genetics (ASHG), "American Society of Human Genetics Social Issues Committee Report on Genetics and Adoption: Points to Consider," *American Journal of Human Genetics* 48 (1991): 1009, 1009–10.
28. Child Welfare League of America, *Standards for Adoption Service,* (Washington, D.C.: Child Welfare League of America, 1988), § 4.13.
29. Ark. Code Ann. § 9–9–501(8) (Michie 1993); Conn. Gen. Stat. Ann. § 45a–746 (1992); Haw. Code Ann. § 578–14.5 (1993); Miss. Code Ann. § 93–17–205 (1994); Neb. Rev. Stat. § 43–107(2) (1993); Okla. Stat. Ann. tit. 10 § 60.5A(A)(3) (West Supp. 1994); R.I. Gen. Laws § 15–7.2–1(7) (Michie Supp. 1993); Tex. Fam. Code Ann. § 16.032(e) (West Supp. 1994); Utah Code Ann. § 78–30–16(1)(g) (1994); Wis. Stat. Ann. § 48.425(1) (am)(1) (1993).
30. Tex. Fam. Code Ann. § 16.032(1) (West Supp. 1994).
31. Del. Code Ann. tit. 13, § 924 (1994).
32. See, e.g., Ohio Rev. Code Ann. § 3111.35(2) (Baldwin 1987).
33. N.H. Rev. Stat. Ann. § 168–B:14 (1994).
34. Fla. Stat. Ann. § 742.15 (West Supp. 1995); Va. Code Ann. § 20–160 (1995); N.H. Rev. Stat. Ann. § 168–B:13 (1994).
35. Ethics Committee of the American Fertility Society, "Ethical Considerations of the New Reproductive Technologies," 835–45.
36. Lori B. Andrews, *New Conceptions: A Consumer's Guide to the Newest Infertility Treat-*

ments, Including In Vitro Fertilization, Artificial Insemination, and Surrogate Motherhood (New York: Ballantine Books, 1985), 216.

37. See, e.g., Ark. Code Ann. 9–9–217 (Michie Supp. 1993); and Wis. Stat. Ann. § 48.93 (1993).

38. See, e.g., Del. Code Ann. tit. 9, § 925 (West Supp. 1993); and Cal. Fam. Code § 92.03 (Deering Supp. 1994).

39. See, e.g., Ala. Code § 26–10A-31 (West Supp. 1993); and Wis. Stat. Ann. § 48.433 (1993).

40. Other states seem not to let the file be accessed by the resulting child. See, e.g., Idaho Code § 39–5403(2) (1993) (file with the state registrar of vital statistics after the child's birth, available only for research and statistical purposes by court order); and N.M. Stat. Ann. § 40–11–6(a) (Michie 1994) (file with the vital statistics bureau of the health services division of the health and environment department; "kept confidential in a sealed file").

41. See, e.g., In re Linda F.M., 418 N.E.2d 1302, 1304 (N.Y. 1981).

42. Bradey v. Children's Bureau, 274 S.E.2d 418, 420 (S.C. 1981).

43. 630 S.W.2d 614, 615 (Mo. App. 1982).

44. Mills v. Atlantic City Dep't of Vital Statistics, 372 A.2d 646, 650 (N.J. Super. 1977).

45. Ibid., 652.

46. Ibid.

47. ALMA Soc'y v. Mellon, 601 F.2d 1255, 1230 (2d Cir. 1979).

48. In re Roger B., 418 N.E.2d 751 (Ill. 1981).

49. See, e.g., Mills, 372 A.2d 646, 650–651.

50. In re Green, 292 A.2d 387, 392 (Pa. 1972). See, e.g., Rowine Hayes Brown and Richard B. Truitt, "The Right of Minors to Medical Treatment," *DePaul Law Review* 28(1979): 289, 292, 299; and Comment, "Who Speaks for the Child and What Are His Rights?" *Law and Human Behavior* 4 (1980): 217, 223.

51. Comment, "The Right to Refuse Medical Treatment: Under What Circumstances Does It Exist?" *Duquesne Law Review* 18 (1980): 607, 613, 614–15. See, e.g., Walter J. Wadlington, "Medical Decision Making for and by Children: Tensions Between Parent, State and Child," *University of Illinois Law Review* 1994 (1994): 311, 319.

52. But see Ellen Wright Clayton, "Removing the Shadow of the Law from the Debate About Genetic Testing of Children," *American Journal of Medical Genetics* 57 (1995): 630.

53. Dorothy C. Wertz, Joanna H. Fanos, and Philip R. Reilly, "Genetic Testing for Children and Adolescents: Who Decides?" *Journal of the American Medical Association* 272 (1994): 875.

54. Ibid., citing *The Genetic Testing of Children: Report of a Working Party of the Clinical Genetics Society,* Angus Clarke, chair (Edgbaston and Birmingham, U.K.: Clinical Genetics Society, Birmingham Maternity Hospital, 1993).

55. Mary Pelias, "Duty to Disclose in Medical Genetics: A Legal Perspective," *American Journal of Human Genetics* 39 (1991): 347, 347–54.

56. Peter S. Harper and Angus Clarke, "Should We Test Children for 'Adult' Genetic Diseases?" *Lancet* 335 (1990): 1205–6.

57. Wertz, Fanos, and Reilly, "Genetic Testing for Children and Adolescents," 878. Similarly, the statement continues, "Expectations of others for education, social relation-

ships and/or employment may be significantly altered when a child is found to carry a gene associated with a late-onset disease or susceptibility. Such individuals may not be encouraged to reach their full potential, or they may have difficulty obtaining education or employment if their risk for early death or disability is revealed."

58. ASHG and American College of Medical Genetics (ACMG), "Points to Consider: Ethical, Legal, and Psychosocial Implications of Genetic Testing in Children and Adolescents," *American Journal of Human Genetics* 57 (1995): 1233, 1236.

59. Lori B. Andrews et al., eds., *Assessing Genetic Risks: Implications for Health and Social Policy* (Washington, D.C.: National Academy Press, 1994), 276 (hereafter *Assessing Genetic Risks*).

60. The Restatement Second of Torts 2d (1965) § 314 states, "The fact that the actor realizes or should realize that action on his part is necessary for another's aid or protection does not of itself impose upon him a duty to take such action."

61. P. Michael Conneally, "The Genome Project and Confidentiality in the Clinical Setting," in Mark A. Rothstein, ed., *Legal and Ethical Issues Raised by the Human Genome Project* (Houston: Health Law and Policy Institute, 1991), 184.

62. J. K. M. Gevers, "Genetic Testing: The Legal Position of Relatives of Test Subjects," *Medical Law* 7 (1988): 161, 163.

63. See Dorothy C. Wertz and John C. Fletcher, *Ethics and Human Genetics: A Cross-Cultural Perspective* (Heidelberg: Springer-Verlag, 1989); and Wertz and Fletcher, "An International Survey of Attitudes of Medical Geneticists Toward Mass Screening and Access to Results," *Public Health Reports* 104 (1989): 35–44.

64. Before *Safer v. Estate of Pack,* 677 A.2d 1188 (N.J. Super. 1996), I had found only one case in which a duty to warn was found when the patient was not the potential agent of harm. In that case, when a patient was diagnosed as having Rocky Mountain spotted fever, the physician failed to warn his wife that she, too, might be at risk; Bradshaw v. Daniel, 854 S.W.2d 865 (Tenn. 1993). But an argument could be made that the physician had a special duty to the wife in that case because he was communicating directly with her.

65. See, e.g., Tarasoff v. Regents of Univ. of Cal., 551 P.2d 334 (Cal. 1976).

66. See, e.g., White v. United States, 780 F.2d 97 (D.C. Cir. 1987), where the fantasy of a patient, according to the physician, did not reflect a danger. The court found this assessment to be reasonable.

67. See, e.g., Simonsen v. Swenson, 177 N.W. 831 (Neb. 1920); and Berry v. Moench, 331 P.2d 814 (Utah 1958).

68. Such a duty was found in Skillings v. Allen, 173 N.W. 663 (Minn. 1919) (scarlet fever); and in Edwards v. Lamb, 45 A. 480 (N.H. 1899) (septic wound).

69. A duty to tell the patient about risks to relatives or third parties was found and liability imposed in DiMarco v. Lynch Homes-Chester County, 583 A.2d 422 (Pa. 1990).

70. 661 So.2d 278, 282 (Fla. 1995).

71. 677 A.2d 1188, 624 (N.J. Super. 1996).

72. Ibid., 625.

73. Ibid., 626.

74. In the infectious disease cases, if the third party would have gotten the disease anyway,

there was no duty to warn. See Britton v. Soltes, 563 N.E.2d 910 (Ill. App. 1990); Skillings v. Allen, 180 N.W. 916 (Minn. 1921).

75. See "The Duty to Disclose," in George J. Annas, Leonard Glantz, and Patricia A. Roche, *The Genetic Privacy Act* (Boston: Boston University School of Public Health, 1995), 76.

76. The rationale that confidentiality should be breached to prevent financial risks to the relative or to enhance the relative's financial planning would probably not hold sway. See Arato v. Avedon, 858 P.2d 598 (Cal. 1993)(physician had no duty to disclose information that could be relevant to the patient's nonmedical interests, such as his financial interests).

77. National Research Council, Committee for the Study of Human Errors of Metabolism, *Genetic Screening: Programs, Principles, and Research* (Washington, D.C.: National Academy of Sciences, 1975).

78. Bridges v. California, 314 U.S. 252, 263 (1941).

79. DiMarco v. Lynch Homes–Chester County, 583 A. 2d 422 (Pa. 1990).

80. Lisa J. Steele, "When Universal Precautions Fail: Communicable Disease Notification Laws for Emergency Responders," *Journal of Legal Medicine* 11 (1990): 451–480, 451. The particular diseases that merit notification are those (1) that are easily transmitted, (2) that pose serious harm, and (3) for which notification can lead to a medical benefit (459).

81. See, e.g., Ill. Rev. Stat. ch. 410, § 305/9 (West Supp. 1993) (a physician may disclose to a spouse if the physician has first attempted to persuade the patient to make such disclosure or has reason to believe after a reasonable time that the patient has not made such disclosure). In contrast, other states would provide a privilege to disclose to partners generally; Kan. Stat. Ann. § 65–6004(b) (Supp. 1993) (disclosure may be made to a spouse or partner).

82. Doe v. Borough of Barrington, 729 F. Supp. 376 (D.N.J. 1990). (The court found that "the sensitive nature of medical information about AIDS makes a compelling argument for keeping this information confidential. Society's moral judgments about the high-risk activities associated with the disease, including sexual relations and drug use, makes the information of the most personal kind. Also, the privacy interest in one's exposure to the AIDS virus is even greater than one's privacy interest in ordinary medical records because of the stigma that attaches with the disease.")

83. For example, confidentiality in the adoption setting was to protect against the stigma of illegitimacy; ALMA Soc'y v. Mellon, 601 F.2d 1225, 1235 (2d Cir. 1979). (The purpose of confidentiality "was to erase the stigma of illegitimacy from the adopted child's life.")

84. Hague v. Williams, 181 A.2d 345 (N.J. 1962).

85. National Research Council, Committee for the Study of Inborn Errors of Metabolism, *Genetic Screening.*

86. Claude Lévi-Strauss, *The Elementary Structures of Kinship,* rev. ed., ed. James Harle Bell, John Richard von Sturmer, and Rodney Needham (Boston: Beacon Press, 1969), 490.

Chapter 15 The Law of Medical and Genetic Privacy in the Workplace

Mark A. Rothstein

Recent concerns about medical privacy in the workplace are attributable to the exponential growth in and changing nature of the medical information in the possession of employers. They are also related to the growing importance attached to privacy by individuals and the justifiable concern that disclosure of sensitive medical information could lead to the loss of employment and insurance as well as to other harms.

The systematic collection of medical information about employees began only at the turn of the twentieth century. In 1909, for example, Sears, Roebuck and Company initiated a program of physical examinations of applicants and employees to discover and isolate individuals with tuberculosis.[1] It was also about this time (1910–30) that workers' compensation laws were enacted in most states, which required employers to obtain medical information about job-related injuries and later, as coverage was expanded, about job-related illnesses as well.

The use of medical screening by employers increased greatly after World War II as many companies realized that it was in their economic interest to employ workers who not only were in good health at the time they were hired but were also likely to remain in good health. Thus, medical screening became both diagnostic and predictive. In addition, medical examinations became increasingly detailed and sophisticated, and included blood tests, urine tests, X-rays, and other medical and laboratory procedures. By the early 1980s, nearly 90% of companies with more than 500 employees were performing preemployment medical examinations.[2]

The focus of medical screening also began to change in the 1980s. Many employers, facing double-digit annual percentage increases in their health insurance costs, increasingly turned to medical screening in an attempt to keep out of their workforces high-risk individuals (and their dependents) who were likely to incur substantial medical bills.[3] All these tests and reviews of medical records generated an ever-growing collection of medical information about individual applicants and employees.

Employers currently possess or have access to a wide range of detailed and sensitive medical information. The medical information comes from two main sources: information generated by the employer's medical staff, both salaried employees and independent contractors, and information generated in the clinical setting by the individual's own physicians and released to employers. This information is both job-related, pertaining to the individual's physical and mental ability to perform a job, and of a more general medical nature. Job-related information includes occupationally related preplacement medical examinations; periodic medical examinations (including those mandated under the federal Occupational Safety and Health Act of 1970);[4] medical surveillance of employees exposed to hazardous work environments; and substance abuse testing records, psychological testing records, and other records of examinations to determine medical fitness for duty. In the category of general medical data are records from the following sources: preplacement medical examinations to determine general health status (including clinical records released to the employer); voluntary medical health assessments and employee assistance programs; health benefits claims (including those of the employee's dependents) submitted under an employer-sponsored plan; other information related to employee benefits (including workers' compensation, sick leave, Family and Medical Leave Act applications, and requests for reasonable accommodation under the Americans with Disabilities Act of 1990 (ADA)); and the direct provision of health services by the employer, such as annual physical examinations.

Not only has the volume of employer-maintained employee medical information grown tremendously, but the information has become increasingly sensitive. It is not uncommon for medical records to contain information regarding substance abuse treatment, psychiatric conditions, HIV status, reproductive health matters (infertility treatment, abortion, sexual dysfunction), marital problems, and other extremely personal matters. Yet, in spite of this growth in workplace medical information, the law has been slow to recognize the important privacy interests at stake. For example, although the ADA provides that "medical records" must be kept confidential and stored separately, benefits records are not considered medical records and may be stored in personnel or other files that are more widely accessible.

HISTORY OF THE COMMON LAW OF WORKPLACE MEDICAL PRIVACY

The law's seeming indifference to employee medical privacy in the workplace is best understood by a brief review of the history of employment law as it developed in England and changed over time in the United States. In agrarian, patriarchal, feudal England, the master really was the king of his castle. He had plenary authority over not only family members but indentured servants, apprentices, and other workers as well. These individuals usually resided in the master's home or on the master's land, often for their entire lives. It is not surprising, therefore, that master-servant law originally was a part of domestic relations law.

Under the common law (the body of judge-made, case law developed over time), the master was responsible for providing food, shelter, medical care, and protection for all those who resided on his property, including servants. The master was legally responsible for the wrongful acts of all individuals under his authority, and to ensure proper behavior, he had the authority to discipline servants as well as family members. Only the most extreme cases of abuse of servants were legally redressed, primarily through the criminal law.

English traditions of master-servant relationships were brought to colonial America and became the basis for the American law. In the nineteenth century, however, the law took a peculiarly American twist. In a now-controversial treatise published in 1877, a legal scholar named Horace Gray Wood formulated the "employment at will" doctrine.[5] Contemporary scholars differ over whether Wood's rule accurately described the existing state of the law or whether he misinterpreted the cases and therefore created a new doctrine.[6] At any rate, the employment at will rule essentially provides that all employment contracts without a stated duration are deemed terminable at will by either party, without notice, and for any reason.

The employment at will doctrine soon swept the United States, and it remains the starting point for analyzing employer-employee relations. The doctrine was well suited to laissez-faire capitalism; entrepreneurs were free to make changes in their workforces quickly and without incurring liability. It also supported employer prerogatives to control the workplace and all who worked there, including regulation of the private lives of employees, if employers were so inclined. At least in theory, if employees considered their employers' inquiries to be too intrusive, they could always resign and seek employment elsewhere.

Before the turn of the century there were no laws regulating privacy in the workplace. Indeed, the legal theory of a general right of privacy was still being developed. In his treatise on torts of 1878, Thomas M. Cooley first expressed the right to privacy as including "the right to be let alone."[7] This became the basis for the often-cited law review article by Samuel Warren and Louis Brandeis in 1890, in which they argued for judicial recognition of a common law right to privacy.[8]

Even as the legal theory of a right to privacy was being developed in the early part of the twentieth century, many employers believed that they had a legitimate interest in learning the intimate details of their employees' personal lives. For example, in 1914, Henry Ford began offering his employees the unprecedented sum of five dollars per day. To ensure that only upstanding men received such a generous wage, Ford formed the "Sociological Department." This group was composed of investigators who visited the homes of Ford employees to determine, among other things, whether an employee gambled, used liquor to excess, had a dirty home, ate an unwholesome diet, or sent money to foreign relatives.[9] Ford's investigators illustrate the longstanding American tradition of employers inquiring into their employees' private affairs.

The increasing value that American society has attached to privacy and the law of privacy have both developed largely outside the workplace setting. The law evolved into two distinct doctrines. First is the federal constitutional right of privacy, which protects individuals from governmental intrusions into their private affairs. This constitutional right of privacy and related interests, such as liberty and autonomy, have been used to prohibit the government from interfering with personal medical decisions, such as providing and withholding medical treatment, procreation, contraception, and abortion.[10] Because constitutional rights generally protect against governmental and not private interference, the right to privacy in the workplace protects only governmental employees and private sector employees whose privacy interests are being invaded pursuant to a statute or other governmental regulation, such as in government-mandated drug testing.[11] A few state constitutions also contain privacy provisions that apply to private sector as well as government employees.

The second privacy doctrine to develop in this century was the recognition of a common law tort action for invasion of privacy. These actions may be based on a variety of factual situations and apply both to employment and other relations. As it has developed, the tort of invasion of privacy actually consists of four separate types of cases: public disclosure of private facts, intrusion upon seclusion, false light, and appropriation of name or likeness. The first two are particularly relevant to employment.

Public disclosure of private facts is the basis for most invasion of privacy actions arising out of employment. The *Restatement (Second) of Torts* describes the level of invasion of privacy necessary: "Every individual has some phases of his life and his activities and some facts about himself that he does not expose to the public eye. . . . Sexual relations, for example, are normally entirely private matters, as are family quarrels, many unpleasant or disgraceful or humiliating illnesses, most intimate personal letters, most details of a man's life in his home, and some of his past history that he would rather forget."[12] To establish a claim for invasion of privacy based on public disclosure of private facts, the plaintiff must show dissemination or "publication" of private matters in which the public has no legitimate concern so as to bring shame or humiliation to a person of ordinary sensibilities.

In workplace medical privacy cases in which the common law doctrine has been construed, the courts have been inconsistent and, in general, restrictive of employee rights. The publication requirement has been one of the major hurdles for plaintiffs. For example, it has been held that there was insufficient publication where an employee's shipmates were told that he had undergone treatment for alcoholism and where "a few" coworkers were told that the plaintiff was undergoing psychiatric treatment.[13] In contrast, the disclosure by an airline's medical examiner to a flight attendant's supervisor of information contained in a report by her gynecologist was held to be actionable.[14]

Another obstacle to plaintiffs has been the invocation of privilege to justify the disclosure. Employers have been granted a limited or "qualified" privilege to disclose certain facts essential to their business interests. For example, where work was disrupted at a nuclear power plant due to rumors that the reason for an employee's illness at work was radiation exposure, the court held that the employer had a qualified privilege to tell employees that the plaintiff was ill owing to the effects of a hysterectomy.[15] The employer's interest in disclosure was found to outweigh the plaintiff's interest in keeping the reason for her illness a secret. In contrast, another court held that it was a question for the jury whether an employer's disclosure to coworkers of the facts surrounding her mastectomy constituted an invasion of privacy.[16]

The other main basis for a common law action for invasion of privacy in the workplace is intrusion upon seclusion. According to the *Restatement (Second) of Torts:* "One who intentionally intrudes, physically or otherwise, upon the solitude or seclusion of another or his private affairs or concerns, is subject to liability to the other for invasion of his privacy, if the intrusion would be highly offensive to a reasonable person."[17] Courts generally agree that an employer has a legitimate business interest in determining the mental and physical condition of an employee to the extent that the employee's health affects performance. That interest must be balanced against the nature and extent of the intrusion in determining if an actionable invasion of privacy has occurred. One employer was held to be justified in discharging an employee who refused to list the prescription medications she was taking, where disclosure was part of the employer's drug testing program.[18] By contrast, an employee recovered where her supervisors, without her consent, questioned her clinical psychologist about her mental state.[19] Similarly, it was held to be an intrusion upon seclusion for an employer to demand that an employee indicate the reason for his frequent medical appointments and, on learning that he had AIDS-related complex, to disclose this fact to a large group of employees.[20]

The doctrine of consent operates to limit the usefulness of common law invasion of privacy as a remedy in the workplace. If an applicant or employee refuses to answer intrusive questions or to supply personal information, the employer may lawfully refuse to hire the individual.[21] If the individual supplies the information, then he or she will be deemed to have consented and therefore cannot bring an action for invasion of privacy.[22] In essence, there is no common law action for attempted invasion of privacy.

The inconsistency of results among jurisdictions is a second problem with common law approaches in this area. A third drawback to the use of the common law to redress invasion of privacy is a practical one. Although tort law often has a deterrent effect on unlawful conduct, the actions frequently involve unique facts from which generalizations about the scope of lawful conduct are often difficult to make. Neither employees nor their employers may know the bounds of lawful conduct. Furthermore, it is likely that invasion of privacy actions are brought in only a small percentage of the instances in which it occurs because employees do not want to jeopardize their employment, may not learn of the disclosures, or may be unable to obtain a lawyer to take their case. Thus, it is important to identify other sources of protecting employee privacy interests.

STATUTORY APPROACHES

Several state laws have been enacted to regulate employee medical records. Laws enacted in five states and the District of Columbia provide that employees have a right of access to their medical records as part of a more general right of access to employment records.[23] The laws in several other states prohibit medical records from being stored in personnel files or otherwise protect the confidentiality of medical records.[24] Several state workers' compensation laws contain provisions giving employees a right of access to their medical records.

At the federal level, under a regulation promulgated pursuant to the Occupational Safety and Health Act, employees have a right of access to their entire medical files, regardless of how the information was generated or is maintained.[25] Although the Department of Labor has a right of access to the records to assess the safety and health conditions in workplaces, medical records in personally identifiable form are subject to detailed procedures and protections.[26]

THE AMERICANS WITH DISABILITIES ACT

Ironically, the most important law regulating the privacy and confidentiality of employee medical information is not a privacy law at all but an antidiscrimination law. The Americans with Disabilities Act prohibits discrimination in employment against individuals with disabilities.[27] Similar laws prohibiting discrimination in employment based on disability have been enacted in virtually every state, although the remedies are often not as comprehensive as under the ADA.

In enacting the ADA, Congress recognized that to prevent disability discrimination, especially concerning individuals with "hidden" disabilities, it was essential to control employers' access to medical information unrelated to determining whether the individual is capable of performing essential job-related functions. Thus, privacy protections under the ADA stem from a desire to prevent discrimination by prohibiting employers from gaining access to certain nonessential information about the health of applicants and employees.

The ADA divides all medical examinations and inquiries into three stages: preemployment, preplacement, and employment. At the preemployment stage, while the employer is assessing the applicant's qualifications and before any offer has been extended, it is unlawful for an employer or the employer's agent to conduct a medical examination or to inquire whether the applicant has a disability or about the nature or severity of a disability. The only inquiries permissible at this time are whether the individual is able, with or without reasonable accommodation, to perform essential job-related functions. Thus, "traditional" preemployment medical examinations violate the ADA, as does requiring applicants to complete a preemployment medical questionnaire.

Under the ADA, employers are permitted to make "conditional" offers of employment, in which successful completion of a medical examination is a condition of employment. The "conditional offeree" may be required to take what the ADA terms an "employment entrance examination" or what is often referred to as a "preplacement examination." To be lawful, preplacement examinations must satisfy three requirements.

First, if medical examinations are required of employees in a certain job category, all entering employees in the same job category, regardless of disability, must be subject to an examination. Second, information obtained at the examination, as well as all other employee medical information, must be collected and maintained on separate forms and stored in medical files apart from more widely accessible personnel records. With few exceptions, the information in all medical records must be treated as confidential. Supervisors and managers may not be given specific information regarding diagnoses, but they may be informed about necessary restrictions on the work or duty of the employee; first aid and safety personnel may be informed, where appropriate, if the disability might require emergency treatment; and government officials investigating compliance with the ADA must be provided with relevant information on request. Third, employers may not use medical criteria to screen out individuals with disabilities unless the medical criteria are job-related and consistent with business necessity.

Under the ADA, preplacement medical examinations may be of unlimited scope. An employer may require a comprehensive medical examination, regardless of the job duties. Similarly, the employer may make the release of all the individual's medical records a valid condition of employment. Nevertheless, it is unlawful to withdraw a conditional offer of employment for any medical reason except that the individual is unable, even with reasonable accommodation, to perform the essential functions of the job. Medical examinations of current employees must be either job-related and consistent with business necessity or voluntary.

An issue of considerable controversy is whether discrimination against an individual because of an unexpressed genetic condition is unlawful under the ADA.[28] In 1995, in response to considerable urging, the Equal Employment Opportunity Commission, the agency charged with enforcing the ADA, issued an interpretation that when an employer discriminates against an individual because of increased risk of a genetic disorder, the individual is being "regarded" as having a disability and therefore is covered under the ADA.[29] This interpretation extends coverage to individuals who are presymptomatic and to those who are genetically predisposed to disease. It is unclear whether the ADA will also cover unaffected carriers of recessive and X-linked disorders, who may be subject to discrimination by employers concerned about the possible future health care costs of dependents. Moreover, as noted below, merely providing coverage under the ADA to individuals who are presymptomatic or predisposed to genetic disorders is inadequate to ensure the privacy of genetic information.

PRIVACY THEORIES OF THE AMERICANS WITH DISABILITIES ACT

It is important to consider the privacy theories implicit in the statutory scheme of the ADA. The first premise of the law is that by prohibiting preemployment inquiries, individuals with disabilities will not be eliminated from consideration before their abilities are considered. Although this is a doubtful proposition when applied to individuals with obvious disabilities, such as blindness or impaired mobility, it is valuable in the context of discrimination based on genetic traits, especially those whose manifestations are not visible and those that are as yet unexpressed. The ban on preemployment inquiries, however, does not prevent the voluntary disclosure of medical information about an applicant by third parties, such as references, or by the applicant.

Another privacy theory of the ADA is that by permitting the revocation of conditional offers of employment for medical reasons only if they are shown to be job-related and consistent with business necessity, irrelevant medical information will not be used to deny employment opportunities. Nevertheless, post-offer, preplacement medical examinations need not be job-related. Thus, for example, the employer's medical officers may require as a condition of employment that the individual consent to the drawing of blood. The employer need not disclose what tests are being performed on the blood and need not disclose any test results. Accordingly, it is not unlawful under the ADA for the employer to perform genetic testing at this time, although, as discussed in the next section, this may violate a state law. It is also lawful under the ADA for an employer to condition employment on the individual's signing a release authorizing disclosure to the employer's medical officer all of his or her medical records, which could include family histories and the results of genetic tests performed in the clinical setting.

A third privacy theory of the ADA is expressed in section 102(d)(3)(B). Medical information about applicants and employees must be "collected and maintained on separate forms and in separate medical files and [must be] treated as a confidential medical record."[30] The purpose of this provision is to prevent medical records from being stored in personnel files, where supervisors and other individuals would have access to them. This provision, however, has been interpreted as applying only to medical records generated after 1992—the effective date of the ADA.[31] Furthermore, the ADA does not prohibit medical officers who work for the company from disclosing specific diagnostic and other medical information to management.

Disclosure of specific medical findings to nonmedical personnel within a company would violate the 1976 version of the Code of Ethical Conduct of the American Occupational Medical Association (AOMA). "Physicians should . . . [7] . . . recognize that employers are entitled to counsel about the medical fitness of individuals in relation to work, but are not entitled to diagnoses or details of a specific nature."[32] The revision of the code in 1993 by the American College of Occupational and Environmental Medicine (which succeeded the AOMA), however, seems to permit this conduct. "Physicians should . . . [6] . . . recognize that employers may be entitled to counsel about an individual's medical work fitness, but not to diagnoses or specific details, except in compliance with laws and regulations."[33] In effect, the revised code provides that disclosures are ethical if they are legal. The paradoxical result is to establish the minimum standards of the ADA, an antidiscrimination law, as the ethical norm of a medical specialty college.[34]

In general, the ADA attempts to prevent employers from gaining access to some forms of medical information at some stages in the employment process. As noted above, however, limiting access to medical information is really a secondary objective of the ADA. Its major nondiscrimination strategy is to prevent the unlawful *use* of medical information.

This approach has several important consequences as applied to genetic information. First, allowing access to the information facilitates surreptitious discrimination by the unknown number of employers determined to exclude from the workplace all individuals with certain genetic traits, predispositions, or conditions. This is more than a theoretical concern. As recently as September 1995, a lawsuit alleging that the Lawrence Berkeley Laboratory was surreptitiously conducting tests on employees for sickle cell trait, syphilis, and pregnancy received widespread publicity.[35] Similarly, a lawsuit alleging that the Chicago Police Department secretly performed HIV testing on applicants was brought in 1994.[36]

Second, even as to employers that do not discriminate on the basis of irrelevant medical information, the ADA permits the disclosure of sensitive information when there is no compelling reason to do so. The result may be embarrassment, stigma, and ostracism. As the Senate Committee Report on the ADA noted with regard to cancer: "The individual with cancer may object merely to being identified, independent of the consequences [because] . . . being identified as disabled often carries both blatant and subtle stigma."[37]

Third, because employers have access to the results, at-risk individuals may forgo genetic testing because they fear that an adverse result may lead to their becoming unemployable and uninsurable. Indeed, the fear of health insurance discrimination is one of the most common reasons why at-risk individuals decline to undergo genetic testing.[38] Thus, employment discrimination and privacy laws have a close relationship with public health.[39]

STATE GENETIC DISCRIMINATION LAWS

State laws directed at genetic testing and discrimination in employment were first enacted in the 1970s to combat irrational sickle cell trait discrimination that arose from the federal government's poorly conceived and implemented sickle cell screening programs. Florida, Louisiana, and North Carolina enacted the first laws prohibiting discrimination in employment on the basis of sickle cell trait.[40] These laws remain in effect today.

As the prospects increased for more broadly based genetic discrimination in employment, other states enacted genetic discrimination laws. In 1981, New Jersey enacted a law prohibiting employment discrimination based on an individual's "atypical hereditary cellular or blood trait," defined to include sickle cell trait, hemoglobin C trait, thalassemia trait, Tay-Sachs trait, or cystic fibrosis trait.[41] (A new law enacted in New Jersey in 1996 bans discrimination based on "genetic information," which includes information "that may derive from an individual or family member.")[42] As with prior laws, the focus of this law was on the irrational use of genetic criteria to screen out heterozygous, unaffected carriers of recessive disorders. The law might have been premised on the belief that some employers would exclude carriers of disorders such as Tay-Sachs disease and cystic fibrosis based on a desire to avoid the health insurance claims of an affected child. Yet, given the history of discrimination based on sickle cell trait, it is just as likely that the focus of the law was employers who erroneously believed that carriers of recessive disorders were affected. Furthermore, the laws prohibited discrimination but still did not prohibit employers from obtaining access to genetic information.

In 1989, Oregon amended its unlawful employment practices act to prohibit employers from requiring applicants or employees to undergo "genetic screening," although the term is not further defined in the statute.[43] (The law was subsequently amended in 1993 and 1995 to prohibit employers from obtaining or using genetic information, defined as information based on a DNA test.) This was the first statute to go beyond recessive disorders as well as the first to prohibit genetic testing. The law, however, did not prohibit employers from using the results of genetic tests performed in the clinical setting or basing employment decisions on family risk factors.

In 1990, New York enacted a law of the earlier type, prohibiting discrimination based on the carrier state for the recessive disorders of sickle cell anemia, Tay-Sachs disease, or Cooley's anemia (beta thalassemia).[44] (The law was broadened in 1996 to prohibit all genetic discrimination based on "genetic predisposition or carrier status.")[45]

In 1992, Wisconsin enacted a law that prohibits employers not only from requiring applicants or employees to undergo genetic testing but also from using the information from genetic tests in employment decisions.[46] Two other states enacted laws in 1992 based on the Oregon model and focusing on genetic testing. Iowa made it illegal for an employer to solicit or require genetic testing as a condition of employment or to discriminate against any person who obtains a genetic test.[47] Rhode Island prohibited employers from requesting, requiring, or administering genetic tests to an individual as a condition of employment.[48]

New Hampshire's law of 1995 prohibits employers from soliciting, requiring, or administering genetic tests as a condition of employment.[49] It also prohibits employers from using the results of genetic tests to affect the terms, conditions, or privileges of employment. Laws enacted in Arizona and Texas in 1997 prohibit discrimination based on the results of a genetic test.

Even the enactment of a law similar to the most recent ones enacted in Iowa,

New Hampshire, New Jersey, New York, and Wisconsin would not eliminate two serious problems. First, it is extremely difficult to define a "genetic" test or "genetic" information. New developments in genetics have identified a genetic component of some forms of many common disorders, such as asthma, hypertension, osteoporosis, diabetes, hypercholesterolemia, and rheumatoid arthritis. Are routine tests that identify an individual as having such a condition "genetic" tests? Is a pedigree that reveals a family history of a genetic or multifactorial disorder "genetic" information? Although the New Jersey law of 1996 prohibits discrimination based on genetic information derived from family members, "genetic information" includes "inherited characteristics," and it is not clear how broadly this will be construed.

Second, these laws prohibit the unauthorized access to genetic information, but they do not prohibit an employer from making the execution of a general medical release a valid condition of employment. Consequently, if the employer has a right of access to all the individual's medical files (under the ADA this is limited to the preplacement stage), then genetic information within the files will be revealed. Minnesota is the only state that prohibits such broad disclosures, and this is not done through specific genetic legislation. Minnesota prohibits all non-job-related medical examinations at any stage of the employment process and limits employers' access to applicant and employee medical records.[50]

INFORMATION FROM HEALTH INSURANCE CLAIMS

To be sure, the close connection between employment and health insurance has important implications for genetic privacy in the workplace. This issue is discussed at length in Chapter 16, on insurance, and in Chapter 23, on policy recommendations. An important privacy issue related to health insurance needs to be addressed: how private medical information, including genetic information, may be obtained by employers in the course of paying health insurance claims.

During the 1970s, many larger corporations with rising health costs realized that, with a stable workforce, increases in experience-rated premiums for employee health insurance could be predicted by applying an inflation factor. Commercial insurers actually were eliminating little risk for companies that were so large they neither needed nor benefited from the risk-pooling feature of commercial insurance.

The result was a growing use of self-insurance, whereby employers directly assume responsibility for health care expenses. Some self-insured companies still contract with insurers for "stop loss" coverage for large claims or for claims processing. By 1993, 85% of employers with 5,000–40,000 employees and 93% of employers with more than 40,000 employees were self-insured. In fact, 37% of employers with 50–199 employees also were self-insured, despite serious questions about whether such small groups are able to spread the risk adequately.[51]

Employers obtain several advantages from self-insurance. They save the profits of the commercial insurers, they can retain and use the earnings on amounts paid to insurers and held as claims reserves, and they pay no tax on premiums. Most important, in an era of increasing state regulation of health insurance, self-insured plans are exempt from state insurance laws and regulations, including state laws limiting policy cancellations and rate increases, and mandating high-risk insurance pools and the coverage of specified services and conditions. This exemption from state insurance law is pursuant to the preemptive effect of the federal Employee Retirement Income Security Act of 1974 (ERISA).[52]

As a practical matter, self-insured employers may be self-administered or they may use a third-party administrator to handle claims. Under the former arrangement, claims by health care providers are submitted for payment to the benefits department of the company. Typically, claims contain the employee's name as well as a code or description of the specific diagnosis or procedure. Thus, at least the employer's benefits department inevitably learns of the specific medical conditions of the employee or the employee's covered dependents.

The disclosure of sensitive medical information may cause stigmatization of the individual or even more tangible harm. It is not necessary for the results of particular diagnostic tests to be known by the employer for adverse treatment to result. For example, if an individual undergoes genetic testing for Huntington disease, even if the result of the test is not disclosed, the employer knows that the individual is at a 50% risk of the disease. Similarly, reimbursement for an annual colonoscopy for an employee under age 40 may not be approved in the absence of a notation that the individual was at risk of inherited susceptibility to colon cancer.

Adverse consequences may attach to employees even in the absence of individually identifiable records. For example, employers that want to save health care payments may obtain a printout of all of the serious medical conditions for which employees are being treated and the average cost of each illness or procedure. The employer then might decide to alter the self-insured health benefit plan to reduce or eliminate the coverage for these conditions or procedures. Although this action might well violate state health insurance laws as to commercially purchased insurance, in general, self-insured employers are free to amend or even terminate their plans at any time so long as the notice provisions of the plan are satisfied. Discrimination in health benefits is permissible under the ADA so long as it is based on valid actuarial principles and is not a subterfuge for disability discrimination.

The federal Health Insurance Portability and Accountability Act of 1996 provides additional protection against discrimination in health benefits. Neither a commercial health insurance policy issued to an employer-sponsored group nor a self-insured employer health plan may treat genetic information as a preexisting condition for purposes of a limitation on or exclusion from benefits. Also, genetic information may not be used to limit or restrict the "amount, level, extent, or nature of the benefits or coverage for similarly situated individuals enrolled in the plan."[53] The act, however, does not limit access to genetic information.

The use of a third-party administrator may eliminate some of the direct disclosure of information, but during the utilization review process (in which data from health benefits claims are analyzed) or at other times individually identifiable information is often revealed. A case in 1995 involved an employee who was the manager of his company's employee assistance program. Before he had a prescription filled under the company's drug plan, he asked his supervisor, the head of the company medical department, whether the company was able to identify what prescriptions individual employees had filled. When he was assured that the company did not get such information, the employee had his prescription for AZT (azidothymidine), an antiviral drug used to treat AIDS, refilled under the company plan. When the pharmacy chain submitted its mandatory utilization report, which included a list of the names of all employees and the medications they were taking, the employer's medical department, including this particular employee's supervisors, learned that he was HIV-positive, a fact that they then indiscriminately shared. The jury's award of $125,000 for invasion of privacy was reversed by the Third Circuit Court of Appeals. The court held that the employer's "important interests" in the prescription information outweighed the "minimal intrusion" into the plaintiff's privacy.[54]

Without a method to control information on health insurance claims, health-based discrimination in employment remains a distinct possibility—to say nothing of the intangible harms caused by compromising medical privacy.

CONCLUSION

A combination of historical events, legal doctrines, practical considerations, and an imbalance in power between employers and employees has operated to undermine employees' interests in medical privacy in the workplace. The most important law to address broad issues of employee medical privacy is the federal Americans with Disabilities Act. In attempting to prevent discrimination against individuals with disabilities, the ADA controls, to a limited extent, the type of medical information available to employers at certain times during the employment process. The ADA, however, permits employers at the preplacement stage to perform unlimited medical examinations and to insist upon access to all of the employee's medical records.

Thus far, 12 states have enacted legislation to prohibit discrimination in employment on the basis of genetic testing or genetic information. In general, the laws have had little or no practical effect. To begin with, there is the increasingly insoluble problem of defining what is a genetic test or what is genetic information. In addition, so long as employers have access to the medical records of employees, there is a risk of stigmatization and possible loss of employment or health insurance. This, in turn, operates to discourage at-risk individuals from undergoing genetic testing in the clinical setting.

Any attempt to provide meaningful privacy protection for employees must address the problem of employer access to information on health insurance claims. The problem is exacerbated by the pervasiveness of self-insurance among large employers. The focus of the law must shift from controlling the use of medical information to controlling access to the information. The essence of medical privacy is the right of the individual to decide who, if anyone, has the right of access to the individual's person and the individual's medical records. This right has never been afforded adequate protection by the law. In the new era of genetic information, this right must be recognized.

NOTES

1. Diana Chapman Walsh, *Corporate Physicians: Between Medicine and Management* (New Haven: Yale University Press, 1987), 39.
2. National Institute for Occupational Safety and Health, *National Occupational Exposure Survey* (Washington, D.C.: Government Printing Office, 1985).
3. Mark A. Rothstein, *Medical Screening and the Employee Health Cost Crisis* (Washington, D.C.: BNA Books, 1989).
4. 29 U.S.C. §§ 651–78 (1994).

5. Horace G. Wood, *A Treatise on the Law of Master and Servant* (Buffalo, N.Y.: W. S. Hein, 1877).

6. Mayer G. Freed and Daniel D. Polsby, "The Doubtful Provenance of 'Wood's Rule' Revisited," *Arizona State Law Journal* 22 (1990): 551; Jay M. Feinman, "The Development of the Employment at Will Rule," *American Journal of Legal History* 20 (1976): 118.

7. Thomas M. Cooley, *A Treatise on the Law of Torts; or, The Wrongs Which Arise Independent of Contract* (Chicago: Callaghan, 1879).

8. Samuel D. Warren and Louis D. Brandeis, "The Right to Privacy," *Harvard Law Review* 4 (1890): 193.

9. Allan Nevins, *Ford: The Times, the Man, the Company* (New York: Charles Scribner's Sons, 1954), 554–56.

10. Cruzan v. Director, Missouri Dep't of Health, 497 U.S. 261 (1990) (medical treatment); Skinner v. Oklahoma, 316 U.S. 535 (1942) (procreation); Griswold v. Connecticut, 381 U.S. 479 (1965) (contraception); Roe v. Wade, 410 U.S. 113 (1973) (abortion).

11. See National Treasury Employees Union v. Von Raab, 489 U.S. 656 (1989).

12. *Restatement (Second) of Torts* § 652D (1977).

13. Ellenwood v. Exxon Shipping Co., 6 IER Cases 1628 (D. Me. 1991) (treatment for alcoholism), reversed in part on other grounds, 984 F.2d 1270 (1st Cir. 1992); Eddy v. Brown, 715 P.2d 74 (Okla. 1986) (psychiatric treatment).

14. Levias v. United Airlines, 500 N.E.2d 370 (Ohio Ct. App. 1985).

15. Young v. Jackson, 572 So.2d 378 (Miss. 1990).

16. Miller v. Motorola, Inc., 560 N.E.2d 900 (Ill. Ct. App. 1990).

17. *Restatement (Second) of Torts* § 652B.

18. Mares v. ConAgra Poultry Co., 971 F.2d 492 (10th Cir. 1992).

19. Leggett v. First Interstate Bank, 739 P.2d 1083 (Or. Ct. App. 1987).

20. Cronan v. New Eng. Tel. Co., 41 FEP Cases 1273 (Mass. Super. Ct. 1986).

21. See Cort v. Bristol-Myers Co., 431 N.E.2d 908 (Mass. 1982).

22. See Luedtke v. Nabors Alaska Drilling, Inc., 768 P.2d 1123 (Alaska, 1989).

23. D.C. Code § 1–632.5(a)(2)(B) (1992); Iowa Code Ann. §§ 91B.1, 730.5 (West Supp. 1995); Me. Rev. Stat. Ann. tit. 26, § 631 (1988 & Supp. 1994); Ohio Rev. Code Ann. § 4113.23 (Page 1991); Okla. Stat. Ann. tit. 40, § 191 (West 1986); Wis. Stat. Ann. § 103.13(5) (West 1988 & Supp. 1994).

24. Cal. Civ. Code § 56.20(a)(c) (West Supp. 1995); Conn. Gen. Stat. Ann. § 31–128a (West 1987); Minn. Stat. Ann. § 181.960(10) (West 1991 & Supp. 1995); N.D. Cent. Code § 44–04–18.1 (Michie 1993). See Lori B. Andrews and Ami S. Jaeger, "Confidentiality of Genetic Information in the Workplace," *American Journal of Law and Medicine* 17 (1991): 75.

25. 29 C.F.R. § 1910.20 (1996).

26. Ibid., Part 1913.

27. 42 U.S.C. §§ 12101–213 (1994).

28. See Mark A. Rothstein, "Genetic Discrimination in Employment and the Americans with Disabilities Act," *Houston Law Review* 29 (1992): 23.

29. *EEOC Compliance Manual*, vol. 2, EEOC Order 915.002, Definition of the Term "Disability," at 902–45, reprinted in *Daily Labor Report*, Mar. 16, 1995, at E–1, E–23.

30. 42 U.S.C. § 12112(d)(3)(B) (1994).

31. Buchanan v. City of San Antonio, 85 F.3d 196 (5th Cir. 1996).

32. American Occupational Medical Association, *Code of Ethical Conduct for Physicians Providing Occupational Medical Services,* Principle 7 (Chicago: American Occupational Medical Association, 1976).

33. American College of Occupational and Environmental Medicine, *Code of Ethical Conduct,* Principle 6 (Arlington Heights, Ill.: American College of Occupational and Environmental Medicine, 1993).

34. See Mark A. Rothstein, "A Proposed Revision of the ACOEM Code of Ethics," *Journal of Occupational and Environmental Medicine* 39 (1997): 616–22.

35. Norman-Bloodsaw v. Lawrence Berkeley Lab., No. C95–3220 VRW (N.D. Cal., filed Sept. 3, 1995). The case was dismissed in 1996 and is on appeal to the Ninth Circuit Court of Appeals. For a further discussion, see Danielle Cass, "Berkeley Lab Sued for Illicit Disease Testing," *Oakland Tribune,* Sept. 14, 1995, A4.

36. Doe v. City of Chicago, 883 F. Supp. 1126 (N.D. Ill. 1994).

37. U.S. Senate, Committee on Labor and Human Resources, *The Americans with Disabilities Act of 1989, S. Rep. No. 116,* 101st Cong., 1st Sess., 40 (1989).

38. See Kimberly A. Quaid and Michael Morris, "Reluctance to Undergo Predictive Testing: The Case of Huntington Disease," *American Journal of Medical Genetics* 45 (1993): 41, 43.

39. See Karen Rothenberg et al., "Genetic Information and the Workplace: Legislative Approaches and Policy Challenges," *Science* 275 (1997): 1755.

40. Fla. Stat. Ann. § 448.075 (West 1981 & Supp. 1995); La. Rev. Stat. Ann. §§ 23:1001–23:1004 (West 1985 & Supp. 1995); N.C. Gen. Stat. § 95–28.1 (Michie 1993).

41. N.J. Stat. Ann. § 10:5–5(y) (West 1993 & Supp. 1995).

42. 1996 N.J. S.B. 695, 854 (1996).

43. Or. Rev. Stat. § 659.010–659.720 (1995).

44. N.Y. Civ. Rights Law §§ 48, 48–a (West 1992).

45. 1995 N.Y. A.B. 7839 (1996).

46. Wis. Stat. § 111.372 (West Supp. 1994).

47. Iowa Code Ann. § 729.6 (West 1993).

48. R.I. Gen. Laws § 28–6.7–1 (Michie Supp. 1994).

49. N.H. Rev. Stat. Ann. ch. 141–H (1995).

50. Minn. Stat. Ann. § 363.02, subd. 1(b)(9)(i)(b), 363.03 subd. 4(b) (West Supp. 1995).

51. A. Foster Higgins & Co., *Foster Higgins Health Benefits Survey, 1993* (1994).

52. 29 U.S.C. §§ 1001–1461 (1994).

53. 42 U.S.C. §§ 300gg(b)(1), 300gg–1.

54. Doe v. Southeastern Pa. Transp. Auth., 72 F.3d 1133 (3d Cir. 1995), *cert. denied,* 117 S. Ct. 51 (1996). In a separate action, Ascolese v. Southeastern Pa. Transp. Auth., 925 F. Supp. 351 (E.D. Pa. 1996), the same defendant was charged with requiring an employee to take a pregnancy test and the defendant's physician with sexual misconduct during her physical examination.

Chapter 16 The Implications of Genetic Testing for Health and Life Insurance

Nancy E. Kass

The advent of genetic testing has focused attention on whether and how health and life insurance companies will use this new technology for the purposes of risk screening. Indeed, an early, explicitly stated focus of the Joint National Institutes of Health–Department of Energy Working Group for the Study of the Ethical, Legal, and Social Implications of the Human Genome Project was the relation between genetic testing and health and life insurance.[1] Several commentators speculated that this new risk-screening tool would lead to increased numbers of persons being denied health and life insurance, with concordant loss of access to particular health care providers and increased public financial burden for health care.[2]

In this chapter, I outline the issues relevant to genetic testing and insurance. After a background discussion on health and life insurance in the United States, including who has insurance and how insurance is currently issued, I discuss the current and potential uses of both genetic tests and genetic testing information by insurance companies. Last, I focus on the implications of insurance companies' use of genetic tests.

Approximately 85% of the American public has some sort of health insurance coverage.[3] Among those insured, approximately 83% have private health insurance, and the remainder have some sort of public coverage.[4] Persons typically gain access to the private health insurance market through their employment, where insurance is provided as part of a group policy. Only 10–15% of private insurance is obtained through the individual market. This is relevant to genetic testing because many of the concerns raised in relation to how insurers might use genetic tests or genetic information would apply to this minority, albeit sizable, segment of the market.

Insurance policies are usually "rated," meaning that different costs are charged to different consumers, depending on the insured person's likelihood of making a claim. In the individual health insurance market, applicants are screened individually for their medical history and health risks. Typically, this process begins with a simple written questionnaire that the applicant completes. A statement or medical record is requested from the applicant's physician for approximately 20% of applicants, usually because of a particular response on a health history questionnaire or because of the applicant's age or other factors.[5] A physical examination is required of only 4% of applicants for individual health insurance. Approximately 75% of individual insurance applicants are approved for coverage. Another 15–20% are approved as "substandard," meaning that either they are charged higher premiums or their coverage will exclude payments for a preexisting condition. Applicants are denied insurance altogether if their chance of disease exceeds three times the risk for others of their age and sex. Approximately 8% of applicants are denied coverage.[6]

Groups also are rated, though not at the individual level. When an insurance company negotiates a contract with an employer, the insurer usually looks at the "experience" of the employee group; that is, the insurer analyzes how many and what types of health insurance claims have been made in the past by the group, as well as the age and sex distribution of the group. A premium rate is determined based on the group's past and predicted future use.

Alternatively, insurance can be community rated. This means that all policyholders within a given geographic area are charged the same rate. When Blue Cross and Blue Shield plans first were created in the 1930s, they used community rating to price their plans.[7] However, when increased numbers of employer groups realized that they could provide insurance more cheaply by experience rating (since their pool consisted almost exclusively of healthy persons), few groups were able to remain competitive if they charged community-based rates. Those who remained in community-based plans were more likely to be the sicker individuals, and as a result, community-based plans were squeezed out of most insurance markets.

It is fundamental to the contemporary insurance market to assess risk. According to one industry spokesperson, "The insurance industry is built upon a basic insurance principle: the ability to appropriately and accurately evaluate risks and, in turn, price the product."[8] The industry wants to be able to predict who is likely to develop a serious disease and whose disease is expected to be prolonged or expensive. Indeed, each of the 50 states and the District of Columbia have legislation known as Unfair Trade Practices acts. These acts prohibit unfair discrimination "between individuals of the same class and of essentially the same hazard in the amount of premium, policy fees, or rates charged for any policy or contract of [life or] health insurance."[9] Unfair Trade Practices acts have been interpreted not only as providing protection against differential treatment for individuals of the same risk but also, more germane to the issue of genetic testing, as justification for rendering differential treatment to individuals of *different* risk. It is the philosophy of the insurance industry that an insurance company "has the responsibility to treat all its policyholders fairly by establishing premiums at a level consistent with the risk represented by each individual policyholder."[10]

The United States does not require individuals to have health insurance, nor does it require employers to provide their employees with health insurance. The insurance industry argues, therefore, that only or predominantly persons who believe they have special reason to need insurance will want to buy it. The industry is concerned about adverse selection, whereby an applicant has information about his or her health unavailable to the insurer and this information might lead the applicant to buy insurance or to buy a greater amount of insurance than he or she would without such knowledge. Insurance companies argue that if they were required to accept all applicants, without being able to screen for preexisting conditions or risk factors (in order, they argue, to "level the playing field"), rates for individual insurance would rise and healthier individuals would choose to stop buying insurance. This concept is difficult to test empirically.

To prevent individuals from being denied coverage from one company and then falsifying details of their medical history as they pursue coverage through a different company, the health, life, and disability insurance industries established a nonprofit database called the Medical Information Bureau (MIB). The MIB serves as a clearinghouse of information to allow insurance companies to share information with one another about insurance *applicants*. If characteristics relevant to risk—such as aspects of medical history or skydiving or alcohol use—are revealed in an application process, details are sent to and stored by the MIB. When someone applies for an individual insurance policy, a background check is conducted with the MIB to ensure that the applicant did not omit information the insurance company would want to have known.

Employers who provide health insurance to their employees have increasingly been "self-insuring" rather than purchasing policies with commercial insurance companies. Self-insuring means that the employer can afford and chooses to be responsible for its employees' health expenses. If an employee makes a claim, the reimbursement comes directly out of the financial reserves of the employer, rather than being paid by an outside insurance company. Self-insuring employers typically have catastrophic coverage so that they are insured against extremely large claims in a given year.

Self-insuring has become more attractive to employers because they do not pay the increasingly expensive monthly premiums on behalf of each employee. Moreover, because self-insured employers technically are employment firms rather than insurance companies, they are exempt under the Employee Retirement Income Security Act (ERISA) from many state taxes and regulations otherwise imposed on insurers.[11] Although estimates vary, approximately 55–65% of employees receiving health insurance in this country obtain their coverage through a self-insurance arrangement.[12]

Since a Supreme Court ruling in 1869, insurance regulation has been considered the domain of state governments.[13] This principle was upheld in another Supreme Court case in 1944 as well as in the McCarran-Ferguson Act of 1945, which legislated the continued regulation of the insurance industry by the states in all cases other than interstate transactions.[14] New Hampshire became the first state in 1851 to have an insurance regulatory body, and all states and the District of Columbia now have an insurance commission, board, or department. Although the original purpose of insurance commissions was to protect consumers from fraud,[15] more recently they have moved into other areas, such as requiring minimum benefits and developing regulations related to the renewal and cancellation of policies.

As mentioned, in accordance with ERISA, self-insuring employers are exempt from state insurance regulation. This means that if, for example, a state passes legislation preventing insurance companies from using genetic tests or information in their risk assessments or requiring insurers to reimburse for genetic tests, self-insured employers would not be subject to such requirements.

Therefore, perhaps two-thirds of employees would not be protected by legislation or regulations intended to safeguard them from certain types of harms.

Approximately 70% of adults have some form of life insurance.[16] Unlike health insurance, the majority (71%) of life insurance policies are sold through the individual market.[17] As with health insurance, individual applicants for life insurance are screened for preexisting conditions or risks, with the amount of scrutiny given to the application related in great part to the amount of insurance sought. Approximately 92% of applicants for life insurance are approved at a standard rate; approximately 5% are approved as "substandard" and approved with a higher premium; and about 3% are denied coverage altogether.[18]

THE USE OF GENETIC TESTS AND GENETIC INFORMATION BY INSURERS

Genetic information could be obtained and used by insurers in one of three ways: insurance companies could conduct genetic tests themselves, for example, by requiring all applicants for insurance to be screened for specific genetic conditions; companies could gain access to results from genetic tests conducted by others, such as private physicians and researchers; or companies could gain access to genetic information that did not come from tests. Complicating this situation is the varied predictive capability of the information obtained. Information could be completely predictive, indicating with certainty or near certainty that the person who tests positive will develop the relevant condition later in life. Such tests are often termed *presymptomatic tests.* Alternatively, the information could indicate that the person tested is at increased risk but not whether the person will develop the condition. Such tests are often termed *susceptibility tests.*

Neither health nor life insurance companies seem to be routinely conducting genetic tests as part of their underwriting process for applicants at this time.[19] This is in part because the tests remain somewhat specialized and expensive and in part because many of the genetic disorders for which they might test are too rare to justify widespread screening. It has been suggested, however, that when the "multiplexing" of tests is possible—that is, the ability to test for multiple conditions as part of a single "panel"—then genetic testing may become more common. Similarly, if genetic testing becomes a more regular part of medical practice, it could also be expected that insurers would use genetic tests more routinely. Indeed, half of the respondents to a survey of medical directors of life insurance companies, when asked to assume the availability of a test with high sensitivity and specificity and general clinical acceptance, reported that they would be interested in using genetic testing, at least in some situations.[20]

Although insurers report that they are currently not conducting testing, they do acknowledge an interest in accessing information collected by others. The assumption on the part of the insurance company is that individuals do not randomly seek genetic tests; they assume that those who have sought genetic testing in the past are those who know themselves (because of a family history, for example) to be at increased risk. Insurers fear that adverse selection would occur if individuals were allowed to withhold from insurance companies information about their testing history. Sometimes insurance companies secure access to such information from the response to a question on the health history questionnaire of applicants; for example, a simple question asking an applicant if he or she had seen a health care provider in the past five years and, if so, for what reason might lead an applicant to disclose that he or she had sought genetic testing. Alternatively, a response on the health history questionnaire about a completely unrelated condition (e.g., asthma) might cause the insurance company to request a copy of the applicant's medical chart from the applicant's physician. Because the record is typically copied and forwarded to the company in its entirety (that is, rather than the sections of the chart exclusively concerning the applicant's history of asthma being forwarded), any mention in the patient's chart, even peripherally, of genetic testing would be available to the insurance company. Moreover, physicians sometimes document in the medical chart if their patients tell them they have been enrolled in a research study. If the note in the chart further described the project as being related to genetic testing, that might be cause for the insurance company to ask the applicant additional questions before issuing the insurance policy. As one medical director wrote, "Insurers today do not do any genetic testing. . . . On the other hand, insurers do want to know the results of tests that have been done by others, for cause, on individuals who are applying for insurance."[21]

Insurance companies also have underwriting guidelines for at least some genetic conditions, although it is not clear to what degree these are based on actuarial data.[22] And certainly insurance companies routinely elicit information that is "genetic"—that is, information that relates to the applicant's family history. The vast majority of life insurance companies, for example, ask all applicants the age and cause of their parents' deaths.[23]

Although any conclusion must remain somewhat speculative, it is reasonable to assume that insurance companies, absent further regulation, will in future conduct at least some genetic testing on their own; it is already true that companies seek access to existing genetic testing information that was collected by others. What implications does this pose for individuals with a genetic condition and for other members of society?

Decreased access to insurance. The first and probably most significant implication of insurers using genetic information in their risk-screening process is that more people would be denied health and life insurance coverage. Approximately 7% of those who currently do not have health insurance in this country are considered "medically uninsurable."[24] This figure undoubtedly would rise if insurance companies engaged in more widespread genetic testing. A basic tenet of President Bill Clinton's unsuccessful Health Security Act proposal for health reform in 1994 was that "no health plan may deny enrollment to any applicant because of health . . . status, nor may they charge some patients more than others because of age, medical condition, or other factors related to risk."[25] It was clear to the president and to others who included this provision in alternative health reform proposals that risk screening contributes to the number of Americans who do not have health insurance.

In the absence of genetic screening, most persons destined to get genetic conditions are currently mixed in among all others as part of the existing pool of insured persons. If, however, it were possible to identify those who were susceptible to or predicted to develop costly genetic conditions, these people invariably would be eliminated from the pool, consistent with risk-screening practices for other serious and costly medical conditions. At the least, this would limit their choice of providers and decrease their access to certain specialists; at worst, it could mean a lack of access to health services altogether.

Life insurance. The moral differences between health and life insurance continue to be debated. Should society guarantee equal access to both coverages? If not, why not? It has been argued that health insurance is a fundamental need, whereas life insurance is more of a luxury. But to some degree this depends on in what light life insurance is being considered. Life insurance could be seen as economic security for an individual's dependents, security that gives these dependents their livelihood and prevents them from becoming the public's financial responsibility. Conversely, life insurance could be considered simply another financial investment—almost a windfall—where purchasers buy significantly larger policies than might be judged necessary. To the degree that one believes life insurance is important for a secure economic future for one's family, limiting access through the allowance of genetic screening by insurance companies deprives individuals of this benefit. Moreover, given that life insurance is sold almost exclusively in the voluntary market (which insurers describe as being most prone to adverse selection), risk screening is more prevalent for life than for health insurance, making access to life insurance potentially more threatened than access to health insurance.

The threat to personal autonomy. Genetic tests are available for medical conditions for which there are no or limited treatments. This means that the decision whether to learn whether one is destined to have—or is at increased risk for—a certain condition is a matter of personal choice. Counseling programs have been established to help individuals who may be at risk for certain conditions for which no intervention is available decide if they want to learn whether they carry a gene mutation associated with a particular health condition later in life. Inherent to such counseling programs is the assumption that valid reasons exist both for wanting the information and for not wanting the information perhaps years in advance of becoming symptomatic.

Mandatory genetic screening—or "conditionally mandatory" screening,[26] that is, screening required as a condition of obtaining health insurance—would deprive individuals of this right to personal autonomy. No longer would the consequential psychological decision about whether to take a genetic test be left to the individual. Already instances exist whereby insurance is denied to children of persons with Huntington disease until the children agree to be tested for the gene mutation and then test negative.

Public health. If insurance companies increasingly seek to use genetic information in their risk-screening process, either by asking applicants whether they have been tested on their own or by requesting copies of applicants' medical records, individuals will have an incentive to avoid testing until it is medically necessary. Obviously, once a patient presents with symptoms and a diagnostic test is warranted, the test may have little additional impact on whether a person is considered insurable. Yet what is in many ways a great *advantage* (certainly, a unique feature) of genetic tests is their ability to predict conditions (or susceptibilities to conditions) years before the conditions manifest themselves. There may be great public health benefits to obtaining predictive information early. For example, on learning of an increased risk of disease, individuals might be able to modify their behavior or other environmental factors and thereby alter the timing or course of onset of a disease. If one's access to health or life insurance were limited severely as a result of acquiring such information early or from sharing such information with one's physician, such public health benefits could not be realized.

It must be noted that this discussion should in no way be understood to suggest that individuals falsify insurance applications. Insurers can cancel a policy if it can be proven that the insured person misrepresented facts at the time of application, that the misrepresentation was material to the approval of the application, and that the insurer would not have issued the policy if all of the facts had been known.[27] This means, for example, that if someone denied knowledge of a genetic predisposition to a condition and it was later discovered that he or she had participated in research demonstrating that he or she carried an increased risk, the insurance company could legally cancel the policy.[28] (All policies include an incontestability clause, essentially a statute of limitations, after which time challenges to the original application cannot be made. The period of incontestability ordinarily is two years for individual policies and one year for group policies.)

What is uncertain is how, legally, an applicant who has tested positive on either a presymptomatic or predisposing test should answer if asked on an insurance application if he or she has been diagnosed previously with a medical condition. Strictly speaking, the applicant has *not* been diagnosed with the condition, for symptoms have not occurred and care has not been sought. Yet neither the courts nor individual states have been consistent on what constitutes a preexisting condition, leaving the definition to the discretion of individual companies.[29] The Health Insurance Portability and Accountability Act of 1996, discussed below, defines preexisting conditions for the purpose of employer-based health insurance. There is no evidence to suggest that the definition used by the act would be used by insurers in the nonemployment context, however.

Research. In many types of research volunteers are asked to undergo genetic testing as part of the research protocol. The purpose of the research may be to map a gene, to follow the natural history of a condition, or to understand the transmission of a condition or trait within a family. In recent years, investigators have begun to include in their delineations of possible risks and benefits in informed consent procedures that research volunteers may experience the harm of insurance discrimination because of their participation; that is, the research may be the first time they are tested, and if a trait or a presymptomatic condition is discovered, it may harm or preclude their access to health or life insurance.

Although it is extremely unlikely that a research investigator would release genetic information directly to an insurance company without the knowledge or consent of the research volunteer, companies might still obtain such personal and, in this context, damaging information in two ways. First, as described above, being enrolled in the research may prompt individuals during the course of their clinical care to mention the research to or to raise a question with their physician. Most physicians keep detailed notes of discussions with patients from regular visits, and it is very possible that a seemingly innocent note would be written in a patient's chart documenting a discussion concerning the patient's participation in a (named) genetics study. Although the company would rarely be able to learn of this participation directly from the investigator, if the note exists in the chart, it is visible to the company whenever they have any other reason to review the patient's medical chart. This might happen during an application for insurance if the individual reported another, unrelated risk factor about which the company wanted further explanation or because the patient made a claim for another medical procedure, such as minor surgery. In either case, as mentioned above, a medical practitioner rarely photocopies only those sections of the medical chart specifically relevant to the condition or medical claim in question. Rather, the simplest and typical procedure is to copy the entire medical record and forward it to the insurance company.

Although the applicant or insured person is required to sign a release of information before this transaction can occur, no insurance applications or claims are processed if permission for release is not granted. Applicants may not realize when they authorize the release of information how broad and inclusive the information that exists about them may be. If an insurance company learns through this route that the applicant had participated in a genetics study, further questioning would undoubtedly ensue, which already would be more questioning than the applicant would have undergone had he or she not participated in the research.

When applying for insurance, individuals are not only asked specific questions about individual medical conditions but also are typically asked a series of general questions about their medical history. For example, applicants might be asked in a general way if they had seen a doctor, been hospitalized, or had any medical tests in the past five years and, if so, to provide details. It is possible that someone who had been enrolled in a research study in which genetic testing was conducted might answer yes to such a question. The applicant might further describe, perhaps believing that it would abate a company's concerns, that the testing had been conducted "only" as part of research and not because the applicant had been experiencing symptoms or because a doctor thought a test was medically indicated. Although underwriting procedures are somewhat haphazard, the insurance company could very well not issue the insurance policy until the applicant had agreed either to have the research records released to the insurer or to be tested by the company.

The denial of access of coverage disproportionately to persons who participate in research is a problem. The principle of justice is violated for the individuals who participate. It is unfair for one group of persons, who may not be experiencing any symptoms and indeed may even have been recruited into a study to serve as a "control," to be singled out for more scrutiny and perhaps less insurance than someone who had decided not to volunteer. Certain studies even have certificates of confidentiality from the federal government that allow them greater authority to refuse to provide information to outside parties. Thus far, genetic testing has not been considered a "sensitive area" thereby protected by such certificates.[30]

Moreover, if it becomes clear that those who participate are disproportionately harmed, fewer people will volunteer for medical research. In general, medical research is thought of as a public good, and much of it is funded by the federal government for this reason. In research, a few individuals are asked to give their time and personal information to contribute to a larger whole. To then punish these volunteers will undoubtedly eliminate the chance that others will volunteer in the future. As such, the public good of research cannot be realized because of a predominantly private sector interest.

Employment. Between 1980 and 1990, the cost to employers of providing medical and dental insurance increased by more than 150%.[31] By 1993, health insurance benefits comprised 7% of employee wages and benefits.[32] As a result of these stifling increases and because most employer health insurance plans are rated by the experience of the group, it is to an employer's advantage to have as healthy a workforce as possible. This has led some employers to offer health promotion plans at work, which could be beneficial for job productivity as well as insurance costs, but in other instances it has led employers to try to eliminate detectable and expensive risks from their insured employee pools. Indeed, increasing numbers of employers are engaging in medical screening in an attempt to keep high-risk individuals out of the workforce.[33]

As described above, between half and two-thirds of employees with health insurance receive their health insurance through self-insured arrangements. ERISA prohibits both commercially insured and self-insured employers from discriminating against an employee to deny the employee benefits under a covered welfare plan; this includes firing or not promoting an employee because the employee would generate more health care costs for the employer. Applicants for employment are not covered by these ERISA protections. Thus, according to ERISA, it would not be illegal for an employer not to hire an otherwise qualified applicant because it was expected that the applicant would make more expensive than average health care claims. (Some protections from the Americans with Disabilities Act are relevant, however. These are discussed below.)

This is not to say that, once employed, someone covered under a self-insured plan can assume that all health expenses will be covered. Indeed, the courts have held that employers can change their benefits precisely in response to an employee's claims to treat an expensive condition and that they do so within the limits of the law. The case of McGann v. H & H Music Co. involved a man, John McGann, who was employed by a small company in Texas.[34] At some point after McGann learned he was infected with HIV he began to make claims using his employer-based health insurance. Because the employer policy was experience rated, the premiums for the entire group were raised considerably the following year. The employer responded to this increase by switching from traditional indemnity insurance to self-insurance. By virtue of self-insuring, the employer was able to modify the insurance plan even after a covered employee had begun to submit claims. Therefore, whereas the employer's previous indemnity plan had provided coverage of up to $1 million for any medical condition, the new self-funded plan provided coverage of up to $1 million for all medical conditions except AIDS, for which a limit of $5,000 coverage was imposed.

John McGann (and, later, his estate) brought charges alleging that ERISA had been violated on the grounds that ERISA prohibits employers from discriminating against any insured person who is exercising the rights to which he or she is entitled under self-insurance. The court of appeals ruled in favor of McGann's employer. The court acknowledged that the employer had changed its policy directly in response to McGann's claims and also acknowledged that, as far as anyone knew, McGann was the only employee of H & H Music to be HIV-infected. Nonetheless, the court ruled that the practice of changing benefits *even after an employee had been making claims* was allowable under ERISA, so long as it was designed to apply to a class of individuals (that is, to all HIV-infected employees) rather than singling out any individual by name for a limitation of benefits.

The McGann case received a great deal of publicity because it so clearly highlighted the vulnerability of employees in self-insured arrangements. The result has been calls for ERISA reform,[35] including proposals that self-insurers be required to treat all medical conditions identically (that is, to have a single, consistent coverage limit for all conditions, rather than being able to cover one condition for one amount and another condition for a lesser amount); also, reform should make it impossible for benefits to be changed after an insured person has already been making claims. Once individuals begin to make claims, it is unlikely that they will be able to obtain coverage elsewhere; at the same time, they typically will not have sought alternative coverage earlier because, according to the "old" policy, their health care needs were covered.

The Americans with Disabilities Act (ADA) was passed in 1990 and took effect for most employers in 1992.[36] It was not the intent of the ADA to limit the discrimination routinely practiced by insurance companies. Nonetheless, the ADA does protect job applicants from employers who might otherwise want to use disability or perceived disability as a reason for not hiring an applicant, even if the employer's justification was that the prospective employee's medical history would cause insurance premiums to increase. Indeed, until an offer of employment has been made, the ADA forbids employers from inquiring about any aspect of the job applicant's medical history other than those directly relevant to the performance of employment. Once an offer of employment has been made, employers not only can demand a full medical examination but also can require the prospective employee to release previous medical records to the employer. Nonetheless, an offer of employment cannot be withdrawn for medical reasons (including, obviously, that those medical reasons would increase insurance or health claim costs) unless, again, the medical reason is germane to the nature of the employment.[37]

Further protections are available through the Health Insurance Portability and Accountability Act of 1996. Before passage of this bill, job mobility was inhibited for persons with genetic and other medical conditions. Indeed, a Gallup poll conducted in 1991 revealed that 19% of respondents reported that fear of losing health insurance benefits kept them from changing jobs, and a *New York Times/CBS News* poll found that the loss of health insurance prevented 30% of respondents or someone in their household from changing jobs.[38]

The Health Insurance Portability and Accountability Act is intended to help people who have had health insurance through work keep that insurance if they leave or lose their jobs. It does *not* increase access for persons who have been uninsured. Under the act, employer-based health insurance policies can have preexisting condition waiting periods for no longer than 12 months (for health maintenance organizations the waiting period cannot exceed two months). A preexisting condition is defined by the act as a condition that was diagnosed or treated in the past six months and specifically excludes genetic susceptibility without a diagnosis from the definition. Once an employee has satisfied the preexisting condition waiting period (that is, once he or she has worked for a given employer at least 12 months), he or she can change jobs and will *not* have a waiting period at the next job. This change should be helpful for persons with genetic conditions who have experienced "job lock"—the unwillingness to change jobs because they would not qualify for health insurance at the new place of employment. Also, if a person leaves a job where he or she had health insurance and wants to apply for an individual health insurance policy, he or she first must buy continuation coverage pursuant to the Consolidated Omnibus Budget Reconciliation Act (COBRA) of 1985 for 18 months, continuing his or her previous coverage.[39] After 18 months of COBRA coverage, the employee can buy an individual plan and, again, not be subject to any preexisting condition exclusions or waiting periods. Although this change potentially increases access for those who would like the flexibility to leave their jobs, there are no price controls on individual policies. Therefore, although individual insurance policies must be made available to a person who leaves a job where he or she was covered, those policies could be priced at unaffordable rates.

LEGAL REFORM

Because of the problems associated with access to health insurance for people with medical conditions or risk factors, several states have proposed or passed reform regulations or legislation. In some instances, the regulations are directed specifically to genetic conditions; in others, they apply to all medical conditions. Legislation related to genetic conditions first focused on preventing insurers from denying insurance if an applicant carried a recessive trait (e.g., sickle-cell, thalassemia-minor, hemoglobin C, Tay-Sachs), following the rationale that the trait did not lead to an increased likelihood of using health care services.[40] Such legislation, however, assumed that if there was an actuarial justification for rating persons differently, then such rating was acceptable. Not until relatively recently did legislation attempt to address this latter issue.

Probably the most comprehensive legislation was passed in Wisconsin. A Wisconsin law of 1991 prohibits health insurers from requiring an individual to obtain a genetic test, requiring an individual to submit the results of a genetic test conducted elsewhere, or conditioning the provision of health insurance coverage, benefits, or rates on genetic testing.[41] A handful of other states have passed legislation incorporating at least some of these protections, and yet others have proposed comparable bills. That there is a recent trend to protect against *genetic* discrimination has raised the question of whether people with genetic conditions or traits deserve special protection compared with persons with other medical conditions or risks. On one hand, it has been argued that genetic risks are special, in that they confer risk much earlier, even from birth, and so the magnitude of discrimination with genetic conditions is potentially much greater. On the other hand, a medical risk is a medical risk, and if it becomes symptomatic, persons need health (or life) insurance equally, regardless of the origin of the disease.

Broader reform is needed to ensure greater access to health insurance for all persons with medical conditions or risk factors. As described above, preexisting condition exclusions could be universally prohibited (rather than only when insured persons changed jobs); mandating universal (even if not providing universal) health insurance; and significantly reforming ERISA, so that self-insured employers could not change benefits once claims have been initiated and would be subject to the same requirements as other insurance providers. Although ERISA reform specifically would need to occur at the federal level, many other types of health reform could be and have been approached at the state level.[42]

In Europe and Canada, where health insurance coverage is universal, questions concerning the appropriate use of genetic screening by insurers focus almost exclusively on life insurance. Of note, the sentiment is for life insurance companies to be prohibited from testing individuals for genetic conditions as well as from asking individuals questions about personal histories of genetic testing. The World Medical Association adopted this position in 1992.[43] In Canada, it has been proposed that underwriting be prohibited for life insurance policies below a certain size, with the size being based on the applicant's financial status.[44] In 1989, the European Parliament declared that insurance companies have no right to demand genetic testing as a condition of eligibility for insurance, nor should insurers have the right to be informed either of any previous test results or about genetic data the applicant or policyholder may know of.[45] Finally, several European countries have explicitly prohibited the use of genetic testing information by insurance companies, whereas in others, insurance companies have adopted a voluntary moratorium.[46] At the same time, practices in Europe, though interesting and important for American policy makers to observe, may not be in sync with the legislative agenda of the United States.

CONCLUSION

With the rise of more sophisticated genetic technology, and with no abatement in the number of uninsured persons, Americans have clear choices to make about how health care will be financed in the future and how differently to consider life from health insurance. New genetic technology may highlight the prevalence of risk factors among so many persons that screening and exclusions begin to seem ridiculous; alternatively, the technology simply may be incorporated into existing insurance practices, resulting in exclusions for even more people. Until reforms are implemented, individuals should seriously consider the implications of a positive genetic screening test, even if only a susceptibility-conferring test, on their ability to access both health and life insurance before agreeing to be tested in any setting.

NOTES

1. U.S. Department of Health and Human Services and U.S. Department of Energy, *Understanding Our Genetic Inheritance: The U.S. Human Genome Project: The First Five Years*, NIH publication no. 90–1590 (Bethesda, Md.: National Institutes of Health, 1989).
2. Nancy E. Kass, "Insurance for the Insurers: The Use of Genetic Tests," *Hastings Center Report* 22 (1992): 6–11; Thomas H. Murray, "Genetics and the Moral Mission of Health Insurance," *Hastings Center Report* 22 (1992): 12–17; Harry Ostrer et al., "Insurance and Genetic Testing: Where Are We Now?" *American Journal of Human Genetics* 52 (1993): 565–77; NIH-DOE Working Group on Ethical, Legal, and Social Implications of Human Genome Research, *Genetic Information and Health Insurance: Report of the Task Force on Genetic Information and Insurance* (Washington, D.C.: National Institutes of Health, 1993).
3. U.S. Bureau of the Census, *Statistical Abstract of the United States: 1995* (Washington, D.C.: Government Printing Office, 1995).
4. Ibid.
5. U.S. Congress, Office of Technology Assessment, "AIDS and Health Insurance: An OTA Survey" (staff paper, February 1988), 25.
6. Office of Technology Assessment, U.S. Congress, *Medical Testing and Health Insurance* (Washington, D.C.: Government Printing Office, 1988).
7. Sylvia A. Law, *Blue Cross: What Went Wrong?* (New Haven: Yale University Press, 1976).
8. Harvie Raymond, assistant vice president of the Health Insurance Association of America, "HIAA Statement on Genetic Testing and Genetic Information," Testimony before the Senate Cancer Coalition, U.S. Senate, Sept. 29, 1995, 3.
9. See, e.g., Md. Code Ann., art. 48A, § 223(a)(1) (Michie 1995).

10. Karen A. Clifford and Russel P. Iuculano, "AIDS and Insurance: The Rationale for AIDS-related Testing," *Harvard Law Review* 100 (1987): 1806.

11. Employee Retirement Income Security Act, 29 U.S.C. § 1101 *et seq.* (1994).

12. Dale A. Rublee, "Self-Funded Health Benefit Plans," *Journal of the American Medical Association* 255 (1986): 787–89; Lawrence O. Gostin and Alan I. Widiss, "What's Wrong with the ERISA Vacuum?" *Journal of the American Medical Association* 269 (1993): 2527–32; Ostrer et al., "Insurance and Genetic Testing."

13. Paul v. Virginia, 75 U.S. (8 Wall) 168 (1869), as cited in A. L. Mayerson, "State Laws and Health Insurance," *Private Health Insurance and Medical Care,* conference papers (Washington, D.C.: U.S. Department of Health, Education and Welfare, 1968), 20.

14. United States v. S.E. Underwriters Ass'n, 322 U.S. 533 (1944); 15 U.S.C. § 1101 (1994).

15. Lewin and Associates, *Nationwide Survey of State Health Regulations* (contract no. HEW-OS-73–212, Sept. 16, 1974).

16. Ad Hoc Committee on Genetic Testing/Insurance Issues, "Background Statement: Genetic Testing and Insurance," *American Journal of Human Genetics* 56 (1995): 327–31.

17. American Council on Life Insurance, *Life Insurance Fact Book, 1990* (Washington, D.C.: ACLI, 1991).

18. Ad Hoc Committee on Genetic Testing/Insurance Issues, 1995.

19. Ibid.; U.S. Congress, Office of Technology Assessment, *Cystic Fibrosis and DNA Tests: Implications of Carrier Screening* (Washington, D.C.: Government Printing Office, 1992).

20. Jean E. McEwen, Katharine McCarty, and Philip R. Reilly, "A Survey of Medical Directors of Life Insurance Companies Concerning Use of Genetic Information," *American Journal of Human Genetics* 53 (1993): 33–45.

21. J. Alexander Lowden, "Genetic Testing," *Science* 265 (1994): 1509.

22. Jean E. McEwen, Katharine McCarty, and Philip R. Reilly, "A Survey of State Insurance Commissioners Concerning Genetic Testing and Life Insurance," *American Journal of Human Genetics* 51 (1992): 785–92.

23. McEwen, McCarty, and Reilly, "Survey of Medical Directors."

24. Randall R. Bovjberg and C. F. Koller, "State Health Insurance Pools: Current Performance, Future Prospects," *Inquiry* 23 (1986) 111–21.

25. *The President's Health Security Plan: The Clinton Blueprint* (New York: Times Books, 1993).

26. Ruth Faden, Nancy Kass, and Madison Powers, "Warrants for Screening Programs: Public Health, Legal and Ethical Frameworks," in Ruth Faden, Gail Geller, and Madison Powers, eds., *AIDS, Women and the Next Generation: Towards a Morally Acceptable Public Policy for HIV Testing of Pregnant Women and Newborns* (New York: Oxford University Press, 1991), 3–26.

27. J. H. Blaine, "AIDS: Regulatory Issues for Life and Health Insurers," *AIDS and Public Policy Journal* 2 (1987): 2–10.

28. The exception to this, of course, would be if regulations were passed specifically exempting any information gathered through research for eligibility purposes.

29. See Bower v. Roy-Al Corp., 109 Cal. Rptr. 612 (Cal. 1973); and Cardamone v. Allstate Ins. Co., 364 N.E.2d 460 (Ill. App. 1977).

30. Public Health Service Act, 42 U.S.C. § 241(d) (1994). Special protection will be granted "sparingly" to research projects of a "sensitive nature where the protection is judged necessary to achieve the research objectives." Examples of the types of research that may qualify are those that collect "information relating to sexual attitudes, preferences, or practices; alcohol, drugs, or other addictive products; illegal conduct; information that if released could reasonably be damaging to an individual's financial standing, employ-ability, or reputation; information that would normally be recorded in a patient's medical record, and the disclosure of which could reasonably lead to social stigmatiza-tion or discrimination; information pertaining to an individual's psychological well-being or mental health." Researchers who have obtained a certificate of confidentiality "may not be compelled in any Federal, State, or other local civil, criminal, administra-tive, legislative or other proceedings to identify [research participants]."

31. U.S. Chamber of Commerce, *Employee Benefits, 1989 Edition* (Washington, D.C.: Gov-ernment Printing Office, 1989).

32. U.S. Bureau of the Census, *Statistical Abstract, 1995*.

33. Mark A. Rothstein, *Medical Screening and the Employee Health Cost Crisis* (Washington, D.C.: BNA Books, 1989).

34. McGann v. H & H Music Co., 946 F.2d 401 (5th Cir. 1991), *cert. denied sub nom.,* Greenberg v. H & H Music Co., 506 U.S. 981 (1992).

35. Gostin and Widiss, "What's Wrong with the ERISA Vacuum?"

36. 42 U.S.C. § 12101 et seq. (1994).

37. See Mark A. Rothstein, "The Law of Medical and Genetic Privacy in the Workplace," Chapter 15 in this volume.

38. Philip F. Cooper and Alan C. Monheit, "Does Employment-Related Health Insurance Inhibit Job Mobility?" *Inquiry* 30 (1993): 400–416.

39. The Consolidated Omnibus Reconciliation Act of 1985 (P.L. 99–272) mandates that persons who had been receiving their health insurance through work be offered the option, when ceasing employment, of continuing with the same insurance policy for up to 18 months at their own expense.

40. See, e.g., Md. Code Ann. art. 48A, § 223(b)(4) (1986).

41. Karen H. Rothenberg, "Genetic Information and Health Insurance: State Legislative Approaches," *Journal of Law, Medicine and Ethics* 23 (1995): 312.

43. Deborah L. Rogal and W. David Helms, "State Models: Tracking States' Efforts to Reform Their Health Systems," *Health Affairs* 12 (1993): 27–30.

43. World Medical Association, *Declaration on the Human Genome Project,* adopted by the 44th World Medical Assembly, Marbella, Spain, Sept. 1992, as cited in Mark A. Roths-tein and Bartha Maria Knoppers, "Legal Aspects of Genetics, Work, and Insurance in North America and Europe," *European Journal of Health Law* 3 (1996): 23.

44. Rothstein and Knoppers, "Legal Aspects of Genetics."

45. Ibid.

46. Ibid.

Chapter 17 Genetic Information in Schools

Laura F. Rothstein

Although little genetic information is being systematically collected or used in educational settings, this could change at any time. Well meaning but unthinking school officials could adopt programs of genetic screening or genetic classification of students. School officials also could acquiesce in commercial pressures by facilitating the collection of genetic information about students. The possibility of using genetic information in schools, obtained or maintained for any reason, raises a variety of important ethical, legal, and social issues that are poorly addressed by current policy.

WHY SCHOOLS WOULD ACQUIRE, HAVE, OR USE GENETIC INFORMATION

Educational purposes. A school could acquire, have, or use genetic information for four main reasons. If a school has genetic information about a condition such as dyslexia or fragile X syndrome, it may be able to provide appropriate educational programming for a particular child. If the school personnel believe that the basis for a child's weak academic performance is genetic, then the school may be able to intervene more appropriately in programming the child's education. Arguably, if problems are identified before a child begins school, difficulties can be anticipated and planned for.[1] Diagnosing dyslexia through nongenetic means usually occurs only once a child is about eight years old. If diagnosis were to occur at a much earlier age through genetic testing, it is believed that interventions would be much more effective. Early speech and language therapy and physical therapy may be positive interventions for children with fragile X syndrome.

The second purpose for using genetic information is that where conditions relate to potential behavioral and disciplinary problems, the school can provide more appropriate behavior management or observe a particular child more closely in anticipation of problems.[2] In most cases, behavior will also affect educational development because it will affect the child's ability to focus and understand. Children with fragile X syndrome have been shown to have positive behavior changes when treated with folic acid.[3] Benefits also have been shown to derive from taking methylphenidate (Ritalin), dextroamphetamine (Dexedrine), and pemoline (Cylert). Identifying fragile X syndrome as the basis for certain behaviors also may ensure that appropriate behavior management techniques (e.g., "time outs") are used.

The third educational purpose relates to conditions that involve health impairments. The benefit of knowing such information is that the school can provide appropriate related services, such as diagnosis and physical therapy, for children whose health or physical ability has been adversely affected. If public health agencies were to provide population-wide information about the incidence of certain types of health impairment in a state based on genetic screening at birth, schools would be better able to budget and plan for related services in anticipation of the entry of these children into public schools.

The fourth reason relates to accountability. Schools must measure abilities and performance to meet the mandates of school excellence expectations as well as to obtain funds under special education laws.[4] Having a genetic marker for certain conditions may in theory assist in better measuring students' eligibility for special education and for determining which students should and should not be held to certain performance expectations.

Noneducational purposes. Schools may in turn be able to provide genetic information to other social service agencies for public health services and planning. If public health officials were convinced that genetic screening of children promoted public health, then schools would be the ideal setting in which to conduct such screening. In almost every state schools already screen children for various public health purposes, including conducting screenings for tuberculosis and scoliosis, as well as dental, vision, and hearing tests.[5]

Public health screening agencies could plan for appropriate interventions in response to the information they obtained through screening. It could be argued that schools are the logical screening and intervention point for many public health issues because (with the exception of children in home schooling) they are the one institution in which everyone is mandated by law to participate. Though not educational in nature, such programs as comprehensive vaccination efforts benefit society as a whole.

By screening all individuals of school age for certain conditions, public service providers could plan for future needs and requirements.[6] For example, if children were screened for certain cancers, the medical community could plan for the required services. If there were comprehensive screening for various late-onset genetic disorders, such as Alzheimer's disease, society at large could make preparations for the number of individuals expected to develop the disorders. Not only could society at large make general preparations, but in some cases, individuals with the genetic marker could begin planning for services.

Schools might also facilitate genetic testing and screening by others for monetary reasons. It is not hard to imagine commercial enterprises providing financial and other incentives to schools to allow them to gain access to children or the names of children with certain genetic traits. In a case involving the Genentech Corporation, schools facilitated the acquisition of information about children who were unusually short for their age. The school board approved the school nurse's provision of information about children's heights, which Genentech then used in marketing its human growth hormone.[7]

There are risks associated with commercial interests joining forces with the schools. Even assuming that the schools' motives are entirely benign, in most cases the administrators who grant permission to carry out such evaluations probably do not appreciate the consequences. One need only think of how television sets and commercial programming have found their way into many schools to realize that financially strapped schools are not averse to exploring opportunities for economic support. This in turn brings to mind the *Jurassic Park* problem: when commercial interests use science, they are unlikely to think through the moral and ethical implications of what they are doing.[8]

PROBLEMS WITH CURRENT POLICIES REGARDING GENETIC INFORMATION

Lack of informed consent. Testing or screening for genetic information by entities conducting federally funded research must be performed pursuant to federal guidelines.[9] Many states have implemented further mandates. A basic requirement of these guidelines is informed consent. Informed consent requires the researcher to explain the purpose and procedure of the research, the foreseeable risks or discomforts, the possible benefits to the research subject or others, the confidentiality of the information obtained, the compensation and medical treatment available should injury occur, the names of research contacts, and information about voluntariness.[10]

The informed consent "safeguard" has a number of problems. Paperwork for informed consent will probably be inadequately completed by those doing and facilitating genetic screening and testing programs. It is questionable whether parents really would understand the "risks, benefits, efficacy, and alternatives to the testing" and whether they will be given "information about the potential variability, . . . treatability . . . , information about the subsequent decisions that will be likely if the test is positive . . . , and information about any potential conflicts of interest of the person or institution offering the test."[11] Testing and screening children raises additional questions about the role the children themselves should have in giving consent or permission.[12]

Although obtaining information about a child's genotype through analysis of epithelial cells in buccal swabs is not physically risky to the child, there are substantial risks relating to discrimination (against the child and other family members), stigmatization, and other psychological and personal harm. Are these risks being disclosed? Does the law require that they be?

Regardless of legal requirements, private companies that engage in genetic testing and screening facilitated by schools should disclose any potential conflicts of interest. Do they manufacture products (such as drugs) or provide services (such as counseling) for which an individual with the tested-for genetic marker would be a potential consumer? If so, are they disclosing this information to the individual? Is this a conflict of interest? If so, should such a conflict merely be disclosed or should it be prohibited?

The biggest problem with the informed consent requirement is that it may not be applicable in school settings because federal human subjects guidelines apply only to federally funded research. There is no comparable protection for privately funded research facilitated by schools. In addition, even where guidelines apply, there is little recourse for any violation. It will be little comfort to the parent of a child whose genetic profile is available on the Internet to know that federal funding for the project is being discontinued because the company violated human research protocols.

Genetic markers are unlike other conditions that can be identified through testing, screening, and evaluation programs. The presence of a certain genetic marker may mean not only that the child is directly affected but also that other family members may be either affected or heterozygous carriers of recessive or X-linked disorders. This could have serious repercussions for other relatives in a variety of ways.[13] As discussed elsewhere in this volume, genetic information could be used as the basis for denying health or life insurance. Although various health conditions may be used to deny insurance for the affected individual, genetic markers have the potential to identify other individuals as having the same characteristic, thereby increasing an insurance company's motivation to deny coverage.

Inappropriate responses by schools. In addition to the problem of discrimination, a number of concerns are related to social and familial responses to genetic information. This involves the conduct of parents and other family members toward the child with the genetic condition as well as toward other children.[14] These issues are discussed at length in chapter 14. Of concern here is the response of the educational agency.

The first issue is the accuracy of the information. Schools may be under political or economic pressure to adopt unproven testing technologies. Even pilot programs should not be implemented without a thorough consideration of the methodology and the potential costs and benefits to the individuals tested and their families.

Second, it is essential that educational agencies understand the difficulty of using even accurate information about genetic conditions to predict the expressivity of the condition.[15] Does having a certain genotype mean that it will be expressed? What is the age of onset? What is the range of severity of the resulting condition? Is it treatable or likely to be treatable in the future? What other factors (environmental, social, psychological, and other genetic conditions) might be relevant in answering any of these questions?[16] Without adequate responses to these questions, any educational intervention would likely be inadequate or inappropriate.

In addition to the educational intervention for the children themselves, what systems are in place to provide counseling and parental education about the options for responding to the identification of a genetic condition?[17] For example, if a child is identified as having fragile X syndrome and the condition has already expressed itself in educational delays and behavior problems, is the school prepared to respond appropriately? Will it provide educational intervention, such as speech therapy and behavior management, as well as recommending drug therapy? Will it also provide counseling for the parents about the long-term effects of the condition, the side effects of the drugs, and how to go about getting financial coverage to pay for drugs and other interventions not provided directly by the schools? Are schools and health care providers prepared to advise parents that by encouraging certain drug therapies, they may risk insurance problems and even employment discrimination?

The fourth concern relates to the long-standing problem of labeling and the self-fulfilling prophecy. By identifying a genetic factor in a child's educational development, will the school and the parents begin to have lowered or different expectations for the child?[18] For example, if a child is identified as having the allele for dyslexia, will this change (even unintentionally) the school's steering of the child toward college preparation or away from certain careers? Similarly, a school may inappropriately base its educational programming on the presumed consequences of a genetic marker. The result may be that the expectations of the student are not sufficiently high, and the self-fulfilling prophecy will occur. For example, a child identified as having the allele for fragile X syndrome or dyslexia may be placed in a remedial program before it is clear that the child needs it. There is, of course, the dilemma relating to the value of early intervention. A child who is dyslexic will almost certainly benefit from intervention before age five or six, the earliest age at which dyslexia is currently identified by evaluation techniques other than genetic testing. It is thus essential that more be known about how particular conditions are expressed before applying educational programming that may be inappropriate for a particular child.

The fifth concern is the danger that always inheres when a test or technique seems to be a clear identification of a problem.[19] It is critical that educators look at such factors as environment, home life, and nutrition before assuming that the sole or even primary reason for a particular level of development results from a genetic predisposition. This is particularly important because many conditions relevant to school-age children, such as learning disabilities and behavior disorders, may be multifactorial. Thus a combination of genetic, environmental, and social factors may be required for a certain condition or behavior to manifest. As with IQ testing, there is a danger that too much will be made of a test that seems to indicate clear and certain information about a child's intelligence, behavior, or abilities.[20]

A sixth concern related to educational response is that the needs of those children who lack the identifying genetic marker will not be adequately addressed. A child who is developmentally delayed or whose behavior is inappropriate and who has not been identified as having a genetic marker to explain the condition may not receive the same attention and intervention as the child whose condition seems to be genetically related. The genetic condition may seem more "real" to the school and thus more likely to merit intervention.

Privacy and confidentiality. Genetic information is unlike other information, including other forms of medical information, that is routinely kept in school files. Not only is it sensitive and stigmatizing about the individual child, but it can reveal information about relatives and their genetic traits.

Before any program authorizes or facilitates the collection of genetic information about schoolchildren, it must be demonstrated that the information is directly related to a legitimate educational purpose and that the benefits of collecting and using the genetic information outweigh any potential harms. Such a policy differs from public health screening in schools by recognizing the unique nature of genetic information. Schoolchildren and their parents should not be coerced directly or indirectly into permitting access by third parties to extremely private and potentially stigmatizing information. The possibility that genetic information could be improperly disclosed is a compelling reason for not obtaining the information in the first place. As discussed below, current policy is inadequate to ensure that improper disclosures will not occur.

For example, genetic testing for common learning disabilities might not seem to raise serious privacy and confidentiality problems. Nevertheless, some cases of learning disability are associated with disorders of chromosomal number, including Klinefelter syndrome and Turner syndrome.[21] Individuals with Klinefelter syndrome have the karyotype 47,XXY, and their phenotype is male, although they carry an extra female chromosome and are frequently sterile and have other reproductive problems. Individuals with Turner syndrome are phenotypically female and have the karyotype 45,X. They often have reproductive problems as well as other disorders. Conditions like these would carry a great deal of stigma if information about them were to be disclosed.

These concerns are not merely hypothetical. A case decided in 1996 involved a 12-year-old girl whose severe emotional and behavioral problems were caused by an underlying condition of hermaphroditism. Unhappy with her daughter's educational plan, the mother requested a due process hearing, at which time the hearing officer entered a protective order prohibiting the disclosure of the girl's confidential records. Nevertheless, the superintendent of the school district and other members of the school board allegedly discussed the girl's medical condition and educational placement with a newspaper reporter. Although thus far the court has ruled only that the Family Educational Rights and Privacy Act (discussed in more detail later) may be the basis for a civil rights action, the facts surrounding this case illustrate the danger of having such sensitive information in the hands of school officials.[22]

If a school were to perform genetic testing or screening or facilitate such evaluation, where would the records go? Would they become part of the student's school records?[23] Would they become part of the child's medical records? If a private entity were doing the evaluation, would that entity be the sole custodian of the records?

Not only who has custody of this information is important but what that custodian can do with it. Will a private testing entity with information about certain genetic markers be able to use this information to market services (e.g., counseling) or products (e.g., drugs)? Will such an entity be permitted to sell lists of individuals identified with certain markers to other private entities? Will insurance companies or employers have access to this information? What safeguards will there be to ensure that this information is not given to those who are not permitted to have it, particularly in the light of access on the Internet? What remedies will be available if violations of policy or legal requirements occur?

Stigma and discrimination. Related to the issues of privacy and confidentiality are issues of stigma and discrimination resulting from identifying individuals as having genetically related conditions.[24] When a Florida community learned that a family had three sons with AIDS resulting from blood transfusions, the hostility was so severe that some residents burned down the family home. Although genetic conditions are not "contagious" in the same way that AIDS is, it is not difficult to imagine a scenario in which it becomes known that a teenage boy has the allele for fragile X syndrome or Huntington disease and parents forbid their daughters to date the boy.[25]

Other stigmatizing and discriminatory actions could well result from knowledge about certain genetic conditions. A teacher or a school counselor, knowing that a student has the allele for amyotrophic lateral sclerosis (Lou Gehrig's disease), might be less likely to encourage or counsel that student into certain professions, such as medicine, because the student may be expected to have a shorter life or diminished ability by age 40.

Will other family members (e.g., siblings, cousins) be entitled to access to this genetic information if it is necessary to perform genetic linkage studies?

What if they do *not* want to know? How is that interest to be protected without safeguards on keeping such information confidential?

Finally, there is a danger that only the negative aspects of having certain genetic markers will be considered, whereas in fact certain genetic conditions that have negative consequences may also have benefits. For example, the mutation for sickle cell trait is also believed to be beneficial in protecting against malaria; the mutation for cystic fibrosis may be protective against cholera. Although individuals with attention deficit hyperactivity disorder (ADHD) are impulsive, "popular books and lectures about ADHD often point out positive aspects of the condition. Adults see themselves as creative; their impulsiveness can be viewed as spontaneity; hyperactivity gives them enormous energy and drive; even their distractibility has the virtue of making them alert to changes in the environment."[26] If a genetic marker for ADHD were to be identified, the negative as well as the positive effects of using drug therapy as a response should be considered.

Although federal legislation responds to some of the benefits and concerns related to knowledge about an individual's genetic status, existing policies must be adapted to account for this new technology and its availability and use, and new policies will probably need to be developed.

LAWS RELATING TO GENETIC INFORMATION AND SCHOOLS

Special education laws. There are currently five main types of laws that relate to the issue of genetic information in schools. The Individuals with Disabilities Education Act (IDEA) requires that appropriate educational programming be provided to all age-eligible children in the least restrictive environment at no cost to the parents. The programming must be individualized and there must be procedural safeguards, which include notice and impartial hearing and a review process in place. States that obtain federal funding under IDEA must meet these requirements. All states have elected to do so.[27]

Under IDEA, states are required to engage in efforts to seek out and find all children eligible for special education services. These "child-find" mandates might be applied with respect to some conditions that are known to or believed to be related to genetic markers. Unlike PKU (phenylketonuria) screening, which is currently mandated in most states and which has a high positive predictive value, available treatment and screening for such conditions as attention deficit disorder, ADHD, and learning disabilities are much more problematic. Even if genetic markers for these conditions are discovered, the implications for expressivity will not be known for some time, if ever. It is not clear what that will mean for the purposes of "child-find" mandates. The same is likely to be true for genetic markers for fragile X syndrome and for markers that may relate to some mental illnesses and behavior and predispositions to addictive behavior.[28]

Will schools have an obligation to conduct screening for markers in those cases where expressivity would likely affect a child's education? Will they have an obligation to coordinate with other agencies under the infant and toddler child-find mandates of the IDEA? These questions raise significant legal and ethical questions, but also questions about resources. Will funding be available to conduct comprehensive genetic screening? Should it be?

Discrimination laws. The second type of law is disability discrimination law. The Americans with Disabilities Act (ADA) of 1990 and section 504 of the Rehabilitation Act of 1973 are statutes prohibiting programs subject to their mandates from discriminating against otherwise qualified individuals on the basis of disability. Title II of the ADA applies to state and local governmental agencies, which means that public schools are subject to the ADA. Title III applies to public accommodations operated by private entities. This covers most private schools. The majority of schools are covered by section 504 of the Rehabilitation Act, which applies to recipients of federal financial assistance. Most public schools receive such assistance through a variety of pass-through funding programs from the states. Private schools are often subject to section 504 by virtue of funding for school lunch programs, Head Start, and so forth.[29]

Both the ADA and the Rehabilitation Act protect individuals with substantial impairments of major life activities, those having a record of such an impairment, or those who are regarded as having such an impairment.[30] The ADA also protects individuals who associate with someone who is considered to be disabled under the ADA.[31] Certain conditions that are genetically based are clearly covered by both nondiscrimination laws. For example, a child with Down's syndrome or cystic fibrosis is almost certainly protected against discrimination by the schools. It is far from clear, however, whether there is coverage for a child with a genetic marker for a condition that is not necessarily severe (such as polydactyly), that has variable expressivity or penetrance (such as fragile X syndrome), or that is late onset (such as myotonic dystrophy) or for a child who is an unaffected carrier of a recessive or X-linked disorder.

Although some advocates have recommended a clarification that both statutes should protect individuals based on certain genetic disorders because such individuals fall within the category of those who are perceived or regarded as having a disability, federal policy makers have yet to directly adopt such recommendations in the context of students.[32] Until the status of individuals with genetic markers for certain impairments is clarified under these statutes, courts may well be inconsistent in their treatment of such individuals as protected against discrimination on the basis of disability.

A child with a genetic marker, such as for Huntington disease, that is known to a school counselor who then counseled the child away from a career as a physician would not be protected under IDEA but might be protected under the ADA or section 504 of the Rehabilitation Act.

Laws regarding school records. The third type of law is educational privacy protection. The Family Educational Rights and Privacy Act (FERPA), which is popularly referred to as the Buckley Amendment, covers access to and accuracy of school records.[33] Under this act, individuals (or their parents in the case of minors) have a right to know what is in their records, have a right to ensure that such information is accurate, and have a right to prevent those without an educational need to know from obtaining those records without permission.

There are a number of problems with this statute as an insurance policy against preventing access to genetic information by various parties. First, FERPA applies only to recipients of federal financial assistance. Second, most courts have not allowed individuals to obtain private remedies for violations of FERPA. Third, it is unclear whether certain genetic information would be classified as part of a student educational record or whether it would be considered a medical record. If it were a medical record, then state laws relating to access to and privacy of medical records would apply. It could be argued that if the genetic information were used as part of an evaluation for educational programming, it would be a school record, but this is far from settled.

FERPA and state medical record laws establish rules related to who has access to these records, procedures for parents of minor children to ensure the accuracy of such records, and timetables for the destruction of certain records. Of grave concern to children whose genetic information might end up in a school record or even a separate medical record maintained in school files would be a waiver that granted parties outside the educational agency access to or copies of certain information.[34] For example, if a parent gave the school permission to send the child's records to an insurance company, the parent may not realize that the insurance company could use certain genetic information that might be in the student's record as the basis for denying the parents health or life insurance.[35]

Laws regarding human research and informed consent. The fourth type of statutory protection involves human subject laws and informed consent laws in the health care system. Federal protection of human subjects from abuses in experimental treatment and research is found primarily under Health and Human Services (HHS) regulations adopted in 1981.[36] Separate but related regulations have been developed for special populations, including children (in 1983), and proposed for individuals with certain types of disabilities.[37] The intent of these regulations is to ensure that when research is conducted on humans, the subjects are not placed at undue risk, that they adequately understand the risks and benefits involved, and that they are competent to make decisions about being subjected to such research and consent to research or evaluation voluntarily.[38]

Each institution conducting such research must establish an institutional review board (IRB) to oversee that these requirements are followed. In addition, a few states have established further regulations and laws applying to research on human subjects.

Some of the problems of relying on the HHS regulations and state law to protect human subjects against abuse related to genetic screening and testing practices are obvious. First, the requirements apply only to federally supported research. These requirements apparently do not apply to privately funded research even if it occurs in schools that receive federal financial assistance. For their part, state laws are too few and two weak. Finally, federal remedies of injunctive relief and withdrawal of federal financial assistance for violations often fail to redress adequately cases of individual harm.

Common law tort and contract actions. State common law tort and contract actions may be available. Although misuse of genetic information could in theory be the basis of a variety of common law actions, such as invasion of privacy, infliction of emotional distress, and breach of contract, this is not a viable avenue for redressing the potential resulting harms. Discussion of these issues is beyond the scope of this chapter, but it should be noted that efforts to prove the elements of these common law actions face severe hurdles. A larger obstacle is the application of immunity doctrines to public educational agencies, which would prevent financial redress, such as lost potential earnings and damages for emotional distress.

CONCLUSION

Current law contains serious gaps relating to concerns about the acquisition and use of genetic information by or through schools. Policy makers need to address a number of questions in evaluating current requirements. Obviously, these also have an impact on ethics policies that various institutions may wish to establish. The following recommendations focus primarily on policy issues to be addressed within the law.

In addition to policy changes relating to ensuring that the nondiscrimination statutes appropriately protect individuals on the basis of genetic markers, a number of areas involving confidentiality and privacy require attention.

Educational institutions should have policies that address when private evaluators can test or screen through the schools. Whether the educational agency does the testing or facilitates it, policies regarding informed consent should be in place. Informed consent should include information about the risks relating to discrimination and the potential loss of insurance or employment based on genetic information. It should also contain information about conflicts of interest. Commercial enterprises conducting genetic research through schools should be required to disclose products or services of the company that may be targeted toward individuals with the conditions being screened for. Appropriate remedies for violations of informed consent requirements also must be available.

School and medical record laws need to be amended to ensure that privacy and confidentiality concerns related to genetic information are met. These amendments should address when parents and students may have access to genetic information and when others may have access to or use the information. The laws should provide adequate protections to ensure the accuracy of genetic information. These policies should indicate when records will be destroyed and who decides about their destruction. As with informed consent policies, school and medical record policies must ensure that procedural and remedial safeguards are in place to provide protection.

New policies could be created at the federal, state, local, or institutional level. At any level, it is essential that decision makers include parents, school personnel, health professionals, social service providers, ethicists, educational psychologists, social scientists, and lawyers. Only when all affected and interested parties bring their concerns to the table will there be a thoughtful consideration of the myriad issues, including appropriate assurances that privacy and confidentiality will be protected.

NOTES

1. See Mike Toner, "Fragile X Defect Gene Discovered: Will Help Find Cause of Mental Disorder," *Atlanta Journal and Constitution,* May 30, 1991, A2.

2. See Peter S. Jensen et al., "Child and Adolescent Psychopathology Research: Problems and Prospects for the 1990s," *Journal of Abnormal Child Psychology* 21 (1993): 551.

3. See Richard J. Simensen and R. Curtis Roger, "Fragile X Syndrome," *American Family Physician* 39 (1989): 185.

4. Dorothy Nelkin, "The Social Power of Genetic Information," in Daniel J. Kevles and Leroy Hood, eds., *The Code of Codes: Scientific and Social Issues in the Human Genome Project* (Cambridge: Harvard University Press, 1992), 183; Dorothy Nelkin and Laurence Tancredi, *Dangerous Diagnostics: The Social Power of Biological Information* (New York: Basic Books, 1989), 109–12.

5. See J. R. Zanga and D. S. Oda, "School Health Services," *Journal of School Health* 57 (1987): 413, 415.

6. Fay A. Rozovsky, *Consent to Treatment: A Practical Guide,* 2d ed. (Boston: Little, Brown), 1990, 327.

7. See Gina Kolata, "Selling Growth Drug for Children: The Legal and Ethical Questions," *New York Times,* Aug. 15, 1994, A1; Ralph T. King, "In Marketing of Drugs, Genentech Tests Limits of What Is Acceptable," *Wall Street Journal,* Jan. 10, 1995, 1, col. 6; and Caroline Berry, "Gene Genie," *British Medical Journal* 306 (1993): 1699.

8. Kolata, "Selling Growth Drug"; Berry, "Gene Genie."

9. Rozovsky, *Consent to Treatment,* chap. 8.

10. 45 C.F.R. §§ 46.116 (1996).

11. Lori B. Andrews et al., eds., *Assessing Genetic Risks: Implications for Health and Social Policy* (Washington, D.C.: National Academy Press, 1994).

12. Rozovsky, *Consent to Treatment,* chap. 5, 565–77.

13. Karen H. Rothenberg and Elizabeth H. Thomson, *Women and Prenatal Testing: Facing the Challenges of Genetic Technology* (Columbus: Ohio State University Press, 1992); Kevles and Hood, *Code of Codes;* Nelkin and Tancredi, *Dangerous Diagnostics;* Dorothy C. Wertz et al., "Genetic Testing for Children and Adolescents: Who Decides?" *Journal of the American Medical Association* 272 (1994): 875; Ellen Wright Clayton, "Screening and Treatment of Newborns," *Houston Law Review* 29 (1992): 85; Diane Loupe, "Fragile X Testing Debated, Special Ed Students Screened, and Diagnosis Helps Cope with Disorder," *Atlanta Journal and Constitution,* Oct. 9, 1993, E1; Barbara Karkabi, "Face to Face with Fragile X," *Houston Chronicle,* Sept. 5, 1993, Lifestyle section, 1.

14. Clayton, "Screening and Treatment of Newborns," 109–23.

15. See, e.g., Jerome Kagan, *Galen's Prophecy: Temperament in Human Nature* (New York: Basic Books, 1994); Nelkin and Tancredi, *Dangerous Diagnostics,* chap. 6; Annette K. Taylor et al., "Molecular Predictors of Cognitive Involvement in Female Carriers of Fragile X Syndrome," *Journal of the American Medical Association* 271 (1994): 507–14; Delores C. S. James, "The Human Genome Initiative: Implications for the Comprehensive School Health Program," *Journal of School Health* 64 (1994): 80; and Carol Rust, "Exploring Windows of the Soul: The Rayid Model: A Guide to Personality," *Houston Chronicle,* Aug. 23, 1994, D1.

16. See Peter S. Jensen et al., "Child and Adolescent Psychopathology Research: Problems and Prospects for the 1990s," *Journal of Abnormal Child Psychology* 21 (1993): 551.

17. In the Institute of Medicine's study *Assessing Genetic Risks,* the issue is raised in the

context of PKU testing. In its Executive Summary, the committee recommends "that states with newborn screening programs for treatable disorders also have programs available to ensure that necessary treatment and follow-up services are provided to affected children identified through newborn screening without regard to ability to pay" (5–6). This recommendation is based on the ethical concerns about screening individuals for conditions in which either no treatment exists or there is no benefit to knowing the information or where treatment exists but is not available because of costs or other factors (260–64, 276–77).

18. See Wertz et al., "Genetic Testing for Children and Adolescents."

19. See Kagan, *Galen's Prophecy;* and Nelkin and Tancredi, *Dangerous Diagnostics,* chap. 6.

20. See Nelkin and Tancredi, *Dangerous Diagnostics,* 112–17.

21. Elaine Johansen Mange and Arthur P. Mange, *Basic Human Genetics* (Sunderland, Mass.: Sinauer, 1994), 222–27.

22. Doe v. Knox County Board of Educ., 918 F.Supp. 181 (E.D. Ky. 1996).

23. See Mary H. B. Gelfman and S. James Rosenfeld, "What You Should Know About School Records," *EDLAW Briefing Paper* (1991).

24. Wertz et al., "Genetic Testing for Children and Adolescents."

25. See Sally Lehrman, "DNA Test in Worker Safety Suit Alarms Geneticists," *Biotechnology Newswatch,* June 20, 1994, 1.

26. Claudia Wallis, "Life in Overdrive: Doctors Say Huge Numbers of Kids and Adults Have Attention Deficit Disorder: Is It for Real?" *Time,* July 18, 1994, 44.

27. 42 U.S.C. §§ 1400 et seq. (1994).

28. Thomas H. Maugh II, "Scientists Identify Hyperactivity Gene," *Houston Chronicle,* May 1, 1996, A2.

29. 42 U.S.C. §§ 12101 et seq. (1994); 29 U.S.C. § 794 (1994).

30. 42 U.S.C. §§ 706(8)(B), 12102(2) (1994).

31. 42 U.S.C. § 12182(b)(1)(E) (1994).

32. Mark A. Rothstein, "The Law of Medical and Genetic Privacy in the Workplace," Chapter 15 in this volume; Joseph S. Alper and Marvin R. Natowicz, "Genetic Discrimination and the Public Entities and Public Accommodations Titles of the Americans with Disabilities Act," *American Journal of Human Genetics* 53 (1993): 26–32.

33. 20 U.S.C. § 1232(g) (1994).

34. See Gelfman and Rosenfeld, "What You Should Know About School Records."

35. See Wertz et al., "Genetic Testing for Children and Adolescents."

36. 45 C.F.R. Part 46, Subparts B, C (1996).

37. See Wertz, "Genetic Testing for Children and Adolescents"; and Martyn Evans, "Conflicts of Interest in Research on Children," *Cambridge Quarterly of Healthcare Ethics* 3 (1993): 549–59.

38. See Rozovsky, *Consent to Treatment,* chap. 8.

Chapter 18 Courts and the Challenges of Adjudicating Genetic Testing's Secrets

Franklin M. Zweig, Joseph T. Walsh, and Daniel M. Freeman

In this chapter we consider foreseeable pressures that may be exerted upon federal and state courts in the wake of genetic information resulting from the Human Genome Project. Writ large, disputes requiring adjudication will be set in motion by a clash of megaforces: molecular genetics' implied insistence that everything be known, out in the open, and brought to market as soon as practicable; and public policy's likely insistence that zones of genetic privacy be honored and protected as a basic good and right of civil society. Social movements for privileged access to genetic information, as exemplified in the search for health histories in the adoption arena, open a third front in the roiling, fertile-for-litigation landscape. The more focused demands for genetic information in civil and criminal courtrooms illustrate some of the more intractable controversies.

The three primary forces of neurogenetic testing, genetic information privacy, and adoption information privileges all involve judges' understanding of molecular genetics and its evidentiary application in motions brought to prohibit or open disclosure of genomic information. Using the example of a death penalty case, we describe the judicial duties likely to confront both federal and state courts as genetic testing becomes a prominent health care technology. Most state and federal approaches to genetic information policy require the courts to grant or deny exceptions to genetic secrecy; manage the dispute resolution of alleged privacy infringements; and allocate remedies to parties. Such delegation to adjudication and enforcement is rooted in the knowledge that no public policy can rationalize the infinite variation of individual disputes raised by genetic testing for diseases numbering in the thousands; account for an infinite number of genetic predispositions; and probe the causes of action alleging gene-based discriminatory treatment, official and private. Inherent powers of the courts will also be marshaled to review regulatory regimes enacted in genetic information statutes.

We examine this moving firmament as a still picture of the expanding universe: knowing that it has been rendered obsolete during the time taken to develop it. We are certain, however, that clients and their lawyers will turn to the courts, and to the 30,000 judges who officiate within them, for interpretation, enforcement, and relief. New private rights of action could virtually guarantee it. We are positive, moreover, that the courts will be challenged to master the complex scientific concepts and facts embedded in molecular genetics and molecular medicine in order to adjudicate effectively the genetic information policy questions now taking form.

FORCE ONE: DEVELOPMENTS IN NEUROGENETIC TESTING

In 1996 the U.S. court system was treated by the peer-reviewed science media to a roller-coaster ride along the diverging tracks of neurogenetic testing's scientific and medical validity. The respected journal *Nature Genetics* offered the tantalizing prospect that molecular biology had discovered a hidden genetic trigger to "novelty seeking" in human personality.[1] "Novelty seeking" is one source of impulsive behavior and risk-taking that millions of presentence reports to criminal courts document routinely among repeat criminals of both the violent and nonviolent types. Two research groups reported that they had linked family histories of "novelty seeking," a cluster of impulsive, risky, and extravagant behaviors, to a genetic marker. A close association was also found between people possessing that marker and high scores on personality tests said to validly document these behaviors.[2] Moreover, American and Israeli research teams had sequenced the gene and found it to be differently constructed among people who tended to score high on tests for impulsiveness, quick-temper, and risk-taking behavior. The two teams had replicated the sequence and agreed that it had fewer repeating DNA base-pair segments among people who were described by the personality tests as being steady, cautious, and risk-averse. The reports were properly sober and cautious. The authors left no doubt, however, that they were onto an important lead on the cutting edge of the neurogenetic frontier. Genetic screening could easily follow or psychometric tests found to correlate with the genetic tests might be used as surrogates for them.

By contrast, at the end of 1995, the respected *Journal of the American Medical Association* (*JAMA*), joined by four medical specialty societies and the American Society for Human Genetics, called for a moratorium on genetic testing for Alzheimer's disease.[3] Alzheimer's disease is another mental condition familiar to civil courts charged with competency determination and appointment of guardianships for hundreds of thousands of mainly older Americans thought to have lost their minds to neurofibulary tangles and plaques that shut down their brains.[4]

For both personality and Alzheimer's genetic predispositions relevant to prosecution or litigation, courts rightly may ask what it takes to obtain a valid and reliable genetic test.[5] To be admissible at trial, the evidence produced by such tests must, under the doctrine enunciated by state jurisdictions following the famous Frye rule, find acceptance by the scientific communities relevant to them.[6] Under the much newer Daubert doctrine enunciated for federal courts and others that elect to adopt it, judges are required to screen evidence for its scientific validity before it is presented to a jury.[7] Using Daubert, courts may inquire along at least four standards in their determination: (1) the proposition tested; (2) the tests adduced and their error rates; (3) peer review status of the research producing the evidence; and (4) acceptance by the relevant scientific communities. Why, courts will want to know, should evidence of the presence of the novelty gene be admissible and evidence of the presence of the Alzheimer's disease gene be inadmissible in light of the journal's report?

Courts with overwhelming criminal caseloads certainly would welcome the prospect that impulsive conduct might be predictable.[8] The prediction of dangerousness has been a major problem in every jurisdiction, and genetic testing might make it more reliable. Impulsive violent crime might be specifically treated, possibly through gene therapy, more likely through "magic bullet" medication to help criminals become productive citizens, empty our jails, and lower the overwhelming criminal caseloads that clog almost every court in the nation. Treatment might then find a place in federal and state sentencing guidelines, tempering citizen demands for criminal punishment and retribution that have resulted in ever-harsher hard-time sentences, and increasingly crowded jails. Capital crime death sentences might be relaxed with reliable mitigation gradients and a showing that treatment could be effective. If the nation's 30,000 judges could have been polled in response to the *Nature Genetics* article, perhaps they might have concluded prospects for a golden age of criminal justice loomed. Judicial embarrassment about neurogenetics in their eugenic form began nearly a century ago in the United States when Oliver Wendell Holmes, Jr., opined in a decision upholding Virginia's sterilization law that "three generations of imbeciles are enough."[9] The *Nature Genetics* articles might begin to cast away the shadowy ghosts of such prejudice and form an illuminated gateway to a more benign era of forensic molecular medicine for which we all yearn. Yet *JAMA*'s publication of the consensus request for a moratorium for Alzheimer's disease gene tests was a reminder that such a golden era continues to elude. Alzheimer's disease carries an enormous stigma, one that judges have considerable past experience with and high expectations of future management for.[10] This stigma is one reason the four sponsoring medical societies and the American Society for Human Genetics declared that they would shun genetic tests to predict or confirm the disease even though the isolation of the suspect gene had become a routine laboratory procedure for perhaps half of all cases.

Once a person is known or believed to suffer from Alzheimer's, he or she is at risk for social consequences ranging from benign neglect to active financial and personal victimization. Official agencies and insurers pay special attention to persons who might harbor even the potential for Alzheimer's, often regarding the predisposition as well as the disease as a death warrant and possible indicator of risk factors that, in their view, cost health care providers millions of dollars. The diagnosis of Alzheimer's is itself a signal event, a labeling through medical records that can set in motion the snuffing out of one's civil self, even if the individual never contracts Alzheimer's. In the circumstances, the report's sponsors seemed to say, genetic tests for Alzheimer's are not valid under scientific or moral standards. Judges may well ask how these tests can survive as evidence in the courtroom, even if they are introduced for constructive legal purposes. Should a medical moratorium be accompanied by a legal one, or are other important interests served by admitting in a particular case valid genetic evidence that fails to satisfy medical genetic screening standards?

JAMA's consensus report also stated that the diagnostic dilemma facing our society as well as the courts is that Alzheimer's disease, like virtually all neurogenetically influenced conditions, can be polygenic, that is, the result of the operation of many genes for which a single test result can be misleading.[11] Powerful as genetic test information can be in certain cases, it may or may not predict Alzheimer's.[12] Some people who have the gene in its mutant form do not develop the disease, and some people lacking it in the mutant form become ill.[13] Even the offensive genes operate in a biological and social environment influenced by many factors. Patterns in that complex interaction have not yet been discovered.[14] The pathways that cause Alzheimer's exceed the ability of medical genetics to describe, understand, or treat. The research that has yielded the test has not produced a treatment. A host of additional complications and qualifications thus led *JAMA* to recommend that laboratories and clinics abandon use of the primary test for the so-called Apolipoprotein E-4 gene. If polygenic understanding of a complex phenotype is invalid in Alzheimer's, the so-called novelty gene must also be viewed through a similar lens.[15]

The disclosure of a positive Alzheimer's genetic test weighed against its uncertainties and its consequences, moreover, seems neatly to justify the second force pressing on the courts and described in some detail below: the movement to draw a zone of privacy around genetic test information and forbid its use in important decisions by powerful organizations.[16] At first blush, tests to document the so-called novelty gene, the dopamine receptor gene D4DR replicated by two research teams half a world away, appear to be irrelevant to a criminal defendant's privacy. If the test's scientific validity could be proved in service to its admissibility at trial, defense counsel might have a useful explanatory tool with which to achieve a genetic equivalent of the insanity defense. Prosecutors may have a surrogate for motive with a positive test, and the defense may widen the shadow of doubt with a negative one. Public records laws and open court files guarantee criminal defendants' disclosure related to the crime charged. If the defendant is convicted, such information could be introduced at the penalty phase trial in a capital case to adduce mitigating evidence that might result in a prison term instead of a death sentence. Zones of privacy in such cases are nonexistent. But the disclosure of genetic information even in criminal cases is complicated by the fact it extends to persons far beyond the defendant. The defendant's genetic test may provide information about noncriminal relatives. Publication of criminal case medical evidence records containing genetic test results strips the privacy away from law-abiding family members by exposing intimate shared inheritances that have the power to label them indelibly.[17] A short case study involving such evidence, and the arguments mustered with the evidence in hand, will illustrate such complex challenges facing the judiciary.

The Chase Tragedy: An Example of Neurogenetic Tests Moved, Denied, and Granted in a Capital Murder Case Involving the Death Penalty

At age 37, Jeffrey Chase, Jr. ("Jeffrey"), was charged with murdering his parents, Jeffrey Chase, Sr., 72, and Anna Chase, 71.[18] Police discovered the bodies of the Chases in their home on a Sunday morning in response to a 911 call made by Jeffrey. The father's body was found in the garage and that of the mother in the master bedroom. Both parents had been shot several times with a small-caliber pistol. The murder weapon was never found. Jeffrey, bleeding from a wound to the head, was also found at the home. He claimed to have found the bodies of his parents just before he was knocked unconscious by an intruder.

Jeffrey's lifelong history of mental disorders and criminal activities sowed suspicions in the minds of the police and prosecutors. Jeffrey was born in 1957 and was adopted at four months. Almost nothing is known of his biological parents. His adopting parents had no biological children, and Jeffrey was their only child. Jeffrey Chase, Sr., was an executive with the Boy Scouts of America and Anna Chase worked as a schoolteacher.

Jeffrey appeared to be a normal child until age two, when he began to display physically aggressive behavior toward other children. He was expelled from the second grade for attacking a smaller child with a nail. For the next several years, Jeffrey's parents placed him in several residential treatment centers and a number of public schools. In the course of such placements, Jeffrey received many psychiatric and psychological evaluations. Different diagnoses focused on different mental infirmities: by the time he was 12, Jeffrey was described in a composite summary as manifesting "some sociopathic and some schizoid features." One social worker labeled him "quite dangerous, especially to little children."

When Jeffrey was 15 he was arrested for shoplifting. His pre-sentence report emphasized "apparently intractable impulse control problems—Jeffrey admits to a string of unrestrained shoplifting offenses over which he claimed he had no control." The following year, Jeffrey was arrested and charged with abducting and assaulting a four-year-old girl from his neighborhood. Although sexual contact was not involved, the girl was choked, suffered broken teeth, and was emotionally traumatized. Jeffrey was tried as an adult and found guilty of kidnapping and assault with intent to murder; at 17, he was sentenced to life imprisonment with a five-year concurrent prison sentence. Under state law, he faced a maximum of 30 years' imprisonment with parole eligibility. Jeffrey remained in a juvenile detention center until he was almost 19, when he was transferred to an adult prison to complete his sentence.

Jeffrey's incarceration in an adult prison was characterized by repeated rule infractions and fighting with other inmates. His rule violations included possession of illegal drugs and disobeying correctional officers. On one occasion his assault on a guard led to an indictment and prosecution. He was found guilty and sentenced to two additional years' incarceration. A presentence report at this time described him as a "consummate, violence-prone con-artist."

While Jeffrey was in prison, his parents maintained a supportive role. They kept in touch and sent him money. In spite of his poor prison record and lack of effort toward rehabilitation, Jeffrey accumulated sufficient "good time" credits to be released from prison just shy of 21 years' incarceration. He evidenced fear about living beyond prison walls. By the time of his release in April 1994, Jeffrey had spent practically all his juvenile and adult life either in a juvenile institution or an adult prison. Although he had been incarcerated for 21 years, his parents, now both retired, agreed that Jeffrey could reside with them. The brief arrangement fared badly from the beginning.

Jeffrey refused to work. He was uncooperative and continuously argumentative. The elder Chases became afraid of Jeffrey's unrelenting string of hostile outbursts and drinking-related rages. His postrelease counselor requested law enforcement vigilance after a home visit and interview. Approximately a month after his release, Jeffrey's parents were dead.

Jeffrey was indicted on two counts of first-degree murder and under applicable state law faced the death penalty if convicted. Two trial court-appointed psychiatrists examined Jeffrey and found him competent to stand trial. Jeffrey thereafter entered a plea of not guilty. Following a four-week trial, Jeffrey was convicted of murder in the first degree.

A Neurogenetic Defense Limited by Privacy and Adoption Considerations

Jeffrey was entitled not only to a guilt-phase proceeding to convict or acquit but, if convicted, to a penalty-phase proceeding to sentence him to death or incarceration. Before the guilt-phase trial, the defense had moved the court to order a complete medical evaluation, including brain assessments, and confirmations of Jeffrey's earlier diagnoses of attention deficit hyperactivity disorder coupled with conduct and antisocial personality disorder. These motions were granted, and the evidence was presented at trial.

Before the trial counsel also requested a complete neurogenetic screen to link Jeffrey's violent history to genetic causation. The defense motion for neurogenetic tests would have totaled $45,000 in laboratory costs and would have included tests for Huntington disease, Alzheimer's disease, bipolar (manic depressive) disorder, monamine oxidase deficiency disorder, nitrous oxide synthase deficiency, and chromosomal abnormalities involving an extra Y chromosome, along with a test for the dopamine receptor gene D4DR to be coordinated with psychometric tests originated at Washington University in Saint Louis. This motion was opposed by the prosecution and denied without a hearing in a terse opinion from the bench that the requested genetic tests were experimental and not accepted biomedical technologies. Moreover, the court ruled, the defense could not—even under its arguments taken in their best light—show that the requested tests had been accepted by the relevant scientific communities as proper tools for forensic inquiry.

At the guilt-phase trial, Jeffrey's counsel first presented an insanity defense. As a secondary defense, counsel argued that Jeffrey was guilty but mentally ill, the defense successfully used to place President Ronald Reagan's attacker, John Hinckley, Jr., in a mental hospital rather than prison. The jury found Jeffrey to be neither, and after eight hours deliberation convicted him of murder in the first degree.

This set the stage for a penalty-phase trial, under which the trial judge would receive the same jury's recommended sentence—death by lethal injection or life imprisonment without the possibility of parole. The court traditionally attached great weight to the jury's penalty verdict and only rarely imposed its own sentence. The penalty-phase trial was usually conducted within two weeks of the guilt-phase trial. Defense counsel, however, appealed under a special action to the state's supreme court for a three-month delay necessary to conduct the neurogenetic tests denied in connection with the earlier trial. The appeal was granted, and the trial court was ordered to reconsider its denial of the genetic test battery in a hearing. The state supreme court justified its order as a U.S. constitutional requirement that any relevant evidence be permitted in order to prove mitigation in face of the death penalty.[19]

Accordingly, and complying with the state supreme court's remand, the trial court conducted a hearing *in limine* (to determine the admissibility of evidence). The defense argued its motion for neurogenetic testing with the support of six expert witnesses, three of whom were distinguished and three of whom had an extensive record of similar, yet frequently unsuccessful testimony in recent years. The hearing consumed eight days. The state's attorney opposed the neurogenetic test battery as a waste and a sham, and presented, as expert witnesses, the medical director of the state's crime lab and a distinguished professor of neurobiology. Prosecution experts countered their defense witness colleagues. They discounted the genetic tests as mere research and discredited the requested psychometric tests as invalid because they had not been standardized with a national sample.

In the course of the hearing, a surprise emerged. Experts for both sides coincidentally agreed that a proper testing procedure required the inclusion of Jeffrey's natural parents and any siblings. With virtual expert stipulation about the necessity for a family link in the genetic testing chain, the defense quickly amended its genetic testing motion to request a court order to find and test Jeffrey's birth parents.

The court took the amended motion under advisement. A written opinion was issued two weeks later. It granted the defense motion for the requested neurogenetic tests of Jeffrey, including the psychometric tests, but it refused to order tests of his natural parents, even if they could be found. To do so, the court concluded, would be to grant an unwarranted information access exception to the state's adoption information blackout law. The only motions granted by any court in that jurisdiction to pierce the adoption information veil had been two instances of need for tissue matches, one for an extraordinary life-saving procedure in a woman's breast cancer case, the second to secure a compatible tissue type in a child's liver transplant crisis. In the present case, the court opined, mitigation could be sufficiently attempted by means of the defense's requested tests of Jeffrey alone. The court refused to order birth parent tests on other grounds as well: an impermissible invasion of their privacy, if they could be found; and the risk of mental and emotional stress resulting from positive tests but no symptoms related to one or more of the disorders for which Jeffrey sought mitigation of the death penalty. Under no conditions, the court stated, could the conduct of a test be justified and the results withheld from the person tested.

Defense counsel implemented the order for Jeffrey's tests and appealed the denial of the birth family's tests. He had only half a loaf. Without confirming familial data, even Jeffrey's positive tests could be characterized as coincidental. As the National Research Council had proclaimed in two panel reports concerning genetic identification data, "a match without a number is meaningless."[20] The family was the closest thing the defense could get to Jeffrey's number. The state's criminal offender gene databank might one day offer statistical parameters to support a causal genetic argument. But it was thousands of samples behind in the first round of simple identification information, and there was no chance that it would produce mitigating epidemiological evidence. Life-threatening circumstances had justified the judicial grant of a health information exception to the state's adoption blackout statute before. Jeffrey was certainly in a life-threatening situation. The state, moreover, had enacted no real health information or genetic test disclosure statutes. It had only a legislative commission poised to study the matter.

The court had adopted the prosecution's objections in its refusal to order birth family genetic tests. It concluded that Jeffrey's natural parents possessed a zone of genetic privacy regarding their neurogenetic information. That right of privacy, however, could not be founded in any express state law. The state's medical records statutes strongly favored disclosure and minimized confidentiality. The state had no constitutional right to privacy. On the contrary, its public records laws were among the most fully disclosing in the nation. And its courts had a long history of compelling disclosure when the ends of justice were to be served. Thus, defense counsel regarded their quick appeals of the trial court's ruling to be promising.

This time, in spite of defense counsel's vigorous arguments, the state's supreme court denied the appeal. In a brief statement, the appellate body affirmed the trial court's discretion to forego the parental tests based solely on a rational nexus related to the intentions and provisions of the adoption information blackout statute. The appellate body did not reach the argument involving genetic test information privacy, saying that issue would wait for another day. The appellate court approved the rationale marshaled in the trial court's record without further comment, and it only briefly referenced opposing counsels' extensive memoranda. Fifteen weeks after his conviction, Jeffrey Chase went on trial for his life or his lifelong incarceration.

Arguing Jeffrey's Mitigating Disorders Evidence Before the Jury

At the penalty-phase trial, the prosecution argued through its expert witnesses that in spite of lifelong medication for his attention deficit hyperactivity disorder, Jeffrey always knew right from wrong. His willful, reckless, and ultimately fatal criminal acts were choices, freely calculated, absent internal or external coercion. From the psychosocial evidence adduced earlier and the genetic testing evidence adduced solely for this trial, and from direct examination by forensic psychiatrists, the prosecution determined that Jeffrey was poised to make his criminal choices but not predestined to do so. The prosecution used Jeffrey's case to make a bright line distinction among predisposition, coercion, and predestination. Jeffrey was merely predisposed, but absent a cognitive impairment or other factor that compromised his ability to judge right from wrong, he was neither coerced nor predestined. To bolster its case, the prosecution cited Jeffrey's "more than passing scores" on two versions of the Moral Decisions Equivalence Scale, an animated interactive cartoon validated for ethical choices and coordinated with a blood-activation brain scan.

As to predisposition, Jeffrey's dopamine receptor gene, D4DR, sequenced with 27 triplet repeats at the very high end for impulsivity. Jeffrey scored in the 98th percentile on psychometric tests indicating propensity for violent preferences—the universal interpersonal volatility and conflict preparedness index. Detailed summaries of Jeffrey's behavior during incarceration were analyzed by content to portray underlying themes.

From the combined data, the prosecution asserted that Jeffrey's conduct was a knowing choice of behavior that was satisfying to his oppositional behavior and temperament. Admittedly, he evidenced a lifelong pattern of antisocial personality disorder under standard psychiatric diagnostic categories, but Jeffrey's choice to kill his parents could have been resisted and his behavior conformed, if not transformed.

Jeffrey's defense team asserted to the jury that he was afflicted by a variant form of mental illness, multiple personality disorder syndrome, a usual form of traditional insanity. The team asserted that Jeffrey's acts always were compelled by genetic predisposition to violence, upon which was built storms of bipolar disorder; that his violent acts always occurred in the manic phase; that the neural abnormalities arising from the predisposition was proved by chromosome 11 mutations in the family of genes coding for serum cortisol overproduction; that too much cortisol in turn capacitated forebrain pathways for constant hypervigilance resulting in attention deficit hyperactivity disorder and compulsive lashing-out behaviors; and that pervasive treatment with the drug Ritalin had resulted, paradoxically, in an additive, chemically induced, violent effect. Jeffrey's violence was coerced by his liver's responses to a post-Ritalin attention deficit hyperactivity disorder control drug, 2-hydroxy-methylphenidate, that, according to Food and Drug Administration announcements, in some people led to liver cancer. In Jeffrey's case, cancer did not develop, but he did manifest a particularly potent by-product liver response to Ritalin that clouded judgment.

Even if Jeffrey could distinguish between right and wrong after a criminal, violent act, he could not do so during the dual assault of genetically predisposing and medicinally induced substances. With recent findings that certain mutations in D4DR and a companion gene on the long arm of chromosome 17, 43PM, are highly associated with type 1 simple schizophrenia, it could be said that Jeffrey manifested a persistent prepsychotic predisposition state. Although this was not active insanity as traditionally defined, it was an aberrant mental state closer to mental illness than to mere personality disorders. Jeffrey, arguably, was either innocent by virtue of insanity or guilty but mentally ill. Moreover, Jeffrey's genetic tests disclosed a risk factor: mutation 12 of the ApoE-4 gene, indicating that first-order plaques in the limbic system could form presymptomatically to create Alzheimer's disease–induced sporadic violence. Jeffrey may have committed homicide. With this combination of factors, however, he was so afflicted and tortured that these disorders mitigated against the death penalty. In many ways, prison was a harsher penalty, the defense argued, for a person so unable to bring his daily impulses under control.

The jury that had deliberated for only eight hours over Jeffrey's guilty verdict in the first trial took four times as long to decide his sentence. The presiding judge's postverdict debriefing of the jury disclosed that the jurors had understood his instructions thoroughly and had engaged the issues closely. They had digested the evidence. All told, they determined that the aggravating factors of the crime outweighed the substantial mitigating factors presented at the penalty-phase trial. The state's jury rules required a unanimous verdict using the preponderant weight of the evidence standard. The 12-person jury agreed that it would not report that it could not agree on a verdict (a "hung jury") for one week. The first vote was evenly split. In successive, agonizing votes, the jurors gradually moved toward unanimity. Consensus was fueled under pressures that Jeffrey's conduct might lead to further deaths in prison; the need for his special protection in prison as well as that of others; and the requirement for special facilities incarceration at a cost of up to $40,000 a year. The jury opted for the death sentence. The judge imposed it.

Jeffrey appealed the sentence, substantially based upon the argument that the absence of the opportunity to discover his birth family's genetic tests deprived him of essential mitigation evidence at trial, evidence that could have been obtained in the absence of a specific, statutory right of genetic privacy.

Adjudicating Motions Regarding Genetic Tests in the Absence of Statutory Authority

Perhaps the jury's verdict would have turned out differently if the defense's motions to find and test Jeffrey's birth parents had been granted. The question will haunt any presiding or reviewing judge. The trial court found itself—as will many courts over the next decade—stymied by the nation's ambiguity with respect to policy on genetic testing information. With the exception of a few pioneering state statutes, genetic information, like genetic tests themselves, is virtually unregulated as we approach the twenty-first century and the completion of the Human Genome Project's mission. Courts experience all of the tensions inherent in a metapolicy environment: social institutions, interest groups, and individuals are engaged in animated struggles to define the issues, determine guiding principles, and recommend a course of action to implement their findings. Although this formative time is understandable, it offers scant comfort to the judicial officers who preside in real cases in real time.

The danger to detached, dispassionate, even-handed adjudication is that courts are required to rule on subject matter and associated procedures that break new ground. In State v. Chase, the court assumed a right of genetic information privacy for Jeffrey's birth parents and possible siblings in justifying its discretion to not grant an exception to the adoption information shield law. Such a decision arguably treads upon the legislature's policy-making realm. But if the legislature is silent and fails to act, the court has little choice. Such inadvertent judicial policy activism challenges adjudication in the genetic context perhaps as strongly as any other issue.

Nevertheless, the courts cannot escape such duties even in the face of the ambiguous policy environment. Rulings on motions are crucial to the resolution of all criminal and civil cases. Genetic test evidence complicates such cases by its very nature and by the unsettled nature of privacy and information access policies incident to it. But one still wonders whether the outcome would have been different for Jeffrey Chase had his case been tried under a clarifying genetic information statute, in a state with a statute that has come to grips with the issue or under one of the several proposals introduced in Congress.

FORCE TWO: DEVELOPMENTS IN GENETIC TEST INFORMATION PRIVACY

Several bills were introduced in the 104th Congress (1995–96) to create a national uniform genetic test information policy. Protections would vary widely, from mere rhetoric to new private rights of action. Disclosure would vary markedly, from limited channeling to absolute prohibition with enumerated exceptions.

Preemptive federal genetic privacy protection bills, whatever their model, would provide access to state and federal courts by jointly allocating subject matter jurisdiction. This means that an aggrieved party could bring a lawsuit in state or federal court. Because most cases are filed in the largest 110 metropolitan courts operated by the states and their federal district court counterparts, these courts would become the magnets for genetic privacy cases. Already under great caseload pressures from burgeoning criminal dockets and civil lawsuits, these courts would face a managerial challenge from imposition of a greater workload amid bleak prospects for an increased judicial workforce.

All of the bills would require judges to determine what a genetic test is and is not. This means knowing what a gene is and is not and how the technology works for describing gene structure and function. It may well be that genetic tests could be defined differently in different forums. If so, the term *genetic information* could take on many variations and colorations. All that would require judicial interpretation. As was thoroughly highlighted above in State v. Chase, these many variations and colorations render cases ever more complex. They become novel, nontraditional subject matter for most sitting judges. Legislatively induced potentials for judicial challenge may be inferred from the widely varying enactments and proposals described by Philip R. Reilly in Chapter 20 of this volume. When other rights, privileges, and policies, such as adoption information privacy—changing in their own orbits—are added to the prosecution or litigation calculus, the courts may be severely challenged by the evidentiary novelty of genetic testing as well as the potential volume of relevant cases.

FORCE THREE: DEVELOPMENTS IN ADOPTION INFORMATION BLACKOUT POLICY

In State v. Chase, Jeffrey's adoption was arranged through a licensed agency to whom a teenage mother had turned for help in 1956. Professional social service tradition and state law have maintained an extremely restrictive information policy in most jurisdictions. Although important changes are taking form in some states, adoption information typically flows in one direction only: from the prospective adoptive parents to the agency and from the birth mother to the agency.[21] Agency files are privileged fortresses from which little information is released, immunized from disclosure by a safe-harbor status specified in state law. Notification of an adoptive child's availability is made suddenly, and delivery is typically accompanied only by the age and race of the mother and sometimes the father. What the adoptive parents see for the first time in the agency office is the child they get. Trial adoptions are discouraged. Birth parents and adoptive parents almost never meet; the adoptive child is not permitted knowledge of or contact with his or her biological mother and father. Stringent preadoption screening tests the adoptive parents' tolerance for the extreme background ambiguity imposed and for the ability to cope with the unexpected as the child matures. No warranties are given; the child whose disabilities emerge in the years following adoption become the adoptive parents' burden. Indeed, many agencies omit or prune background information; its classified status rivals national defense secrets; its volatility is regarded as extreme.

The Chases' tolerances for ambiguity were tested early. Something was wrong with the child as early as 18 months when he would not sleep through the night, seemed to have an inexhaustible supply of big-muscle energy, and developed extreme and extended reactions of rage over minor frustrations. By the time Jeffrey was two, according to presentence reports prepared with respect to a kidnapping charge 16 years later, tantrums occurred three or four times a day, frequently over his inability to perform small motor tasks, such as coloring pictures. By the time he was three, mother and father were taking turns staying up at night with Jeffrey. He was more likely than not to delight in destructive and even pain-inducing acts—from propelling balls through windows to pulling the dog's ears until it yelped.

As a professional social service worker, the father appealed to the Red Feather agencies for help. The adoption agency offered a few counseling sessions, but the Chases developed the uncomfortable feeling that the agency regarded Jeffrey's problems a result of their shortcomings. At the same time, everyone who knew the Chases regarded them as steady, caring, exhausted parents. If the schoolteacher mother was a little forbidding in her behavior standards, the child guidance clinic (that era's outpatient psychiatric clinic) noted, she was balanced by the scout leader father's general sense of optimism and jocularity. Jeffrey was diagnosed at four years old as "severe acting out of undetermined origin."

The Chases decided not to test the adoption agency's iron-clad confidentiality policy in order to help the child guidance clinic obtain sorely needed background information. The clinic's psychiatrist listened supportively as Jeffrey was ejected from one kindergarten after another for uncontrollable behavior and attacks on other children. But nothing changed, and the adoption health history blackout persisted as Jeffrey was told on turning nine that he was adopted but that he was chosen by the Chases and that they knew nothing more about his biological parents than he knew. The records of several institutions to which Jeffrey later was committed for "incorrigibility" indicated his deep anger over having been "thrown away." Jeffrey could barely read and write. He was "kept back" and was still in the fourth grade by age 12. At age 11, Jeffrey was diagnosed as having "hyperkinesis/hyperactivity disorder." The modern version of that diagnosis would be "attention deficit hyperactivity disorder with conduct disorder and associated uncoded impulse control disorders."

Even though attention deficit hyperactivity disorder is widely thought to have important family linkages that transmit it through the genetic chain, the health care information lurking in Jeffrey's background could not be retrieved.[22] Jeffrey's counsel in State v. Chase could not obtain the necessary confirming pedigree studies, clinical tests, or genetic tests. The court's ruling against granting an exception to the state's adoption blackout law simply ended the matter and, arguably, short-changed the nature and quality of the penalty-phase trial evidence.

This would probably not have been the case if Jeffrey had been put on trial in Connecticut in 1996, for a year earlier Connecticut rode the crest of adoption information reform. In its adoption information reform statute of 1995, Connecticut repealed decades of earlier law and replaced it with an entirely new policy.[23] The new law shifts its central organizing principle from the state's right to monopolize preadoption information to an adult adopted person's right to obtain such information. Exceptions were also shifted: from exceptions to release information about natural parents to exceptions under which the state could retain the information. The statute emphasizes the priority with which the state accords adopted persons' genetic information access and attempts to balance birth parents' privacy rights against such access. The General Assembly has fashioned a two-way street for the exchange of information—reciprocally between adoptive children and natural parents.

"It is intended," the Connecticut statute instructs in the first of its enumerated preamble explanations, "to make available to adult adopted persons and adult persons whose genetic parents have had their rights terminated information about their background and status; to give the same information to their adoptive parent or parents; and, in any case where such adult persons are deceased, to give the same information to their adult descendants, including adopted descendants." This paradigm shift from rationed to unrestricted information is conditioned, to be sure. Privacy is protected by written consent requirements. But the state must provide certain background information and assistance. Moreover, the moving party is the individual, whose rights are secured with a simple written request. And the state is charged to facilitate in favor of adoption background information supply rather than fortify its secrecy.

Connecticut has also fashioned a special role for the courts. It delegates them as overseer of state agencies' comportment with the new adoption information law's intentions and provisions. It provides an expedited docket with designated reports to be sought by and furnished to either the probate or superior court. In ambiguous situations, the court is directed to appoint a guardian *ad litem* (for the purpose of litigation) to give constructive consent for adoptive information, especially in cases where a birth parent appears to be incompetent or cannot be located. Such constructive consent is to be introduced to the court, after investigation, unless the guardian ad litem "concludes that it would not be in the best interest of the adult person to be identified for such consent to be given."

Other limitations apply in cases of incompetency or disappearance, but the thrust of the policy is to give the courts a flexible and timely engine for facilitating the adopted person's or natural parents' access to information. This special role for the courts, it should be noted, is not the passive one usually associated with rulings on motions for exceptions to secreted adoption information. Stressing over and over the genetic connection among the parties, the Connecticut statute activates the judicial role.

In so doing, Connecticut may well have positioned Jeffrey Chase's trial court to take a different course—one favoring at least a judicially impelled inquiry into his natural relatives and the opportunity to obtain their consent for genetic and other testing. In so doing, the Connecticut statute further challenges the court's duties and crafts a bright line: genetic relationships are important, and the information attending them is to be pursued vigorously. Whether such a policy principle can rest easily with federal momentum favoring privacy of genetic information remains to be seen. The looming conflicts between open access and restricted disclosure will likely be played out in court.

PREPARING FOR THE GATHERING STORM

How the courts should prepare for such adjudication challenges is a ripe question, one whose time came in the summer of 1995 as geneticists moved to restrain testing for Alzheimer's disease; as researchers prepared for final publication their reports of the "novelty gene"; as Congress busily introduced information privacy bills founded on widely differing models and a dizzying array of state-based statutes; and as Jeffrey Chase's lawyers were frantically trying to marshal information to save his life.

Meeting in Snow Library in Orleans, Massachusetts, for a "Working Conversation on Genetics, Evolution and the Courts," 37 federal and state trial and appellate judges, scientists, and lawyers developed a beginning judicial branch agenda to anticipate the next decade's adjudication challenges. Many of the challenges discussed earlier light up the case types expected to emerge from the Human Genome Project:

- discrimination cases based on the dissemination of genetic testing information to official and private entities;
- personal injury cases involving genetic testing and prenatal and adult gene therapy;
- orders assessing genetic diseases and predispositions in court-ordered health care cases;
- privacy infringement cases involving personal genetic information records;
- claims to integrate ethical considerations, and the "natural law" of religion, with constitutionally derived patent laws and decisions;
- motions for injunctive relief based on irreparable harm to health, life, or species posed by gene therapy and biotechnology regimes;
- civil rights relief sought in the concurrent jurisdiction of various titles of the Americans with Disabilities Act of 1990, the Civil Rights Act of 1964, and various other federal and state laws for perceived discrimination based on inherited genomic construction;
- criminal jurisprudence of claims challenging the validity of individual responsibility based on conceptions of free will, the cornerstone of Anglo-American law;
- the judicial review of administrative regulation of genetic testing methods, genetic counseling services, and gene therapeutic technologies;
- special adjudication issues presented by specially vulnerable, dependent, and custodial populations, including litigation regarding gene data banks;
- cascading episodes of DNA forensic technology review as it evolves from RFLP (restriction fragment length polymorphism) profiles to polymerase chain reaction–based tests to polymarkers to STSs (sequence tagged sites) and STRs (single tandem repeats) to mitochondrial DNA sequencing to direct genomic sequencing;
- and others, including claims for a bewildering array of declaratory judgments, that will develop as our society transitions into the 21st century armed with a full quiver of new genetics-based testing and therapy tools.

Cases like these will challenge the courts for at least the coming decade. The Working Conversation met again in 1996 to map specific responses for managing these complicated cases. High in everyone's mind was the coming clash between scientific progress and the preservation of privacy. That clash attracts many other public policy issues, such as adoption, resulting in multidimensional challenges for the years ahead. The Working Conversation has begun to contribute to the judicial branch's ability to understand and manage ELSI (ethical, legal, and social implications)-related cases of intensifying complexity. As the Human Genome Project enters its second trimester, much remains to be done if the courts are to adjudicate confidently the chaotically transacting forces illustrated by the wrenching case of Jeffrey Chase—criminals, families, law enforcement institutions, legal services, health care authorities, child-serving agencies, courts, and legislatures, all caught midstream among the crosscutting forces of the genomic age.

NOTES

1. Jonathan Benjamin et al., "Population and Familial Association Between the D4 Dopamine Receptor Gene and Measures of Novelty Seeking," *Nature Genetics* 12 (1996): 81; Richard P. Ebstein et al., "Dopamine D4 Receptor (D4DR) Exon III Polymorphism Associated with the Human Personality Trait of Novelty Seeking," ibid., 78.
2. C. Robert Cloninger et al., "Mapping Genes for Human Personality," *Nature Genetics* 12 (1996): 3.
3. American College of Medical Genetics/American Society of Human Genetics Working Group on ApoE and Alzheimer Disease, "Consensus Statement: Use of Apolipoprotein E Testing for Alzheimer Disease," *Journal of the American Medical Association* 274 (1995): 1827.
4. Kenneth L. Davis, ed., "Neuroscience and Socioeconomic Challenge of Alzheimer's Disease," *Neurology* 43, no. 8 (supp. 4) (1993). See, especially, John P. Blass, "Pathophysiology of the Alzheimer's Syndrome," ibid., 45–51. Also, generally, U.S. Congress, Office of Technology Assessment, *Losing a Million Minds: Confronting the Tragedy of Alzheimer's Disease and Other Dementias* (Washington, D.C.: Government Printing Office, 1987).
5. The answer is not straightforward. Genetic testing is an unregulated compartment of the health care industry, falling outside of the Food and Drug Administration's jurisdiction and escaping, largely, the ambit of the Clinical Laboratory Improvement Act. See Lori B. Andrews et al., eds., *Assessing Genetic Risks* (National Academy of Sciences, Washington, D.C.: National Academy Press, 1994), especially chap. 4, "Issues Related to Laboratories." Creeping between regulatory regimes amid great pressures for genetic test commercialization, magic bullets, and snake oil can be confused one for the other by even well-meaning health care providers.
6. United States v. Frye, 293 F. 1013 (D.C. Cir. 1923).
7. Daubert v. Merrell Dow Pharmaceuticals, Inc., 509 U.S. 579 (1993).
8. The contending schools for explaining the genetic, socioenvironmental, and psychologi-

cal foundations of violence are well described in Robert Wright, "The Biology of Violence," *New Yorker,* Mar. 13, 1995, 68.

9. Buck v. Bell, 274 U.S. 200, 207 (1923).

10. Franklin M. Zweig et al., "Securing the Future for America's State Courts," *Judicature* 73 (1990): 296.

11. Mark Patterson and John A. Todd, "Multifactorial Inheritance: A Complex Issue," *Trends in Genetics: Special Issue on Multifactorial Inheritance* 11–12 (1995): 463.

12. Margaret A. Pericak-Vance and Jonathan L. Haines, "Genetic Susceptibility to Alzheimer Disease," ibid., 504.

13. American College of Medical Genetics/American Society of Human Genetics Working Group on ApoE and Alzheimer Disease, 1828.

14. Ibid., 1829.

15. In spite of the excitement, however, subdued voices counsel that the society as well as the courts would do best to take a step back from the reduction of all causation to genetics and the determination of all root sources of behavior as brain proteins. See, e.g., Steven Weinberg, "The Rise of Neurogenetic Determinism," *Nature* 373 (1995): 380. Also see Dorothy Nelkin and M. Susan Lindee, *The DNA Mystique: The Gene as a Cultural Icon* (New York: W. H. Freeman, 1995).

16. Robert Gellman, "Genetic Engineering Symposium: Washington Perspectives on Genetics and Privacy," *Dickinson Journal of Environmental Law and Policy* 3 (1994): 71.

17. Andrea L. Bonnicksen, "Review Essay: Commentaries on the Uses and Abuses of Genetic Knowledge," *Journal of Health Politics, Policy and Law* 20 (1995): 795.

18. State v. Chase is taken from an actual case prosecuted in Delaware during 1994 and 1995. Jeffrey Chase is a pseudonym adopted for the purpose of retaining as much privacy as possible for the persons connected with this case. No doubt a keen investigator could determine the actual identities without difficulty. Our purpose is to illustrate the human dilemmas and issues confronted. To that end, we have added facts not evident in the actual case, and we have added factors to enrich our exploration of the combined neurogenetic, adoption, and privacy dimensions of the real case. Although these additions have been made as artfully as possible, the people and events described have been sufficiently modified so as to qualify as a hypothetical and not an actual, accurate case study.

19. See Penry v. Lynaugh, 492 U.S. 302 (1989).

20. National Research Council, *DNA Technology in Forensic Science* (Washington, D.C.: National Academy Press, 1992); National Research Council, *DNA Technology in Forensic Science: An Update* (Washington, D.C.: National Academy Press, 1996).

21. D. Marianne Brower Blair, "Lifting the Genealogical Veil: A Blueprint for Legislative Reform of the Disclosure of Health-Related Information in Adoption," *North Carolina Law Review* 70 (1992): 681; "Note, Adoption Nightmares Prompt Judicial Recognition of the Tort of Wrongful Adoption: Will New York Follow Suit?" *Cardozo Law Review* 15 (1994): 1687.

22. Russell A. Barkley, *Attention Deficit Hyperactivity Disorder: A Handbook for Diagnosis and Treatment* (New York: Guilford Press, 1990), 227–28.

23. Conn. Gen. Stat. Ann. § 19–5–301 et seq. (West 1995).

Part Five Ethics and Law in the United States and Abroad

Chapter 19 Justice and Genetics: Privacy Protection and the Moral Basis of Public Policy

Madison Powers

Recent and anticipated discoveries in genetics and the race to extend our capacities for genetic testing present unprecedented challenges to our thinking about individual privacy and the means for its protection. Moreover, rapid changes in the financing and delivery of health care and new developments in computer-based information technologies provide independent reasons for the propelling of health care issues to the forefront of public policy debates in the United States.[1] One motivating force behind this revitalized interest in privacy protection is the awareness that although an increase in health information available to medical researchers and caregivers can be used for great good, it can also have adverse economic and social consequences for individuals and groups.

Nowhere are such concerns greater than in the area of genetics. The collection, aggregation, and analysis of genetic information may be used to prevent or delay the onset of disease, alleviate the burden of illness, or assist people in planning their futures, but genetic information can be used for a variety of other, more controversial purposes not directly related to research or the delivery of appropriate medical care.

Such information can be used to determine suitability for employment, set eligibility for government benefits, limit access to insurance, or otherwise allocate health resources.

Many secondary uses for genetic information are controversial precisely because they can contribute to the stigmatization and oppression of individuals and groups or play a role in expanding or contracting the range of opportunities available to some segments of society. Accordingly, the analysis of the ethical issues that inform choices among public policy options requires consideration of the potential uses, the expected benefits and harms associated with each use, and the set of overlapping and competing interests at stake in each context. Moreover, any attempt to balance these competing interests can be appreciated only from within a larger theoretical context in which questions of justice receive explicit attention. Public policy, therefore, can never stray far from the concerns of political philosophy.

I first examine competing interests that need to be considered in formulating a comprehensive genetic information policy. I then present a theoretical framework for thinking about the most effective means to privacy protection, arguing that no one policy option is adequate to all contexts and that the kinds of privacy rights that ought to be legally recognized will vary depending on contextual differences. This chapter defends the general thesis that the evaluation of public policy options designed to protect genetic privacy inevitably involves a consideration of the underlying principles of justice governing the basic structure of our political and economic institutions.

THE INTERESTS AT STAKE

Debates about the importance of privacy protection policies are often portrayed as involving an underlying conflict between the interests of society and the individual. The defense of strong privacy protection policies is framed largely in terms of concerns about averting the harms to individuals that may occur when other persons or institutions gain access to an individual's genetic information. Individual interests widely cited on behalf of privacy protection policies are contrasted with various societal interests in making more information readily accessible to other individuals or institutions for the sake of the public good. As we shall see, the arguments often turn out to be far more complicated than this traditional picture suggests.

Nonetheless, a consideration of some individual interests directly affected by others having access to personal genetic information provides a useful starting point for thinking about genetic information policy. Some of the main interests of individuals secured by genetic privacy protection policies can be classified under four general headings.

First, an important interest many individuals have in genetic privacy protection is the protection of their social and economic well-being. A person's general life prospects often depend on limiting the access others may have to sensitive or personal medical information. Such information, if revealed, can have profound adverse social and economic consequences, including the loss of employment opportunities and insurability. Although it is controversial how much genetic information is, or will be used, as a basis for employment or insurance decisions—and, indeed, whether such information differs fundamentally from other kinds of health information—there are ample grounds to believe that the risks to social and economic interests of individuals justify a heightened degree of concern for the protection of genetic privacy.[2]

Unlike information derived from many other types of medical tests and evaluations, information obtainable from genetic tests can reveal a more comprehensive picture of each individual's current medical condition, his or her risks for developing an inheritable disease, or genetic predispositions for developing other medical conditions not caused directly by genetic factors alone. Moreover, as new genetic discoveries are made, available DNA samples can be reanalyzed to learn additional information about a person and existing data can be used for purposes substantially different from those for which consent was initially given.[3] This potential of genetic testing to reveal new information not contemplated at the time of consent for testing ensures that one can never be certain of the final nature of, or potential uses for, information at the time of testing. More important, perhaps, is the fact that the individual has less ability to take additional steps to mitigate potential adverse consequences of disclosures if he or she has no basis for anticipating what genetic samples can reveal and no ability to exercise continuing control of the samples.[4] In addition, much genetic information has the potential to be misleading or incorrect in particular cases, because it often relies on probabilities for whole populations. Consideration of genetic information by itself ignores other personal and environmental factors that also influence health outcomes. How individuals are affected by an inherited condition varies widely, and the age of onset of some conditions for which some individuals are at an increased risk (such as cancer) may vary considerably. Access to an individual's genetic information, therefore, may cause others to overreact or unjustifiably alter their responses to the individual. Even if some genetic markers do not perfectly predict disease, mental or physical dysfunction, or occupational risk, the widespread belief that they do may reliably foretell social stigma or discrimination in employment and insurance.

A second set of interests at stake in any genetic privacy policy choice can be described under the heading of an individual's psychological interests. The dissemination of highly sensitive personal information to others may result in severe emotional distress due, for example, to the perception of social stigma or the loss of respect by others. Even if the economic consequences of disclosure of genetic information could be eliminated, many individuals simply will not want information about their medical and psychological predispositions or conditions to be known by others. Their concern may be to avert equally significant adverse consequences for social standing and sense of self-worth. Indeed, the ability to control information about the most intimate aspects of oneself is often central to the ability to remain insulated from excessive scrutiny and the invidious judgments of others.[5] For example, although there is no inherent reason why someone should feel ashamed or embarrassed by the fact that he or she has a genetic risk of developing an inheritable psychiatric condition, others falsely may conclude that the individual is lacking in intellectual abilities, is emotionally unstable, or poses an added risk to the physical safety of others. The dissemination of genetic information of this sort can profoundly affect an individual's very self-concept and capacity for functioning in society.

A third set of interests individuals may have in limiting access others have to genetic information can be called relational interests. Because a selective sharing of information is frequently an essential element of what distinguishes one's deepest personal commitments from the variety of relations with others, inability to control access to personal information may inhibit a person's ability to form and maintain the desired intimate relationships with others.[6] For example, when genetic information obtained from one patient or subject is revealed to other family members by researchers or caregivers rather than by the subjects or patients themselves, the ability of persons to shape their most intimate relationships is compromised, and the trust and patterns of usual communication within families can be compromised.

A fourth, crosscutting set of genetic privacy interests comprises the interests individuals have in the protection of their autonomy. Although disclosures of genetic information can undermine the economic, social, psychological, and relational interests of individuals, the potential harms to those interests are of two distinct kinds. On one hand, individuals may experience harm to their well-being, their autonomy, or both. If, for example, the presence of genetic information in a medical record prevents an individual from obtaining adequate health insurance his or her economic and (ultimately, medical) well-being may be adversely affected. But even if no loss of, or decrease in, insurance coverage results, an individual may experience a loss of autonomy, or the ability to make and act on his or her own choices. For example, the presence of the genetic information in a medical record may effectively deter a person from changing employment for fear of an inability to obtain adequate insurance to cover future medical needs.

Indeed, the ability to make a variety of medical and other personal choices without substantial interference by others often depends on the protection of informational privacy. If, for example, learning one's own genetic status creates legal duties or economic pressure to make such information available to employers or insurers, then an individual's autonomy within both medical and nonmedical spheres of life may be undermined. Individuals might find their choices of employment limited by employers who wish to avoid legal liability for potential work-related fetal injuries, even if the employee has no plans to have children. Others may find their reproductive freedom compromised by a concern that a decision to have children who may develop heritable medical conditions may cause their employer to impose limits on the insurance coverage available to their families. The lack of assurances that privacy will be protected also may deter persons from seeking beneficial medical testing and treatment for themselves.

The predominantly individual interests cited thus far are often contrasted with a variety of societal interests advanced by policies favoring greater access to individual genetic information by researchers, health care providers, family members, public policy makers, or private institutions. Among the most significant of these societal interests are the promotion of scientific research, public health or safety, and economic efficiency.

However, the interests at stake in the analysis of privacy policy options frequently intersect in three other ways. In some cases, arguments either for restricting or increasing (someone's) access to genetic information rest on there being a substantial harmony of individual and social interests. In a second range of cases, the arguments reveal a conflict between someone's need for increased access to another's genetic information, based on some societal interests promoted by the access, and a need to restrict access, also based on a societal or group interest promoted by the restriction. Finally, some interests putatively advanced by greater access to genetic information turn out to be largely parochial interests of particular segments of society rather than a genuinely public interest.

Consider first cases in which potentially conflicting interests can be harmonized. Individual patients, as well as society as a whole, often share an interest in making genetic data more readily available to medical researchers and caregivers. Research conducted as a result of access to data obtained from both population screening and individualized genetic testing may provide the knowledge basis needed for enhanced patient decision making. Knowledge of genetic susceptibilities may allow patients to make more informed decisions about examinations, diet, behavior, and exposures to environmental hazards. Individuals may benefit from the knowledge gained from genetic research in making such reproductive decisions as preconception planning, preimplantation diagnosis, or deciding whether to terminate a pregnancy.[7] Thus, both society as a whole and individual patients ultimately stand to benefit from public policies that ensure that genetic information is made available for research purposes. But this harmony of interests is likely only if other limitations on access to genetic information are in place.

Some researchers worry that stringent privacy protection policies can have the undesirable effect of reducing the available data crucial for research. In at least some instances, however, stringent privacy protection policies can have the contrary effect. Privacy protection for individuals can serve the broader societal interests in advancing medical research when, for example, barriers to persons seeking genetic testing are removed by policies that assure subjects that the information obtained will not be made available for unrelated purposes. Privacy protection policies that restrict access by those who can limit eligibility for insurance or employment, as well as policies that guarantee that the data will not be disclosed to persons outside the research context without explicit consent, can provide assurances necessary to maintain public trust in the process by which researchers gain access to test results.

In other cases, the primary justification for public policies designed to restrict access to genetic information may lie in societal interests rather than the purely individual interests served by some restriction. The use of genetic screening to track the incidence of genetic conditions or carrier states within populations is an example. Whether a screening program is a net social benefit or harm will depend on the further uses of the data obtained. If the tracking of disease or carrier status is used to provide individuals with information that they can use to enhance patient choice or improve patient outcomes for themselves or their children, then the positive benefits, both to affected individuals and to society generally, can be considerable. If, however, the consequence of collecting genetic information is the stigmatization or marginalization of certain groups, the harms to societal interests may dwarf the expected societal benefits. The protection of privacy arguably matters in such cases for reasons not directly related to any identifiable harm that may result to any particular individual whose privacy is diminished, but rather in virtue of the harm to the interests of society generally. Though less widely appreciated in the United States than in Europe, the less tangible interests everyone has in maintaining social solidarity, preserving trust in public institutions, and limiting destructive social cleavages may provide some of the most compelling arguments on behalf of those privacy protection policies designed to combat group stigmatization or marginalization.[8]

Finally, consider an example of some interests often characterized as societal, which may in fact be more accurately described as the interests of a segment of society that stands to benefit from access to genetic information. One familiar argument is that employers or insurers need to know genetic information for the promotion of such societal interests as economic efficiency or public health. The claim is that society benefits from decreased occupational risks to health and a more efficient organization of the workforce. As more is learned about inherited predispositions to certain types of disease and their relation to environmental exposures to substances in the workplace, employers may be able to identify prospective or current employees who are at greater medical risk in certain types of work.[9]

However, putative gains in public health or efficiency achieved by reconfiguring the composition of the workforce, rather than by reducing workplace hazards, may neither promote the most efficient use of labor resources nor offer the most cost-effective means for reducing morbidity and mortality associated with occupational hazards. Employers may be able to decrease workplace hazard abatement costs and reduce their financial liability from tort litigation or workers' compensation for work-related illnesses through selective hiring and placement practices, or reduce the costs of health insurance benefits for their employees by eliminating medically costly employees and reducing available employee health insurance coverage for certain conditions. But it is not obvious that the use of exclusionary employment practices and targeted benefits programs best serves either of the advertised societal goals. These are, of course, empirical matters, but the point is that it is an open question whether important societal interests, such as the promotion of public health or economic efficiency, are arrayed on the side of increasing, rather than restricting, access to genetic information.

In conclusion, not all interests supporting the restriction of access to genetic information are based on individual interests championed at the expense of societal interests, and not all interests that support a more relaxed genetic information policy rest on an appeal to societal interests. Interests of both kinds can be marshaled on behalf of any imaginable genetic information policy option. Moreover, some aspects of a comprehensive genetic information policy rest on the assumption that sometimes there is a substantial harmony of interests rather than a fundamental conflict, and some conflicts that may appear to pit the interests of the individual against those of society are actually conflicts among individual interests.

A PRAGMATIC APPROACH TO PRIVACY POLICY

However the variety of societal and individual interests in making genetic information more readily available to some parties are ultimately weighed against interests in restricting access, it seems that privacy protection matters, if at all, for a wide variety of reasons dependent on the context. Many who have defended the moral importance of privacy have tried to find *the* underlying interest that explains why privacy matters in all cases.[10] The brief survey of arguments thus far raises deep doubts about the wisdom of that reductionist enterprise.[11] Many diverse interests are likely to be implicated by any loss of privacy, and although many of those interests tend to cluster, in many cases the importance of privacy protection depends on differing constellations of interests, both social and individual.

The complexity of the pattern of interests at stake in the development of any plausible genetic information policy has profound implications for how we think about privacy rights. If no one interest uniquely accounts for the significance of privacy, then it is unlikely that a single privacy protection policy will be adequate for all contexts, and it is likely that a differing bundle of legally recognized rights, duties, and institutional arrangements will be required for each context. Consequently, a pragmatic approach to privacy protection will be required to accommodate the diverse set of interests at stake in a variety of research, clinical, and administrative contexts.[12]

Essential to the pragmatic approach is a recognition that the kinds of information that ought to be protected from access, the degree and nature of the protection needed, and the institutional arrangements that determine the contingent importance of privacy will vary, depending upon the kinds of harms threatened by a loss of privacy and the vulnerabilities of persons under any given set of economic and social arrangements. The implication is that, when harm to some important interest is threatened as a consequence of someone's having access to genetic information, the policy maker has available at least two types of policy options. Either access to genetic information may be prohibited or restricted through the creation and enforcement of a system of legal rights and duties, or the institutional arrangements themselves may be changed, such that incentives for some to gain access to genetic information to the detriment of others are reduced or eliminated.

Consider first the traditional privacy policy approach involving the creation and enforcement of legal rights. The most stringent types of privacy rights are rights of informational self-determination. Such rights rest on the assumption that in some cases the only feasible way of protecting the interests that give rise to privacy concerns is to create a right to control what information is generated or a right to control subsequent disclosures of, or uses for, information once it is generated and revealed to designated persons for specific purposes.

For example, in cases in which the specificity of certain tests is an issue, such as those used in carrier screening, there is a substantial risk that couples identified as at-risk through population screening will be falsely labeled. Thus, the potential for increased anxiety and unwarranted interference with reproductive plans augments the case for an individual's right to control what information gets generated.

In addition, the case for stringent control rights is even stronger when it involves institutions that collect and store genetic information that may be used for medically unrelated purposes, including access by law enforcement officers, other governmental agencies, and those with commercial interests. It simply may not be reasonable to require individuals to rely on institutional safeguards or the good intentions of the custodians of the information to protect their interests once control is surrendered.

Stringent rights of informational self-determination, however, may be less well justified in other instances, for example, when they would prevent transmission of individual data to regional cancer registries, exclude use of data from persons who are dead or untraceable, and make retrospective studies of health records impossible.[13] Or in the case of genetic registries or research data banks, for example, the arguments for rights to individual control may be less compelling, at least if certain further conditions are satisfied. If, for example, access to genetic information for research can be limited by building a wall between research data banks and records used in the delivery of medical services (which have a wider audience and hence greater potential for harm from disclosure), and the informational practices are vigilantly monitored by institutional review boards, adequate privacy protection may be available without granting individuals a degree of control that would make research virtually impossible.

However, even if special rules for genetic privacy protection are desirable in some research contexts, there are three reasons to think a genetic information policy, distinct from other more stringent medical information policies, would be inadequate in the long run. First, to the extent that genetic testing becomes integrated into routine medical practice, genetic information will become a part of all medical records and thus made available to the wide audiences to which medical records are now available. Second, because blood and tissue samples from any medical context can yield genetic information, it is exceedingly difficult to regulate many nonresearch data banks separately and apart from the rest of medical practice. Third, to the extent feasible, public policy should leave it to individuals to decide what information they are most concerned to keep private. These considerations suggest that the adequacy of any genetic privacy policy will include substantial attention to the improvement of medical privacy protections generally.[14]

In other contexts, however, reliance on a purely rights-based model of privacy protection will likely be inadequate or inefficient, given the magnitude of the interests at stake and the potential for evading enforcement. Policy makers may need to consider options that reconfigure existing institutional arrangements, especially when the institutional arrangements themselves are responsible for making widespread access to genetic information—and the consequent harms to important interests—more probable.

Consider how policy makers might address concerns about the potential adverse consequences of unregulated access to personal genetic information by employers and insurers. Policy options include legal prohibition of access to individual genetic information by employers and insurers and modification of the system of health insurance so that the need for access to information about medical risks is eliminated. Arguably, the objectives underlying both policies include protection of the economically vulnerable in a market economy and the reduction of a major source of inequality of opportunity. The policy maker's task is to consider which option is best suited to achieving these objectives.

The choice between creating new legally enforceable rights of privacy and adopting institutional reform depends on a number of considerations. For example, if laws restricting employer access to genetic information reasonably require exceptions that allow employer access for purposes other than the determination of insurance eligibility or coverage decisions, then restrictions may be difficult to enforce or easily circumvented. If the financial viability of insurance plans offered by employers or other insurers depends on access to information about medical risks generally, prohibition of one type of risk-related information may not produce an economically stable environment adequate to guarantee solvency and continuity of health insurance. In light of such considerations, policy makers must take seriously the possibility that the most feasible alternative for protecting the interests at stake may be the elimination of a risk-based insurance scheme. For only then are the powerful incentives for undermining the privacy of individuals effectively eliminated.

Many other factors, of course, are relevant to the choice of policy options involving such substantial modifications of existing institutional arrangements. However, two objections to treating institutional reform as a component of a pragmatic approach to privacy protection should be addressed.

First, it might be objected that viewing fundamental institutional change as an instrument of genetic information policy is a somewhat counterintuitive understanding of what privacy protection involves. But privacy, as it has been understood throughout this chapter and elsewhere, simply is a matter of limited or restricted access to information, however that restriction is achieved.[15] Rather than achieving the goal of reducing access to genetic information through a system of legally enforceable rights, the same desired effect may be achieved by making access to such information economically worthless (or nearly so). A health care finance policy that eliminates the market incentives for gaining access to genetic information can be as effective an instrument of genetic privacy protection policy as legal prohibitions. If privacy, or restricted access to information is the policy objective, changes in market dynamics no less than legal prohibitions can be a part of the solution.

Second, it might be objected that the two proposals represent qualitatively different kinds of policy options, with insurance reform involving direct state intervention into the domain of private market transactions in a way that the creation of privacy rights does not. However, this claim rests on a confusion. Any genetic privacy protection policy is a market intervention by the state, no less than proposals to change the system of health care financing. For genetic information, like any other kind of information, has market value, and the legal creation of individual privacy rights effectively eliminates the status of such information as a commodity subject to market exchange. Both proposals therefore involve an active role for the state in carrying out a clearly redistributive social objective. Although they differ in the nature and extent of their intervention into the market, both nonetheless have their justification, if at all, based on some theory of the appropriate role of the state in bringing about a particular conception of distributive justice.

Indeed, many, if not all, of the most pressing concerns about genetic privacy discussed here raise more fundamental issues of political philosophy, especially questions of distributive justice and the role of the state in affecting patterns of distribution within society. Implicit in the formulation of genetic information policy generally are judgments about how benefits and burdens, opportunities and risks, and perhaps less obviously, decisional authority ought to be distributed within society. The power to control access to genetic information gives competitive advantage to some and disadvantages others. Without limits on the access others have to genetic information many will find that they have fewer choices about the kind of work they will perform, the health services they will receive, the reproductive choices open to them, and the social status they can expect within the culture. Accordingly, the ability to control access to genetic information itself must be seen as an important social resource, and its distribution can profoundly affect the distribution of much of what else matters to the well-being and autonomy of individuals. For genetic information policies can shape how much access individuals have to other valuable social goods, including the ability to make other personal decisions about a range of significant life options.

Policy decisions about the nature and degree of privacy protection to be accorded to genetic information can compound, solidify, and entrench existing social inequalities, or they can have the effect of redistributing valuable resources. An informed and effective genetic information policy simply cannot be formulated in isolation from an awareness of its distributive implications.

CONCLUSION

The pragmatic approach defended in this chapter yields no single answer to the protection of the interests put at risk by the increased access some persons and institutions have to genetic information. The variety of interests at stake and the complexity of the patterns in which those interests intersect make uniformly applicable solutions impossible. However, the pragmatic approach does provide useful guidelines for policy makers. When other alternatives for privacy protection are unreliable, the underlying interests of the individual are substantial, and the interests at stake include important aspects of individual autonomy, individual rights of control, both the generation and subsequent disclosure of genetic information, may be the only feasible policy alternative. In other cases, the best vehicle for protecting the interests underlying our concerns about genetic privacy may require changes in the economic and social institutions themselves. Fundamental issues of justice lie at the core of any policy meant to ensure the protection of genetic privacy.

NOTES

1. National Academy of Sciences, Institute of Medicine, *Health Data in the Information Age: Use, Disclosure, and Privacy* (Washington, D.C.: National Academy Press, 1994); Work Group for Electronic Data Exchange (WEDI), *Report to Secretary of U.S. Department of Health and Human Services* (1992); Lawrence O. Gostin et al., "Privacy and Security of Personal Information in a New Health Care System," *Journal of the American Medical Association* 270 (1993): 2482–93; U.S. Congress, Office of Technology Assessment, *Protecting Privacy in Computerized Medical Information* (Washington, D.C.: Government Printing Office, 1993).
2. Mark A. Rothstein, "Discrimination Based on Genetic Information," *Jurimetrics* 33 (1992): 13; Paul R. Billings et al., "Discrimination as a Consequence of Genetic Testing," *American Journal of Human Genetics* 50 (1992): 476–82; Lawrence O. Gostin, "Genetic Discrimination: The Use of Genetically Based Diagnostic and Prognostic Tests by Employers and Insurers," *American Journal of Law and Medicine* 17 (1991): 109.
3. Bartha M. Knoppers and Claude Laberge, "DNA Sampling and Informed Consent," *Canadian Medical Association Journal* 140 (1989): 1023–28.
4. George J. Annas, "Privacy Rules for DNA Databanks," *Journal of the American Medical Association* 270 (1993): 2346–50.
5. Ruth Gavison, "Privacy and the Limits of Law," *Yale Law Journal* 89 (1980): 346–402.
6. James Rachels, "Why Privacy Is Important," and Charles Fried, "Privacy: A Moral Analysis," both reprinted in Ferdinand Schoeman, ed., *Philosophical Dimensions of Privacy: An Anthology* (New York: Cambridge University Press, 1984), 291–99, 203–22.
7. John Robertson, "Genetic Alteration of Embryos: The Ethical Issues," in Aubrey Milunsky and George J. Annas, eds., *Genetics and the Law III* (New York: Plenum Press, 1985), 115–27.
8. Norway, Ministry of Health and Social Affairs, *Biotechnology Related to Human Beings (Report No. 25)* (1993), 51–58.
9. Lori B. Andrews and Ami S. Jaeger, "Confidentiality of Genetic Information in the Workplace," *American Journal of Law and Medicine* 17 (1991): 75.
10. Jeffrey Reiman, "Privacy, Intimacy, and Personhood," *Philosophy and Public Affairs* 6 (1976): 38.
11. Madison Powers, "A Cognitive Access Definition of Privacy," *Law and Philosophy* 15 (1996): 369–86.
12. I have developed some of these arguments more fully elsewhere. See Madison Powers, "Privacy and the Control of Genetic Information," in Mark S. Frankel and Albert H.

Teich, eds., *The Genetic Frontier: Ethics, Law, and Policy* (Washington, D.C.: American Association for the Advancement of Science Press, 1994), 77–100.

13. E. J. Knox, "Confidential Medical Records and Epidemiological Research: Wrong-headed European Directive on the Way," *British Medical Journal* 304 (1992): 727–28; Editorial, "Protecting Individuals; Preserving Data," *Lancet* 339 (1992): 3.

14. For a survey of legal protections of medical information and their limitations, see Madison Powers, "Legal Protections of Confidential Medical Information and the Need for Anti-Discrimination Laws," in Ruth Faden et al., eds., *AIDS, Women and the Next Generation: Towards a Morally Acceptable Public Policy for HIV Testing of Pregnant Women and Newborns* (New York: Oxford University Press, 1991), 331–58.

15. Anita L. Allen, "Genetic Privacy: Emerging Concepts and Values," Chapter 2 in this volume.

Chapter 20 Laws to Regulate the Use of Genetic Information

Philip R. Reilly

Legislative interest in the threat to personal privacy that is inherent in our rapidly growing ability to collect and store human genetic information is at an all-time high. In 1995, at least 18 bills to regulate the uses of genetic information in employment or insurance were introduced before at least 13 state legislatures.[1] Late that year two federal bills that directly address genetic privacy were introduced[2] and committee hearings were held on a more general health care bill that specifically recognized the importance of this issue.[3] At the close of 1995, statutes to control or limit the use of genetic information in certain ways were on the books in 14 states.[4] Of these, 10 have been enacted since 1990. One, passed in Oregon in 1995, reflects a growing effort to develop a comprehensive approach to the underlying issues.[5]

During 1996 legislative interest in genetic information remained intense. The two most significant developments took place in New Jersey and New York. That June both houses of the New Jersey legislature unanimously passed a bill sharply restricting the right of insurers to use genetic information in underwriting and giving individuals a property right in their genetic information.[6] The Biotechnology Industry Organization and representatives for the pharmaceutical industry (which has a strong presence in New Jersey) then intervened. On September 19, 1996, Governor Christine Todd Whitman of New Jersey returned the bill to the legislature with a conditional veto, advising the lawmakers that she thought the "property" provision could chill biomedical research and harm the state economy.[7]

On August 8, 1996, Governor George Pataki of New York signed a law (that also passed by unanimous vote in both houses) to regulate the practice of DNA-based predictive genetic testing.[8] The New York law mandates that no genetic test be performed unless the patient has signed a consent form and that with a few exceptions the sample must be destroyed within 60 days after testing. The law saves samples from destruction if they are to be used in anonymously conducted research approved by an institutional review board (IRB) for which the investigator has obtained a signed informed consent, but this will in many instances sharply limit the value of the samples.

Given the steady increase in legislative proposals in this area of the past several years and slim possibility that a federal law will be enacted to preempt state lawmaking in this area, genetic privacy bills will continue to proliferate. It is appropriate, therefore, to take stock. What issues do the current laws cover? What issues do they skirt? What achievements can they claim? What are their shortcomings?

In this chapter I present a brief history of state and federal legislative interest in genetic privacy, provide an overview of the current state legislation, summarize current federal bills, comment on the influence of model legislation,[9] and prognosticate concerning legislative trends in this area in the near future. Any discussion of the legislation on genetic privacy must acknowledge that concern for genetic discrimination has unfolded in a landscape dominated by the larger issue of how to protect the privacy of medical records in general. Thus, a subtext of this chapter is to ask whether genetic information merits special attention or whether it is an interesting facet of the larger debate over the privacy of medical records but not one that requires an independent solution.

HISTORICAL BACKGROUND

There have been two large-scale legislative responses to clinical advances in genetic testing: newborn screening laws and statutes to encourage sickle-cell screening. These stories have been told in detail elsewhere.[10] In both cases legislative eagerness to realize the perceived benefits of genetics failed to attend to privacy issues that were inherent to the programs the state laws were designed to implement.

Shortly after it became possible in 1962 to screen newborns at apparently low cost to detect the rare infant (1 in 12,000) with phenylketonuria (PKU), a treatable inborn error of metabolism, most states followed the lead of Massachusetts and enacted mandatory newborn screening laws.[11] Six years later, more than 40 states had such laws. Today, almost all states have a mandatory screening law that in most instances provides for performing between three and seven tests on each child's blood sample to detect treatable genetic disorders.[12] Few of these laws explicitly promise confidentiality of the genetic data that are generated by testing, although in some states regulations, usually issued by the department of public health to implement these laws, do offer a measure of security.[13]

Between 1970 and 1972, some 13 states enacted laws that required certain persons (usually African Americans) to be tested to determine whether they carried the gene for sickle-cell anemia. These well-intended statutes constitute a case study in the failure of lawmakers to appreciate the clinical and ethical issues inherent in genetic testing programs. Some states required sickle-cell testing as a condition of attending public schools; others would issue a marriage license only to those who provided evidence that they had been tested.[14] After sharp and sustained criticism of the law by leading black physicians and legislators, in the summer of 1972 the federal government enacted a law that made substantial funds available to support sickle-cell screening programs that were voluntary, provided that each person tested had reasonable access to genetic counseling services, and promised to protect the privacy of the genetic information generated by the test.[15]

The sickle-cell screening debacle generated the first state laws written specifically to protect the confidentiality and limit the extraclinical uses of genetic information. During the late 1970s and 1980s several states enacted laws that forbade insurers and employers from using knowledge about one's sickle-cell status in underwriting and employment decisions.[16] In 1986, Maryland, a state in which public health officials have examined clinical and ethical issues in genetics, enacted a broad law that required "actuarial justification" for charging persons differentially higher premiums because of a genetic condition.[17]

THE MODERN ERA

The protection of genetic privacy has been a concern among clinical geneticists, bioethicists, and other experts for more than two decades, but during the period extending from the mid-1970s to the mid-1980s there was comparatively little public discourse on this topic and virtually no legislative activity. One prominent exception was the publication in 1983 of a presidential commission report on genetic screening recommending that "genetic information should not be given to unrelated third parties, such as insurers or employers, without the explicit and informed consent of the person screened or a surrogate for that person."[18] The commission was clearly aware of the possibility that genetic data could be abused. But by today's standards even this document places relatively little emphasis on the issue that drives the current interest in genetic privacy—the fear that genetic data will be used on a grand scale to deny access to or increase the cost of insurance for large numbers of people.

By the mid-1980s scientists were beginning to call attention to the ethical and legal problems inherent in our ability to discern genetic facts about individuals. One of the first uses of the term "genetic discrimination" was at a workshop organized under that title by the Social Issues Committee at the meeting of the American Society of Human Genetics in Philadelphia in 1986.[19] Speakers explored many of the themes that have become the focus of the laws and bills I discuss here.

THE FEDERAL INITIATIVE: THE HUMAN GENOME PRIVACY ACT OF 1990

The first major legislation intended to address the issue of protecting the privacy of genetic information was the Human Genome Privacy Act (HGPA), introduced by Representative John Conyers (D–Mich.) on September 13, 1990, seventeen days before the official birth of the federally funded Human Genome Project (but two years after its conception).[20] Modeled after the federal Privacy Act, the HGPA was designed to protect the privacy of all genetic information generated by a federal agency or in projects using federal funds. It would thus have applied to all research projects funded by the National Institutes of Health. It proposed that individuals have the right to inspect, challenge, and correct genetic records, generally forbade unauthorized disclosure of data to third parties and provided remedies for wrongful disclosure, made significant exceptions for law enforcement proceedings, and provided criminal penalties for deliberate abuse of a privacy interest. With minor revisions the HGPA was reintroduced on April 24, 1991, and hearings were held on October 17 of that year.[21] The bill had the backing of some of our nation's leading geneticists, but it never emerged from committee.

STATE LEGISLATION, 1990–92

By 1989, a number of small public interest groups, such as the Cambridge-based Council for Responsible Genetics, and highly motivated individuals (e.g., Harvard physician Paul Billings and his colleagues in Boston, who met informally as the Genetic Screening Study Group) were attempting to interest state legislators in sponsoring laws to regulate the use of genetic information so that it could not be used to deny access of otherwise healthy persons to health care coverage or employment.[22]

One of the first major state initiatives occurred in California, which had already enacted a law intended to forbid insurance discrimination against healthy people who were at increased risk for bearing children with genetic disorders. In 1991, both houses passed a bill that would have established the right of all persons in California, regardless of their genetic characteristics, to be free from discrimination in "obtaining and enjoying the services, facilities, advantages, housing or other accommodations, or employment opportunities of all business establishments."[23] A genetic characteristic was defined as information known to be associated with a disease or risk of a disease in an asymptomatic individual. In vetoing the bill, Governor Pete Wilson expressed concern that the bill would pose an undue cost burden on employers who purchased health care coverage for their employees.[24]

The various state proposals to protect some feature of genetic privacy took three general forms: bills to forbid any disclosure of genetic data by health care providers unless a person had given a written informed consent, bills to forbid the use of certain genetic information by health insurers, or to a much smaller extent, life insurers, and bills to forbid the use of genetic test results in employment decisions. Despite a flurry of bills, only Florida, Montana, and Wisconsin enacted laws attending to one or more of these issues, and no state comprehensively addressed the topic.[25]

STATE LEGISLATION, 1993–95

In spite of extensive public discussions concerning genetic discrimination, during 1993 and early 1994 the major interest shown by state legislators in genetics related to the creation of DNA felon data banks. In 1993, at least 22 bills concerning this topic were introduced in at least 10 states. In 1994, the volume of new bills pertaining to DNA forensics was even higher, and many laws were enacted. In general, these bills require felons convicted of certain kinds of offenses (usually rape or murder, but sometimes also lesser crimes) to provide a blood sample before parole. This sample is subjected to standardized DNA profiling techniques and stored in a digitized form in a data bank that can be remotely searched. The rationale is that violent criminals have a high rate of recidivism. Thus, DNA analysis of biological evidence (e.g., semen on a rape victim or blood at a murder scene) may quickly lead to identification of the perpetrator.[26] By late 1995, more than 30 states had enacted such laws (see Chapter 13). Pursuant to the federal DNA Identification Act of 1994, which makes substantial funds available to cooperating state laboratories, a national advisory board now oversees the development of operating standards in DNA felon data banks, including protocols to protect the privacy and limit the use of the DNA and data derived therefrom.[27]

Colorado, 1994

On June 2, 1994, Governor Roy Romer signed Colorado Senate Bill 94–058, Concerning Limitations on Genetic Testing, a relatively broad effort to regulate the uses of genetic data.[28] The law includes a declaration that genetic information is the "unique property" of the person to whom it pertains, a finding that it "may be subject to abuses" if disclosed to unauthorized third parties, and a statement of intent that information derived from genetic testing not be used to "deny access to health care coverage, group disability insurance, or long-term care insurance." The law defines information derived from genetic testing as "confidential and privileged" and forbids most disclosures unless the person tested has provided "specific written consent." It expressly forbids the use of genetic test results in certain kinds of underwriting but does not prohibit its use in regard to life insurance and individual disability insurance. The law also provides that "any research facility" may use "genetic information in research so long as the identity of any individual to whom the information pertains is not disclosed to any third party." Interestingly, this provision does not require that the research be conducted anonymously, only "in confidence."

California, 1994

The other significant event of 1994 in regard to genetic legislation was the decision by Governor Wilson of California to sign legislation that amended state insurance laws to forbid certain uses of genetic information by insurers.[29] Until January 1, 2002, the new law does three things: (1) it prohibits health care service plans, self-insured employee welfare benefit plans, and nonprofit hospital service plans from refusing to cover an individual on the basis of having a genetic characteristic that may under some circumstances be associated with a disability in that person or that person's offspring; (2) it forbids insurers that issue disability policies for hospital, medical, and surgical expenses from refusing to accept an application for coverage, refusing to issue a policy, canceling a policy, charging a higher rate or premium, or limiting coverage on the basis of a person's genetic characteristics; and (3) it prohibits a life or disability insurer from requiring a genetic test for the purposes of deciding insurability other than in accordance with informed consent and privacy protection requirements.

California law defines "genetic characteristics" as "any scientifically or medically identifiable gene or chromosome, or alteration thereof, that is known to be a cause of a disease or disorder, or determined to be associated with a statistically increased risk of development of a disease or disorder, *that is presently not associated with any symptoms of any disease or disorder*" (emphasis added).[30] That is, the protections offered under the new California laws are limited to otherwise healthy persons. They do not extend to persons with an illness or disability caused by the underlying genetic characteristic.

The amendments pertaining to the underwriting of life and disability income insurance are limited in effect. They do not forbid genetic testing. They require that the insurer disclose information to the applicant about the test and its purposes and limitations, that the insurer obtain a detailed, written, informed consent to such tests, that the insurer promise to keep the results confidential, and that the insurer bear the cost of testing. Most important, the new law requires that "no policy shall limit benefits otherwise payable if loss is caused or contributed to by the presence or absence of genetic characteristics, except to the extent and in the same fashion as the insurer limits coverage for loss caused or contributed to by other medical conditions presenting an increased degree of risk."[31] The life and disability insurers are protected by that portion of the law stating "that nothing in this chapter shall limit an insurer's right to decline an application or enrollment request for a life or disability income insurance policy, charge a higher rate or premium for such a policy, or place a limitation on coverage under such a policy, on the basis of manifestations of any disease or disorder."[32]

THE GENETIC PRIVACY ACT

Early in 1995, George Annas and his colleagues at the Boston University School of Public Health published a model Genetic Privacy Act (GPA).[33] Produced under a grant from the U.S. Department of Energy, thoughtfully drafted, comprehensive, and carefully explained, the model legislation quickly garnered much attention. The "overarching premise" of the GPA is that "no stranger should have or control identifiable DNA samples or genetic information about an individual unless that individual specifically authorizes the collection of DNA samples for the purpose of genetic analysis, authorizes the creation of that private information and has access to and control over the dissemination of that information."[34] Under the GPA, each person collecting a DNA sample would be required to: provide specific information verbally before the DNA sample is collected; provide a notice of rights and assurances before the DNA sample is collected; obtain written authorization that incorporates required information; restrict access to DNA samples to persons authorized by the sample source; and abide by a sample source's instructions regarding the maintenance and destruction of DNA samples.[35]

According to the Boston University team, during 1995 the GPA was used as a model in drafting Oregon Senate Bill 276, which was enacted; for a Maryland bill, entitled the Genetic Privacy Act, which received an unfavorable report from the Maryland Senate Committee on Economic and Environmental Affairs; and for Pennsylvania Senate Bill 394 (Genetic Information Confidentiality Act), which was referred to the Pennsylvania Senate Committee on Public Health and Welfare. It also has served as a model for federal legislation introduced by Senator Mark Hatfield (R–Oregon).[36]

Even without the influence of the GPA, there can be little doubt that during 1995 state legislative interest in genetic discrimination increased dramatically. As of March 31, 1995, at least 118 bills pertaining to genetic data were before the state legislatures. The largest single category again was bills to create DNA felon data banks or to promote the admissibility of DNA evidence. At least 18 bills, however, were introduced in 13 states that sought to limit the use of genetic information by health insurers and/or employers. During 1995, versions of these bills became law in California, Georgia, Minnesota, New Hampshire, and Oregon.[37] By early 1996, 14 states had laws that in some fashion limit the use of genetic information by insurers, of which 10 are of recent origin.

Another approach (considered in Massachusetts, Nebraska, New York, and Virginia) has been to create special commissions to study genetic privacy. In Massachusetts, where hearings were held on such a bill, lawmakers were wary of appointing gubernatorial commissions.[38] The several most interested legislators decided to sponsor a "special committee" to study the issues and to propose legislation on genetic privacy before the end of 1996. Virginia has created a commission to study breast cancer, including predictive testing to determine those at genetic risk for this condition.[39]

NEW YORK BILLS, 1994–1995

During 1994 the New York State Legislative Commission on Science and Technology issued a report summarizing the issues raised by genetic testing and offering several policy options to state lawmakers.[40] These included: (1) "enacting legislation to prohibit the use of DNA-based tests by insurers" and allowing "those persons who have been denied insurance based on actuarial data to use DNA-based test results to prove that their genetic status does not predispose them to future risk of disease"; (2) amending state law to add "genetic predisposition" to those categories such as race, creed, and color that are already broadly protected from discrimination; (3) expanding a section of the state civil rights law to cover persons with genetic predisposition to disease; (4) enacting a broad new medical records confidentiality law; (5) prohibiting insurers from asking about genetic test results; (6) requiring the destruction of biological materials after a brief time; (7) licensing genetic counselors; and (8) creating a statewide advisory body to oversee the proper uses of genetic information.

Assemblyman Ronald J. Canestrari, chairman of the Legislative Commission on Science and Technology, used the report as the foundation for a packet of genetics bills introduced in 1995. Assembly Bill 5796 proposes to amend the civil rights law by forbidding genetic tests without the prior written informed consent of the individual.[41] The bill requires the consent form to include a number of elements, including "a statement that no tests other than those authorized shall be performed on the biological sample and that the sample shall be destroyed at the end of the testing process or not more than thirty days after the sample was taken." The bill also states that "records, findings and results" of any genetic tests performed on any person "shall be deemed the exclusive property of the individual subject of the test." This is a significant break with a long-established commercial practice that the physical records of clinical tests and the used sample become the property of the laboratory.[42]

On May 24, 1995, Assemblyman Canestrari and others introduced four more bills pertaining to genetics. Assembly Bill 7836 proposed to amend the civil rights law to declare that an "otherwise qualified individual shall not be denied the opportunity to obtain and/or maintain employment and/or advancement solely because of a genetic condition, predisposition to a genetically influenced disease, or carrier status for a genetically influenced disease."[43] The bill added "genetic anomaly, genetic predisposition, or carrier status for such anomaly" as protected categories in the state employment discrimination law. This bill did not come to a vote.

A companion bill, Assembly Bill 7839, declared that "employers have no legitimate interest in requiring or requesting a genetic test or test result from an employee or applicant and should be prohibited from requiring or requesting such test except where such a test is shown to be directly related to the occupational environment, such that the employee or applicant with a particular genetic anomaly might be at an increased risk of disease as a result of working in said environment."[44] The bill forbids employers, employment agencies, and labor organizations from discriminating on the basis of genetic status. It was passed by the Assembly but not by the Senate. Another bill, Assembly Bill 7840, would require that persons who desired to practice genetic counseling in the state must be licensed.[45] As written, it could be construed to exclude physicians from that practice. It was not passed by either house.

Also in 1995, the New York Legislative Drafting Commission proposed to create a Genetics Advisory Board to "assess the social impact of any DNA-based genetic test proposed for use in the state by insurers, employers or educational institutions and advise the commissioners of health and education, the superintendent of insurance, the governor and the legislature in relation to the implications of such test on individual liberties, civil rights and social justice for the people of the state of New York."[46] It was not enacted.

OREGON, 1995

On September 9, 1995, Oregon Senate Bill 276, the most comprehensive state law pertaining to the use of genetic information yet enacted, went into effect.[47] Among its key legislative findings are: that "genetic information is uniquely private and personal information that should not be collected, retained or disclosed without the individual's authorization," that "improper collection, retention or disclosure of genetic information can lead to significant harm to the individual, including stigmatization and discrimination in areas such as employment, education, health care, and insurance," and that laws are needed "to protect individual privacy and to permit legitimate genetic research." With some notable public health exceptions (newborn screening, paternity proceedings, and the identification of deceased persons), the new law forbids the collection of genetic information of an individual without first obtaining informed consent. It declares that "an individual's genetic information is the property of the individual" and that no person may retain another's genetic information without first obtaining authorization. It also provides that the individual may request the destruction of the sample at any time, and it requires that a sample acquired for research purposes be destroyed promptly at the completion of the project unless the individual specifically consents to retain it.

The law also requires that samples tested for insurance or employment purposes be destroyed after the purpose for which they were acquired has been accomplished. Section 5 protects persons who control genetic information from compulsory disclosure to third parties except pursuant to certain law enforcement proceedings, by court order, to establish paternity, with specific authorization from the individual, to furnish information to prospective adoptive parents, to furnish genetic data about a decedent to blood relatives, and to identify dead bodies. Section 6 forbids employers from using genetic information to discriminate but permits them to use it to determine a bona fide occupational qualification as may be determined by state regulations. Section 8 forbids the use of genetic information to "reject, deny, limit, cancel, refuse to renew, increase the rates of, affect the terms and conditions of or otherwise affect any policy for hospital medical expenses."

FEDERAL LEGISLATION, 1995–96

There was an unprecedented level of federal legislative interest in genetic privacy during 1995–96. The Genetic Privacy and Nondiscrimination Act of 1995 was introduced by Senator Hatfield and Senator Connie Mack (R–Florida) on November 15, 1995; its companion was introduced in the House of Representatives by Representative Cliff Stearns (R–Florida) on November 29, 1995.[48] These bills proposed to prohibit the use of genetic data in hiring and in determining access to health insurance, and to require other types of insurers who choose to use genetic tests to disclose the results to the applicant. On January 24, 1996, Representative Edward Kennedy (D–Massachusetts) introduced a bill to limit the collection and use by the Department of Defense of individual genetic identifying information to the identification of remains, unless informed consent was provided for other uses.[49] On March 6, 1996, Senator Dianne Feinstein (D–California) introduced the Genetic Fairness Act of 1996, which aimed to place limits on the use of genetic information by health plans.[50] On April 23, 1996, Senator Olympia Snowe (R–Maine) introduced the Genetic Information Nondiscrimination in Health Insurance Act of 1996, which sought to prohibit insurance providers from denying or canceling health insurance coverage or varying the premiums, terms, or conditions for health insurance coverage on the basis of genetic information.[51] It is the companion to the bill introduced by Representative Louise McIntosh Slaughter (D–New York) on December 7, 1995.[52] I do not discuss these bills here because it is likely that a bill introduced by Senator Pete Domenici (R–New Mexico) on June 24, 1996, will be the focus of debate on this topic.[53]

Although all these bills focus specifically on regulating the use of genetic information, the topic was first discussed during hearings on The Health Insurance Reform Act of 1995, introduced by Senator Nancy Kassebaum (R–Kansas).[54] That bill proposed to protect access to health care benefits by a variety of mechanisms, including mandating the portability of health coverage when persons move from one job to another. The use of "pre-existing condition" limitations has historically created a problem for job mobility in that individuals who are covered under a current plan may have to wait anywhere from three months to two years for coverage of a specific condition under a new plan. As genetic testing has become more useful in determining hereditary risk of illness in the future, the concern that such genetic status will be treated as a preexisting condition has grown. Of even greater concern is that genetic information will be used to deny access to health coverage under any conditions; that is, that genetic data will become a tool to remove persons perceived to be at high risk from the pool of covered individuals.

The bill also proposed to make new rules for group market insurance. It sought to forbid an employee health benefit plan from establishing eligibility criteria on the basis of health status, medical condition, claims experience, receipt of health care, medical history, evidence of insurability, or disability.

In its report on the bill, the Senate Committee on Labor and Human Resources noted that it was concerned about "individuals being denied access to health care coverage based on genetic information."[55] For that reason it explicitly interpreted "health status" and "medical history" as used in section 101(a)(B) of the legislation as including information about past, present, or future health status and medical history, including genetic information. Further, it wrote that section 110(a)(1), that portion of the law that would prohibit discrimination in writing private health insurance, should be interpreted to forbid the use of genetic information to deny access to individual health plans.[56] Acknowledging that there was no clear definition of genetic discrimination, the committee made clear that it intended to define the term broadly. It wrote: "This construction is intended to protect individuals who have, or whose family members have, a gene associated with a genetic disorder. It also is intended to protect couples who are healthy, but have the gene or genes for a recessive disorder that might affect their children."[57] A version of the bill became law on August 21, 1996, as the Health Insurance Portability and Accountability Act of 1996. It specifically forbids using "genetic information" in establishing eligibility criteria.[58]

The first federal bill to focus on the issue of genetic privacy since the the Human Genome Privacy Act of 1990 was the Genetic Privacy and Non-Discrimination Act of 1995, introduced on November 15, 1995, by Senator Hatfield and cosponsored by Senator Mack. It recognized the power of genetic information, the risk of harm inherent in improper disclosure, and the need for laws to protect genetic privacy. It proposed to define the rights of individuals whose genetic information is disclosed, define the circumstances under which such data may be disclosed, and "protect against discrimination by an insurer or employer based upon an individual's genetic information."[59]

The bill focused mainly on health insurance, aiming to reach "self-funded health plans and health plans regulated under the Employee Retirement Income Security Act of 1974," the very plans that currently elude state-based regulations. With few exceptions, section 4(a) of the bill forbade disclosure of genetic information, even by subpoena, unless such disclosure is specifically authorized by the individual from whom the data were derived. The exceptions were when the disclosure is required pursuant to a criminal investigation, an inquest, or an investigation concerning child abuse, pursuant to a court order or a legal proceeding to establish paternity, to provide information about a decedent to blood relatives, or for identifying dead bodies. The bill also sought to prohibit the use of genetic information in employment decisions and to extend the protections of the Civil Rights Act of 1964 to persons claiming a violation.[60] Section 6 forbade any health insurer from using genetic information "to reject, deny, limit, cancel, refuse to renew, increase the rates of, or otherwise affect health insurance." As to other insurance underwriting, the bill required that the insurer must obtain written authorization before performing a genetic test.[61] Section 6 forbids any health insurer from using genetic information "to reject, deny, limit, cancel, refuse to renew, increase the rates of, or otherwise affect health insurance." As to all other insurance underwriting, the bill requires that the insurer must obtain written authorization prior to performing a genetic test.[62]

On December 14, 1995, Representative Slaughter introduced the Genetic Information Nondiscrimination in Health Insurance Act of 1995 (HR 2748).[63]

The bill would prohibit insurance providers from: denying or canceling health insurance coverage or varying the premiums, terms, and conditions of health insurance coverage on the basis of genetic information; requesting or requiring an individual to disclose genetic information; and disclosing genetic information without the prior written consent of the individual. The bill, which has 24 cosponsors, has the support of the American Cancer Society and the National Breast Cancer Coalition.[64] Public concern over genetic discrimination has increased sharply as we have become more aware that common diseases of adulthood have a significant genetic component.

The Slaughter bill would forbid the use of genetic data in group and individual health insurance underwriting, including in regard to employee health benefit plans covered by the Employee Retirement Income Security Act (ERISA).[65] Section 2(c)(3) would create a private right of action to remedy violations of the law, including the right of a party alleging injury to sue for monetary damages. The bill was referred for hearings before the Committee on Commerce and the Committee on Economic and Educational Opportunities.

Neither the Hatfield bill nor the Slaughter bill address a fundamental question implicit in any proposal to regulate the uses of genetic information by insurers and other third parties. Does genetic information merit special protection or is it merely a fascinating component of the more global problem of how to protect the privacy of all medical information? The Medical Records Confidentiality Act of 1995 (S. 1360) introduced on October 24, 1995, by Senator Robert Bennett (R–Utah) and 13 cosponsors and referred to the Committee on Labor and Human Resources, represents a more comprehensive approach that would almost certainly cover genetic information.[66]

The goal of this bill is to "establish strong and effective mechanisms to protect the privacy of persons with respect to personally identifiable health care information that is created or maintained as part of health treatment, diagnosis, enrollment, payment, testing, or research processes." Of interest, it seeks to do this while recognizing the compelling need for the "health care community" to "exchange and transfer health information."[67] The bill would make all those who acquire and hold medical information as part of their professional or commercial lives "health information trustees" who would be primarily responsible for protecting the privacy of that information.[68] The bill would give individuals the right to inspect and copy protected health information and file written requests to the trustee to correct errors in the record. If upon review the trustee decides not to amend the record, the individual would have the right to file a "statement of disagreement."[69]

The bill would also require the trustee to establish and maintain appropriate administrative, technical, and physical safeguards to ensure the security of health information under his or her care.[70] The bill would impose strict rules concerning the disclosure of information by trustees.[71] However, it would permit disclosure of protected health information to certified health information services to create nonidentifiable health information, presumably summary in nature, to help discern trends in health care. The bill would also permit disclosures in the interest of public health and for research projects that have been approved by an IRB.[72] Although this bill did not become law, it garnered much interest, a signal that a revised version could soon be enacted.

S. 1360 was not a bill to limit the use by health insurers or others of genetic or medical information. It would have established a system that would make it easier for individuals to monitor the dissemination and use of such information and to correct misinformation.

THE DOMENICI BILL

On June 24, 1996, Senator Pete Domenici introduced the Genetic Confidentiality and Nondiscrimination Act of 1996 (S. 1898), the most comprehensive effort to date to confront the myriad privacy issues raised by advances in genetic testing.[73] Significantly, Senator Domenici is a well-known supporter of government-funded science, and the Los Alamos National Laboratory, situated in his home state, has a major interest in genomic research.

The bill includes a number of provisions that, if enacted, would have a major impact on the operation of diagnostic genetic testing laboratories, the nonclinical uses of genetic information, and the conduct of genetic research. The two key premises are straightforward: (1) the term "genetic information" should be broadly defined, and (2) the individual from whom the genetic information is derived should (with some relatively narrow exceptions) have ongoing control of the use of the tissue sample and information derived therefrom.

The June 24 version of the bill defines "genetic information" as "the information that may derive from an individual or a family member about genes, gene products, or inherited characteristics." The term includes "DNA sequence information including that which is derived from the alteration, mutation, or polymorphism of DNA or the presence or absence of a specific DNA marker or markers." This definition can be read broadly to include information about predisposition discerned from conducting a family history, a routine part of medical care. Another important definition is "insurer," which (unlike most state genetic privacy laws, which address only health insurance) includes entities that write any line of insurance.

Title I sets out rules for the "collection, storage, and analysis of DNA samples." At the moment the vast majority of clinical genetic testing is not based on DNA analysis. Thus, this title would arguably have comparatively little impact on newborn screening, prenatal screening, and most diagnostic tests as currently conducted because they do not depend directly on DNA analysis. However, much more testing will be DNA-based in the relatively near future. The title requires that testing be preceded by a consent process and a written authorization and lays out 11 topics that must be addressed in obtaining the informed consent. Key elements that must be discussed include the information that testing will provide, how a patient might be able to use test results, and the availability of optional genetic counseling.

The bill requires written authorization for the collection and storage of DNA samples and the retention of that authorization for as long as the sample is preserved. The form must include a provision that enables the individual to allow the DNA to be used for "purely academic research" (a term that is not defined further and is difficult to understand) and another that permits "commercial uses." Section 104 declares that a "DNA sample is the property of the individual." This is probably the most controversial provision of the bill, but it may well not be retained. Among other things, it would change how pathologists and other physicians have handled surgical specimens for more than a century. Both professional custom and case law have long held that a patient has no property interest in pathological specimens. Section 104 also requires routine destruction of DNA samples on the completion of genetic analysis unless the individual has directed otherwise in writing.

Title II sets out the ground rules for disclosure of genetic information. Except for a few law enforcement and public health exceptions, disclosure is permitted only on receipt of a written authorization that identifies the recipient and the purpose of the release. Section 202 specifies that a general release of medical records is not to be construed as an authorization for disclosure of genetic information. This could create significant costs associated with reviewing and protecting selected bits of genetic information from within a much larger record.

Title III addresses "genetic discrimination," the issue that has been the major focus of most other state and federal bills pertaining to genetics. Section 302 places strict limits on all insurers concerning the uses that they may make of genetic information in underwriting. Here the precise contours of the meaning of "genetic information" become crucial. The broader the definition, the farther-reaching the impact on the insurance industry.

Title V would regulate research activities involving "genetic analysis" (a term defined as including only DNA-based studies and thus not applicable to tests of proteins or chromosomes). Section 501 requires virtually all genomic studies involving humans to be reviewed by an IRB and sets forth a risk-benefit guideline that could discourage certain kinds of research. It also requires that researchers must bear the costs of psychological counseling of subjects when that need grows out of a disclosure of research findings (even if the person sought the disclosure). Although perhaps not so intended, this could be very costly for the research enterprise, for the bill places no limit on liability for counseling costs.

Title VI addresses the collection and genetic analysis of tissue from minors (persons under age 18). It requires that for conditions that "do not in reasonable medical judgment produce signs or symptoms of disease before the age of 18" that tests be conducted only if "there is an effective intervention that will prevent or delay the onset or ameliorate the severity of the disease," the intervention would be initiated in childhood, and the parent consents to it. Title VII requires that employees at institutions covered by this act be notified of their responsibilities under it.

Title VIII, the enforcement provision, creates a private right of action for any violation of the act, with a specified penalty of actual (proven) damages or $50,000, whichever is greater. Liability for willful violations is $100,000 or actual damages, whichever is greater, and the bill recognizes the court's right to award additional punitive damages. S. 1898 will almost certainly be the focus of the federal legislative debate over genetic privacy in 1997.

No action was taken on the Domenici bill during the 104th Congress. During the autumn and winter of 1996–97, Senator Domenici's staff revised the bill. Domenici introduced it as "The Genetic Confidentiality and Non-discrimination Act of 1997" (S. 422) on March 11, 1997. The 1997 bill has considerably shortened its introductory sections on "findings and purposes" and no longer has a section concerning genetic testing of children. The all-important section of definitions of terms contains a much more precise and improved definition of *DNA sample* that effectively excludes most routine clinical tests, blood banking, and newborn screening from the bill's scope.

The overall structure of S. 422 remains unchanged, and it still contains troubling features. Section 302(e), for example, specifies that a general authorization for release of medical records "shall not be construed as a release of genetic information." To comply with such a rule would require that every record be scanned for genetic information and that such information be redacted before it could be released. This would be time-consuming and extremely expensive, if not impossible, to do.

Title V, which would regulate genetic research, may cause unintended harms. Section 501(a)(2) would require IRBs to evaluate genetic studies with a balancing test that could cause some IRBs to reject research protocols that pose little risk to subjects. Section 501(a)(3)(F) places a limited duty on researchers to disclose findings of clinical relevance to families of deceased persons who were subjects in a study. It would be difficult to comply with this provision. Further, it represents a step toward imposing a duty to contact subjects about the results of research, which I would oppose. Much early research is too uncertain to yield a clear message about clinical relevance. Section 501(b) would require genetic research studies to obtain federal certificates of confidentiality from the Department of Health and Human Services. This greatly expands the original purpose of such certificates, and the responsible agency would have trouble meeting the demand. It is essential that the research community contribute to the discussion of this bill.

CONCLUSION

Given the current political climate, it seems unlikely that the federal government will substantially revise how Americans gain access to health care. Market forces have stopped the inflationary health care cost spiral and those same forces will probably constrain costs for some time. The federal government is not likely soon to significantly alter ERISA, the law that gives self-insuring employers the legal grounds to avoid the reach of many state health insurance regulations. ERISA's preemption provision states that ERISA "shall supersede any and all State laws insofar as they . . . relate to any employee benefit plan."[74]

It is of interest, however, that in its most recent decision concerning ERISA's preemption clause, the Supreme Court departed somewhat from several earlier cases in which it had unambiguously agreed that ERISA had a broad reach. For example, in 1985, in Metropolitan Life Insurance Co. v. Massachusetts,[75] the high court upheld a state rule that all commercial health insurance policies, including those purchased by employers, offer coverage for mental health care. A decade later, the Court upheld a New York law that required hospitals to charge commercial health insurers more for hospital care than it did for not-for-profit insurers, in effect validating a surcharge on private plans to redistribute costs.[76] In so doing the Court sent a signal to the states that, despite ERISA, it would tolerate some policy making that generally affects benefits laws.

A substantial minority of states now have statutes intended to limit the use of genetic information by health insurers and/or give individuals control (by requiring consent for transfer of information) of the use of genetic data compiled about them. These laws are new and it is impossible to measure their effects. The best one can do is to ask what impact they are likely to have. To answer that question one must determine to whom the laws apply and what uses of genetic information they actually restrict. It is important to keep in mind that, thus far, these laws really apply only to health insurers' use of genetic data. I discern no trend to enlarge the scope of these bills to regulate life, disability, or other forms of insurance. Furthermore, the existing genetic discrimination laws are limited to regulating the use of genetic test results. Generally speaking, they do not prohibit insurers or health maintenance organizations from inferring genetic information from medical records or from asking questions about family history.

The states with relevant laws are home to about one-fourth of the population. The laws are irrelevant to Americans who are covered under Medicare and largely irrelevant to those covered under Medicaid. They are of little importance to the roughly 60% of Americans who obtain health care coverage for themselves and their families through employer-based group plans that do not rate the health status of individuals. For otherwise healthy persons in whom a genetic test has suggested an increased risk of developing a disease in the future, the state laws may in theory be valuable in dissuading plan managers from expanding the reach of "preexisting condition" clauses. Practically speaking, however, many factors of much more immediate relevance than the advent of genetic testing are coalescing to limit the reach of such clauses. Further, for many of the conditions that might be anticipated, the onset of illness (if it occurs) is likely to be long after standard preexisting condition exclusion periods have been tolled.

Ironically, the new state genetic antidiscrimination laws may be most relevant to a fraction of the population that is unlikely to need them. The statutes clearly cover persons seeking to purchase individually underwritten health insurance. This class, which numbers about 10–15% of Americans, is steadily declining, largely due to the high cost of purchasing such policies. In general, those who can still afford this option tend to have the resources to obtain the coverage they desire despite negative genetic information. The statutes will make that task a bit easier.

Taking into account the population of the states in which laws have been enacted and estimating the fraction of the population that has health care coverage to which the laws are relevant, I estimate that only 3–4% of Americans could currently perceive a direct benefit from them. If enacted, the Hatfield and Slaughter bills would have a much greater impact, but the political climate does not portend well for them.

We are entering an era when genetic testing will become ever more important in medicine. It is quixotic to think that test information can be sequestered from medical records (as has been done with HIV tests). Within a decade or two genetic information will rarely be gathered about a single disorder. As is the case with many existing biochemical tests, it will be cheaper and will make more clinical sense to amass information through the standard battery. Genetic data will be essential to decisions about reproduction, preventive screening, behavioral choices, prognosis, choice of therapy, and follow-up monitoring. In time such data will be part of virtually all medical records and will be essential to formulating a strategy to maintain health.

As part of the general medical record, genetic information will be accessible to a disturbingly large number of viewers, including, of course, third-party payers and financial staff at health maintenance organizations. How, then, can we use genetic information to maximize human health and minimize the threat of discrimination and abuse? I think that the best course is to secure laws that protect the privacy of all individual medical records and that dissuade providers from using information to exclude selected individuals. The Medical Records Confidentiality Act of 1995 proposes a reasonable approach to the privacy issue. If one added the category of "genetic information" to its list of protected entities, that statute, shorn of unnecessary bureaucracy, could secure most of the goals sought by the more focused genetic discrimination statutes. Various state and federal laws providing for "portability" of health insurance also offer a reasonable approach to solving most aspects of the genetic exclusion program.

NOTES

1. Karen H. Rothenberg, "Genetic Information and Health Insurance: State Legislative Approaches," *Journal of Law, Medicine and Ethics* 23 (1996): 309–16.
2. S. 1416, 104th Cong., 1st Sess., Nov. 15, 1995; H.R. 2748, 104th Cong., 1st Sess., Dec. 14, 1995.

3. S. 1028, 104th Cong., 1st Sess., July 15, 1995. See Senate Report no. 104–156, 20.

4. Kathy L. Hudson et al., "Genetic Discrimination and Health Insurance: An Urgent Need for Reform," *Science* 270 (1995): 391–93.

5. S.B. 276, 68th Or. Leg. Ass., Reg. Sess. 1995, Or. Stat. §§ 659.036, 659.227.

6. New Jersey "Genetic Privacy Act"; Senate Committee Substitute for Senate, nos. 695 and 854. Adopted Mar. 14, 1996.

7. Christine Todd Whitman, "Conditional Veto Message to Senate Committee," Substitute for Senate Bill, nos. 695 and 854, Sept. 19, 1996.

8. New York 219th General Assembly—Second Regular Session (1996) Senate Bill 4293 (Enacted). Signed by Governor George Pataki, Aug. 8, 1996.

9. George J. Annas, Leonard H. Glantz, and Patricia A. Roche, *The Genetic Privacy Act and Commentary* (Boston: Boston University School of Public Health, 1995).

10. Philip R. Reilly, "Genetic Screening Legislation," in H. Harris and Kurt Hirschhorn, eds., *Advances in Human Genetics,* vol. 2 (New York: Plenum, 1995), 319–76.

11. Philip R. Reilly, *Genetics, Law, and Social Policy* (Cambridge: Harvard University Press, 1977), 43–49.

12. Council of Regional Networks for Genetic Services (CORN), *Newborn Screening Report: 1990* (New York: CORN, 1992), 8.

13. Lori B. Andrews, *State Laws and Regulations Governing Newborn Screening* (Chicago: American Bar Foundation, 1985).

14. Reilly, *Genetics, Law, and Social Policy,* 62–86.

15. National Sickle Cell Anemia Control Act of 1972, 86 Stat. 136.

16. Hudson et al., "Genetic Discrimination and Health Insurance," 392.

17. Md. Insur. Code of 1957, art. 48A, § 223(b)(4).

18. President's Commission for the Study of Ethical Problems in Medicine and Biomedical Research, *A Report on the Ethical, Social, and Legal Implications of Genetic Screening, Counseling and Educations Programs* (Washington, D.C.: Government Printing Office, 1983), 6.

19. Social Issues Committee Workshop, "Genetic Discrimination: Rights and Responsibilities of Tester and Testee," *American Journal of Human Genetics* 39 (supp.) (September 1986): 15.

20. H.R. 5612, 101st Cong., 2d Sess.; H.R. 2045, 102d Cong., 1st Sess.

21. Philip R. Reilly, "ASHG Statement on Genetics and Privacy: Testimony to United States Congress," *American Journal of Human Genetics* 50 (1992): 640–42.

22. Paul Billings et al., "Discrimination as a Consequence of Genetic Testing," *American Journal of Human Genetics* 50 (1992): 476–82.

23. Cal. Assembly Bill no. 1888. Introduced Mar. 8, 1991.

24. Jean E. McEwen and Philip R. Reilly, "State Legislative Efforts to Regulate Use and Potential Misuse of Genetic Information," *American Journal of Human Genetics* 51 (1992): 637–47.

25. Fla. Stat. § 760.40 (West 1996); Mont. Code Ann. § 33–18–206 (1991); Wis. Stat. § 631.89 (West 1995).

26. Jean E. McEwen and Philip R. Reilly, "A Review of State Legislation on DNA Forensic Data Banking," *American Journal of Human Genetics* 54 (1994): 941–58.

27. 42 U.S.C. § 3751(b) et seq.

28. Colo. Rev. Stat. Ann. § 10-3-1104.7 (West 1994 & Supp. 1996).

29. Cal. Insur. Code §§ 10123.3, 10140, 10148, 10149, 10149.1, 11512.95 (West Supp. 1996).

30. Cal. Health and Safety Code § 1374.7 (West 1990 & Supp. 1996).

31. Cal. Insur. Code § 10148(e) (West Supp. 1996).

32. Ibid., § 10148(f).

33. Annas, Glantz, and Roche, *Genetic Privacy Act and Commentary.*

34. Ibid., vi.

35. Ibid., §§ 101-105, pp. 9-14.

36. Patricia A. Roche, Memorandum, Nov. 7, 1995, and personal communication, Jan. 8, 1996.

37. Rothenberg, "Genetic Information and Health Insurance," 311-12.

38. Mass. Senate no. 2045 (September 1995). Introduced by Senator Mark Pacheco.

39. Virginia Senate Joint Resolution 372 (1995).

40. New York Legislative Commission on Science and Technology, *DNA Based Tests: Policy Implications for New York State* (Albany: New York State, 1994).

41. New York Assembly Bill 5796. Introduced Mar. 7, 1995.

42. Ibid., § 1.

43. New York Assembly Bill 7836. Introduced May 24, 1995, § 1.

44. New York Assembly Bill 7839. Introduced May 24, 1995, § 1.

45. New York Assembly Bill 7840. Introduced May 24, 1995.

46. New York Legislative Bill Drafting Commission, no. 09302-01-5.

47. Or. Rev. Stat. §§ 659.036, 659.277 (West Supp. 1996).

48. S. 1416, 104th Cong., 1st Sess., Nov. 15, 1995; H.R. 2690, 104th Cong., 1st Sess., Nov. 29, 1995.

49. H.R. 2873, 104th Cong., 2d Sess., Jan. 24, 1996.

50. S. 1600, 104th Cong., 2d Sess., Mar. 6, 1996.

51. S. 1694, 104th Cong., 2d Sess., Apr. 23, 1996.

52. H.R. 2748, 104th Cong., 1st Sess.

53. S. 1898, 104th Cong., 2d Sess., June 24, 1996.

54. S. 1028, 104th Cong., 1st Sess., July 13, 1995.

55. Senate Committee on Labor and Human Resources Report 104-156, 104th Cong., 1st Sess., 1995.

56. Ibid., 20.

57. Ibid.

58. Pub. L. 104-191.

59. S. 1416, § 2(b)(3).

60. Ibid., § 6(c).

61. Ibid.

62. Ibid.

63. H.R. 2748, 104th Cong., 1st Sess.

64. Rep. Louise M. Slaughter, Floor Statement to U.S. House of Representatives, Dec. 14, 1995. Introduction of H.R. 2478.

65. 29 U.S.C. §§ 1001-461 (1994).

66. S. 1360, 104th Cong., 1st Sess., § 2(1).

67. Ibid., § 2(2).

68. Ibid., § 3(7).

69. Ibid., § 102(c).

70. Ibid., § 111.

71. Ibid., § 203.

72. Ibid., §§ 208–9.

73. S. 1898, 104th Cong., 2d Sess., June 24, 1996.

74. 29 U.S.C. § 1144(a) (1994).

75. 471 U.S. 724 (1985).

76. New York State Conference of Blue Cross & Blue Shield Plans v. Travelers Ins. Co., 514 U.S. 645 (1995).

Chapter 21 European Data Protection Law and Medical Privacy

Paul M. Schwartz

Advances in modern genetics and information technology have brought legal protection of informational privacy to a crossroads. Developments in genetic science allow the creation of different kinds of highly sensitive personal data, while information technology encourages the transmission and sharing of personal data on a national and global basis.[1] The critical issue is how the legal order should structure the application of personal genetic data by government and private enterprise alike.

In this chapter I shed light on the question of genetic privacy by taking a comparative perspective, discussing European data protection law in general and its approach to medical information and genetic privacy in particular. After an overview of European informational privacy law, I consider its treatment of personal medical data and then move on to examine European approaches to genetic privacy and European mechanisms for blocking international data exports. The possibility of such European data embargoes indicates how important it is for the United States to pay attention to international developments in data protection law.

Even in countries where universal access to health care is assured, serious concerns remain regarding the use of personal health care data. This phenomenon suggests that even sweeping reform of the American health care system and the institution of universal coverage would not obviate the need for regulation of the use of personal genetic data. The risks of misapplying this information will not simply vanish. Moreover, European trends indicate a preference for ongoing legislative activity through targeted laws directed at specific areas in which personal genetic information will be used. Although some American experts have expressed a preference for enacting a broadly conceived genetic privacy statute, the United States will likely find that no single legislative solution can regulate all uses of personal genetic data. Instead, the best legal response will be through a series of targeted laws.

EUROPEAN DATA PROTECTION LAW

Comparative law provides a novel perspective on similar kinds of legal problems found in different nations and offers the chance for new insights. A comparative perspective is particularly useful in the context of European and American information privacy law because responses in Europe and the United States to a similar range of problems exhibit distinctive differences. The differences begin, in fact, with an essential point of terminology: "data protection" is the term of art that in Europe refers to issues that are more commonly called "informational" or "data" privacy in the United States. Although different European nations employ varying methods of data protection, enough similarities exist for a discussion of a European model of data protection.

The European approach consists of a shared agreement regarding both the appropriate process for regulation and a core group of fair information practices. In contrast, the United States handles the regulation of the use of personal information in a different fashion. These differences are most apparent at the level of process.

European law foresees an active, prophylactic state role to protect individual interests from harms that may arise from the processing of personal information. As a result, most European nations have fairly broad laws that regulate the use of personal information. Such data protection laws can be termed "omnibus" statutes. In Europe, regulation of both the public and private sectors is sometimes found within a single piece of omnibus legislation. These laws establish a comprehensive series of rights and responsibilities that address issues of data collection, storage, use, and disclosure. In addition to such omnibus laws, European data protection employs "sectoral" statutes that regulate a single area of data processing activity. These laws govern narrower fields of processing activity than the omnibus statutes.

Legislative regulation of data processing in Europe tends to take place in an ongoing fashion. Moreover, oversight by independent agencies is considered an essential element for effective informational privacy.[2] Data protection commissions or commissioners usually have oversight responsibilities over wide areas of the use of personal information; their mandate allows them to examine the interrelation of data processing activities and law. They also participate in the development of international measures that affect global information transfers. Considerable diversity exists, however, in the scope of the regulatory power that individual European nations grant to these commissions. Only some of these agencies have the power to license data banks or to issue binding decrees. A second approach is to assign merely advisory functions to such agencies (discussed below).

The European approach to data protection is expressed not only through the adoption of a certain kind of regulatory process but also through attention to a core set of fair information principles. European consensus regarding fair information principles centers on four critical elements (1) the creation of a statutory fabric that defines obligations and responsibilities with respect to the use of personal information; (2) the maintenance of "transparent" processing of personal information; (3) the assignment of special protection for sensitive data; and (4) the establishment of enforcement rights for the individual and effective oversight of the treatment of personal information.[3] These basic principles are set out in existing national laws and in such European-wide documents as the European Union's Data Protection Directive and the Council of Europe's Data Protection Convention. A few words should be said about each of the core substantive principles.

The first principle is the creation of statutes that define obligations with respect to the processing of personal information. Different risks will arise depending on the area of human activity subject to administration through data processing. As a result, European law seeks to craft a varied statutory response to different contexts of personal data processing.

The second element in the European approach is the maintenance of "transparent" processing systems. The notion of transparency rests on a belief that personal information should be used in an open manner that is understandable to individuals. The establishment of secret files can coerce the individual into retreating from social and political activities. In contrast, comprehension of the application of personal information can encourage one's participation in social and political life.

European data protection law also requires the creation of special protection for sensitive data. This principle requires the establishment of greater protection for certain types of information, namely those concerning race, religion, political beliefs, or health. The third core principle has special significance for personal medical and genetic information, which fall squarely into the category of sensitive data.

The final element of European fair information practices begins with a requirement that enforcement rights be assigned to the individual. Such interests provide a remedy in the event of violations of the data processor's obligations and responsibilities with respect to personal information. Finally, as noted above, European countries have created a governmental agency that carries out oversight. These independent authorities monitor the development of processing practices and the implementation of national and international data protection law.

An area of particular relevance for genetic information is personal health care data. Despite guarantees of universal access to health care in Europe, significant efforts have been made to protect personal medical information. Understanding the European difference, however, requires a description of current legal standards for the privacy of medical information in the United States.

Most observers of the legal regulation of the privacy of medical information in the United States agree that it is insufficient. A report by the Office of Technology Assessment concluded, "The present legal scheme does not provide consistent, comprehensive protection for privacy in health care information, whether it exists in a paper or computerized environment." The Institute of Medicine's Committee on Regional Health Data Networks has stated that the "threats and potential harm" from disclosure of health records "are real and not numerically trivial."[4]

The lack of adequate regulation of medical information in the United States is shown most clearly by the compilation and sale of lists of persons with specific conditions or diseases. These data are *not* typically obtained through access to medical records in the control of hospitals or physicians. Rather, such lists are created by pharmaceutical and other companies reaching out to health care consumers through toll-free numbers that offer product information and by exchanging coupons or samples in exchange for filling out a questionnaire.[5] Such contact with individuals is usually made without disclosure of planned future usage of the information gathered in this fashion. Direct marketing companies have advertised lists containing the names of people who suffer from such conditions as epilepsy, bleeding gums, diabetes, high blood pressure, thinning hair, and incontinence.[6]

Such mailing lists, which often contain details about sensitive kinds of medical conditions, are freely trafficked in the United States. Joel Reidenberg, a legal scholar who has studied this area, has criticized the lack of effective regulation of the direct marketing industry. This industry creates and sells lists of individuals not only with medical conditions but with different single and multiple characteristics ranging from denture adhesive buyers to subscribers to Penthouse to "married, middle-aged, 'large-sized' women with children and moderate incomes who purchase particular types of underwear." Yet, as Reidenberg notes, "meaningful notice" of these kinds of practices does not exist for the people on such lists. Robert Gellman has cogently summed up the legal response to the situation regarding lists of health care data: "The use of this health information for marketing is unregulated."[7]

The regulatory failure in the United States occurs in both federal and state law. At the federal level, data protection measures are found in constitutional law, the Privacy Act, and a few statutes that regulate narrow areas of data use.[8] Any discussion of these provisions must begin by noting their extremely limited coverage. Most medical information in the United States is collected and processed by private institutions, which are unlikely to meet applicable constitutional tests for state action or jurisdictional requirements in the Privacy Act or other statutes. As a result, most medical data are entirely outside the protections of either constitutional or federal law.[9]

In addition, notable weaknesses exist in federal measures even within their fields of limited application. The Supreme Court first identified a constitutional right of informational privacy in Whalen v. Roe, a case involving a New York State plan to create a data bank to store information about patients' use of certain prescription drugs.[10] The Supreme Court found that this data bank implicated a right of informational privacy with two facets; these interests are in nondisclosure of personal information and decisional autonomy.[11] Despite this constitutional doctrine's potential for improving health care privacy, lower courts have not always capitalized on this promise.[12]

The limited constitutional protection for medical privacy has not been adequately supplemented by federal statutes.[13] As for state law, even where applicable, it has not overcome the weaknesses in current federal data protection. At the state level, relevant measures include constitutional law, which has sometimes been interpreted as setting limits on the collection and dissemination of medical data.[14] States also possess statutory measures regarding doctor-patient confidentiality and common law tort remedies.[15] Finally, more than a dozen states have enacted laws that limit health insurers' use of genetic information.[16] Yet these provisions have failed to impose a consistent and effective framework on the use of medical information.[17] The current state legislative approaches to genetic privacy, for example, focus narrowly on genetic tests rather than genetic information generated in other ways.[18] In addition, the practice and administration of medicine now increasingly take place on an interstate level, which makes state solutions to data protection increasingly unwieldy.

In Europe, as in the United States, legal protection of personal medical data occurs through the interplay of different kinds of measures. The existence of this detailed regulation is noteworthy in itself. Although European nations vary in their method of financing and dispensing medical services, all these countries share a commitment to universal access to health care.[19] One might expect such a guarantee of health care coverage to lessen the need for laws that protect the privacy of health care information. It might do so by indirectly preventing personal medical data from being used to cut off health care coverage. Yet throughout Europe there exists a strong commitment to create careful limitations on the use of health care information. European data protection for personal medical data shows that more is at stake in this context than guaranteeing health care for all. Europeans view data protection as a human right, and one whose existence helps safeguard the existence of a free society.[20] Even with access to medical services guaranteed, European law remains highly concerned with how personal health care information and genetic data are used by government and private institutions.

The result of this concern is a level of legal standards for the protection of medical information in Europe that, though not without flaws, is generally higher than in the United States. At the same time, the ongoing shift to an electronic environment for the processing of health care data has raised significant challenges to existing European regulation.

The most important European-wide measure for data protection is the Directive on the Protection of Individuals with Regard to the Processing of Personal Data and on the Free Movement of Such Data, , a joint measure of the European Parliament and the Council of the European Union, which requires member countries to establish legislation that conforms with its standards.[21] Citizens of European nations may rely directly on the directive should it fail to be implemented correctly, completely, or punctually into domestic law.[22] This document's goal is to ensure a "high level of protection" within the European Union for "fundamental rights and freedoms, notably the right to privacy." The directive stresses that fair information practices must be in place before member states can permit the processing of personal information, including "data concerning health." Put another way, without sufficient data protection, the processing of personal information, including personal medical data, may not occur. The directive explicitly requires that the data protection law of individual European nations articulate and enforce the core fair information principles I have identified here.[23]

In addition to the Directive on Data Protection, a European-wide treaty also affects the level of protection for medical information within individual nations. This treaty, the Council of Europe's Convention for the Protection of Individuals with Regard to Automatic Processing of Data, is a non-self-executing treaty; its standards do not directly impose binding norms on signatory nations.[24] It does, however, require signatory nations to establish domestic data protection laws that will give effect to the convention's principles. The convention requires that signatory nations only permit the processing of sensitive data, including "personal data concerning health," when "domestic law provides appropriate safeguards."[25] Like the Directive on Data Protection, the convention expresses the core fair information principles and requires that they become part of domestic European law.[26]

The convention's protections have been expanded on by the Council of Europe's Recommendation no. R(81)(1), which provides sectoral regulations for automated medical data banks.[27] A new recommendation, the Draft Recommendation on the Protection of Medical Data, will provide more detailed and in certain respects stronger protections for medical data.[28] Taken together, the directive, the convention, and these two recommendations reflect a considerable European-wide commitment to data protection in the medical domain.

On the domestic level, data protection starts in some European nations with constitutional law. In Germany, for example, an important constitutional right applies to personal information, including medical data.[29] Germany's Constitutional Court has termed this interest "the right of informational self-determination" and has found that it protects the individual from unrestricted collection, storage, application, and transmission of personal data. This right prevents the processing of personal data that would limit an individual's capacity for self-governance. It also compels the state to organize data processing so that personal autonomy will be respected. Thus, the right of informational self-determination both limits certain actions and obliges other activities on the part of the state.[30] Whereas the German judiciary has played an important role in identifying this right, in Switzerland, explicit language in the constitution applies to genetic science (discussed below).[31]

Constitutional safeguards also exist for personal information in the United States. Most European nations, however, unlike the United States, have an omnibus data protection law. Such statutes often regulate the use of personal data in both the public and private sectors.[32] In Germany, the omnibus statute is the Federal Data Protection Law; in France, it is the Act on Data Processing, Data Files, and Individual Liberties.[33]

These omnibus laws are supplemented and strengthened by other general laws and by sectoral measures that contain more precise regulations for individual areas of processing activities. In Germany, for example, the Federal Data Protection Law has played a secondary role in regulating the use of medical data. A more important role has been carried out by the statutory provisions found, for example, in the Social Welfare Code (*Sozialgesetzbuch*), the Criminal Code, and the Cancer Registry Statute of 1994.[34]

Examples from Germany and France illustrate the high legal standard for medical data protection in Europe and the potential for future difficulties. In Section 28(2)(b), Germany's Federal Data Protection Law regulates the possibility of transfers of personal information for direct marketing purposes. It explicitly states that such transmissions are generally forbidden when the data in question relate to "health" (*gesundheitliche Verhältnisse*).[35] This approach is also followed in Germany's Social Welfare Code, which permits information, including medical data, collected in the context of social welfare programs to be processed, stored, and transferred only when a specific legal measure permits such action. This law contains no such provision allowing medical data to be used for direct marketing purposes.[36]

Another use of health care data forbidden in Germany is the transferring of personal patient information to "clearinghouses" without patient consent. These services function as "factoring" enterprises; they purchase charges for private medical services from physicians at a discount and then undertake to collect the amount owed.[37] Germany's highest civil and criminal court, the Federal Court of Justice (the Bundesgerichtshof, or BGH) found that this practice violated the physician's duty of confidentiality as set out in the Civil Code and Criminal Code.[38] The BGH stated that patients must be informed of a physician's intention to transfer patient data to such services and give their consent in writing to this practice.[39]

An area of ongoing difficulty in Germany concerns the use of health identification cards. Beginning in the late 1980s and with an accelerated rate of change in the 1990s, Germany began to reform its national health insurance program, which couples a guarantee of universal access to medical care with global budgetary constraints on physicians and hospitals.[40] These budgetary limits are set through negotiations between the nation's nonprofit sickness funds and physician representatives.[41] When past negotiations failed to contain expenditures effectively, a critical part of the legal response was an aggressive use of data collection and processing to control patient and physician behavior. To further the use of personal data, the Health Reform Law of 1989 required that all patients be furnished with machine-readable health insurance cards by the start of 1995.[42] Strict legal limits have thus far been placed on the type of information stored on this card and on the sharing of data generated through use of this device.[43]

German law does not allow medical information to be stored on the health insurance card. The Fifth Book of the Social Welfare Law enumerates the information that may be stored on this device; these data fall into roughly two categories: information relating to the individual (full name, birthdate, address, insurance number, insurance status, and a machine-readable signature); and information relating to the insurance policy (name of issuing insurance fund and the policy start and end dates).[44]

In spite of these statutory restrictions, the introduction of more technically complex "chip cards" has challenged the effectiveness of this approach. In contrast to the German health insurance card, which usually contains a simple magnetic strip like those found on most credit cards, chip cards are more advanced devices that contain a small silicon chip. A chip card is already capable of storing the contents of a newspaper; in the future, even greater storage capacity will be possible. One day a patient will be able to carry his or her entire medical record, including digitized X-rays, on a plastic card. Chip cards containing detailed medical histories are already in use in Germany, and the data protection issues this technology raises are only beginning to be explored.[45]

Although German law has placed strict legal limits on the type of personal information to be stored on the standard health identification cards, it permits insurance companies to introduce chip cards based simply on the health care consumer's consent.[46] This loophole represents a flaw in German data protection law. Fortunately, data protection commissioners are currently playing a critical role in leading the public and political discussion regarding the acceptability of this device.[47] Understanding this role requires a few preliminary words about the nature of these figures in Germany.

Data protection officials work in Germany at federal and state levels. Compared to other nations, these commissioners carry out an "advisory" approach to data protection. Although binding legal decisions concerning data protection generally rest elsewhere, German data protection commissioners have powers to investigate information processing and to submit formal complaints to the responsible federal ministers. They can also issue appeals to the legislative branches of government and to the media. In addition, the commissioners have a special obligation to help anyone who believes that the government's processing of his or her personal data has caused a hardship to a legal interest.[48]

Data protection commissioners have actively performed their advisory function in the area of medical information. A unanimous resolution of the Federal and State Data Protection Commissioners of Germany at Potsdam in 1994 offers important insights into how chip cards are used in the administration of health care in Germany and how data protection experts envision an optimal response to this use. In the Potsdam Resolution, the data protection commissioners made a number of objections to the use of these devices and articulated principles necessary for their future application.[49]

First, the commissioners noted a lack of safeguards to assure the voluntariness of an individual's decision whether to use a chip card. As examples of "de facto pressure" to choose the chip card, the commissioners pointed to insurance companies' awarding "bonus points" for health care consumers who asked for these cards and increasing the difficulty of paperwork and other administrative procedures for those who insisted on receiving only the standard card. Another shortcoming in the employment of these devices was that they contained no technical means for restricting access to any part of the medical histories stored on them. As a result, all physicians and medical personnel with whom the patient came into contact had access to the complete data on the chip cards.[50]

In the Potsdam Resolution, the commissioners recommended that chip cards not replace the standard health identification card with its more limited personal information. Any use of the chip card as a supplemental device, they insisted, had to be truly voluntary. The difficulty here, as American students of the "informed consent" doctrine will recognize, is that agreement in many such situations involving the administration of health care is neither informed nor freely given.[51] In response to the difficulties with a simplistic reliance on informed consent, the commissioners called for a legal requirement that consent to patient chip cards be valid only if made in writing and after the sharing of complete information about "the goal, contents, and application of the offered card."[52] These are certainly appropriate requirements concerning the policing of informed consent; perhaps even more important, the commissioners also made demands involving the procedures that accompanied the employment of chip card technology.

The Potsdam Resolution considered how this device might be shaped so that its application in the administration of health care would be consistent with ideals of data protection. The commissioners advocated the construction of health care chip cards with built-in access restrictions. Such internal safeguards were to ensure the availability of only "necessary data" for each use of these cards.[53] Finally, "the affected party," namely the health care consumer, should be considered, in the words of one state commissioner, as the "master of his information."[54] The individual was at all times to have access to the complete information on the chip card, to determine which data would be stored on this device, and to decide whether the card would be used in any given circumstance. Finally, the commissioners noted that all health care consumers with chip cards should have free access to card readers.[55]

German law has not yet adopted the recommendations of the data protection commissioners' Potsdam Resolution. Indeed, because of the relentless pace of technological change in this area, new problems are arising even before improvements can be made in the application of chip cards. For example, there is now interest in Germany in establishing a nationwide electronic information infrastructure for the transmission of personal medical data. Different pilot projects are being planned by the newly privatized German telephone company, by various publishing enterprises, and by a major organization of German physicians. Of these data highways for medical information, *Der Spiegel* has tersely observed that such technology would be "practical, but dangerous."[56]

If Germany faces some of the same problems in the field of informational privacy as the United States, it may also have developed a better system for engaging in political, legal, and social debate about these issues. In a recent annual report, the data protection commissioner of Hesse, Winfried Hassemer, emphasizes the importance of the political, legal, and social processes that lead to decisions about the use of medical data. He writes, "Concrete solutions can not be reached merely from a data protection perspective, but depend on a dialogue between all participants." In a similar spirit, the federal data protection commissioner, Joachim Jacob, has pointed to the importance of the data protection agency's "moral-political authority and . . . direct access to Parliament." Federal and state data protection officials in Germany will continue to have an important role in shaping the debate about the use of personal health care data.[57]

Two important developments regarding medical information in France are the passage of a statute regulating the use of medical data for research purposes and the Conseil d'Etat's issuance of a decree concerning access to health care information as part of the reimbursement process. In a major statutory amendment in 1994 to the French omnibus data protection law, French legislators set out restrictions on the automatic treatment of personal information for the purpose of health care research.[58] This statute sets up a new body of data protection oversight, establishes substantive principles for data protection in medical research, and specifies important individual interests that must be respected before personal information can be used in a health care research project.

The new body of oversight is the Consultative Committee on the Treatment of Information for Purposes of Research in the Health Care Sector. Each request to process information for medical research is to be submitted first to this committee of experts, who are then to send the request to the National Commission on Information and Liberties (CNIL).[59] This approach follows the traditional French "licensing" approach to data protection.[60] In the public sector, government bodies must receive the CNIL's authorization before setting up data processing systems that use personal information. In the private sector, the CNIL lacks the power to decide whether data systems are authorized under the law. However, French law requires private processors of personal information to file a declaration with the CNIL "before the commencement of operation." Such a declaration must include a statement that "the processing is in accordance with the law."[61]

Over the past decade, the CNIL's responsibilities regarding licensing and declarations have been streamlined. The French data protection agency has introduced simplified and model declarations that automatically take effect after a certain number of days unless the CNIL takes action. In addition to its licensing duty, the CNIL also issues regulations and assists individuals in the exercise of their interests under the French data protection act. The creation of the Consultative Committee in the 1994 amendment to the French data protection statute has strengthened this approach. As a prelude to the CNIL's review, the Consultative Committee carries out its own examination of requests to establish health care research projects.[62] Such action by a body with special expertise in health care issues will help the CNIL, the French data protection commission, make well-informed decisions in this technically complex area.

In addition to setting up a new body of oversight, the 1994 amendment also establishes important individual interests. Most important is a general requirement that personal medical information that permits the identification of individuals be encoded before transmission to a research project. Although there are exceptions, the law forbids the reporting of research results that permit the direct or indirect identification of concerned parties. The law also grants individuals a right to object to use of their data in any medical research project. Finally, treatment of one's health care information in a research project generally requires the individual to be personally informed of: the nature of the transmitted data and his or her right to access and correct the information; the intended recipient of the information; and the end use (*finalité*) of the information.[63]

This first important development in French data protection law was made through an amendment of France's omnibus data protection statute. A second development has taken place through a change in the Social Security Law. The French legislature amended this statute in 1993 to permit the introduction of a series of detailed numerical codes that would increase the information to which public and private insurers had access during the reimbursement process. The goal was to improve the allocation of financial resources and the administration of health care. The new numerical codes are to be applied to the services provided by physicians (*actes effectués*), the payments to be provided (*prestations servies*), and the illness diagnosed (*pathologies diagnostiquées*). Although insurers already had access to some of this information, the creation of a numerical system allows greater efficiencies in limiting health care costs and supervising health care interventions. The 1993 law specifically required the Conseil d'Etat to establish specific requirements for the application of these statutory provisions; these regulations were to be issued after consultation with the CNIL. Although the Conseil d'Etat is well known to comparative lawyers as the French supreme court for administrative law, it has an equally important role in issuing decrees that interpret and develop statutory measures.[64]

Following the Conseil d'Etat's drafting of a decree that developed and applied the 1993 amendment to the Social Security Law,[65] the CNIL issued an opinion in May 1995 that raised a number of objections to this proposed regulation.[66] Admitting the necessity of a better control of medical expenses and medical services, the CNIL nevertheless warned that this project would lead to the creation of "exhaustive files of personal data containing information of a medical character that touched upon the intimacy of people's private life." In particular, the CNIL expressed concern over the codes for specific diagnoses (*pathologies diagnostiquées*). It requested that the Conseil d'Etat's decree be changed so that only physicians employed by the insurers would have access to codes regarding these diagnoses and would receive them in "a fashion that preserved medical confidentiality." In addition, these codes were not to appear on the "statements of medical services" (*feuilles de soins*), which are generally sent directly to insurers.[67] The Conseil d'Etat is currently reconsidering the language of its decree.

THE APPROACH TO GENETIC PRIVACY

In Europe, as we have seen, specific sectoral measures have supplemented general data protection laws in individual nations. There is usually not one specific law for all contexts of the use of medical data. Rather, European legislators have enacted statutes that regulate specific areas where medical information is used. A similar approach is being followed for genetic privacy.

This regulatory method is of particular interest in the United States, where an ongoing debate has considered the merit of enacting broad genetic privacy laws. In Chapter 23, Mark Rothstein argues that no single law is likely to be able to apply to all kinds of genetic information and the many areas in which these data are used. Although different regulatory methods are being tried in Europe, the general European trend has been in the direction Rothstein prefers, which is the enactment of different laws that structure the application of personal genetic information in a range of areas.

The emerging European response to genetic privacy has generally not been through broadly drafted genetic privacy laws. Rather, with general data protection laws and more specific statutes that apply to health care data in place, European lawmakers have acted on a targeted basis. Specific laws or regulations have been formulated or are under discussion in different nations concerning "genetic fingerprints," prenatal testing, and the application of genetic data to the employment relationship.[68]

The two exceptions to this approach are Switzerland and Austria. Although targeted legislative action has been taken or is planned in these countries, these nations have also responded to issues involving genetic privacy through, in Switzerland, the broader form of constitutional law and, in Austria, a general statute that regulates genetic science. Switzerland's constitution is relatively open to change through popular referendum, and a constitutional amendment has been promulgated concerning the application of genetic science. This provision seeks the protection of "man and his environment . . . against abuses of reproductive and genetic technology." One part of this amendment concerns personal genetic information; it specifically requires the basis of "either consent or a legal authorization" before "examination, registration, or revelation" of "the genetic patrimony of a person."[69]

In Austria, the Genetic Technology Law, or Gentechnikgesetz, regulates how genetic science is applied in a number of areas. This statute sets limits on the genetic engineering of humans, animals and plants.[70] It also contains rules for the use of prenatal testing and the genetic analysis of humans for medical purposes.[71] Finally, the law establishes broad data protection principles for genetic information. This section of the law begins by establishing a basic requirement of secrecy for information gained through genetic analysis. It goes on to require that the individual whose data are analyzed be provided upon request with access to all data concerning him or her. Use of identifiable personal data for purposes other than the one for which they were collected, moreover, is permissible only with the explicit and written consent of the individual to whom they pertain.[72] Finally, any non-anonymous genetic data can be subject to automatic processing only in the establishment in which they were collected, are to be stored separate from other kinds of personal information, and are to be accessible only to a limited number of persons specified in the statute.[73]

Switzerland and Austria are the exceptions that prove the rule regarding the European preference for narrower sectoral regulation of the use of personal genetic information. In contrast to the situation in the United States, however, this targeted European regulation exists with a safety net in place. The safety net is provided by the data protection principles of European-wide and general European domestic law. Yet even the targeted sectoral laws that regulate the use of genetic information in Europe have to cover a broad range of situations and speak in fairly abstract language. Spiros Simitis, the former data protection commissioner of the German state of Hesse and a leading scholar of data protection law, has observed, "As much as it is necessary to define the domain of application of the individual rules as concretely as possible, it cannot be ignored that a precondition to any legal regulation is a certain minimum level of abstraction."[74] Individual European laws that concern specific areas of the use of personal genetic data cannot escape reliance on general principles and use of abstract language. A few examples from German law will illustrate how such general principles are being applied to the use of personal genetic information.

In Germany, the initial response to the issue of using "genetic fingerprints" in criminal trials has been judicial, but the federal legislature is considering a detailed statutory regulation of this area. Beginning in the 1980s, a series of lower criminal courts upheld the use of DNA testing for purposes of identification in criminal trials.[75] Judges permitted this information to be introduced through Section 81a of the Criminal Procedure Code. This provision speaks in general language of the permissibility of ordering "physical examination of the accused" for the "establishment of facts . . . that are of importance for the lawsuit." The Criminal Procedure Code also explicitly authorizes the taking of blood tests and other physical invasions without the consent of the individual "if no apprehension exists of a detrimental effect on [the accused's] health."[76]

More recently, however, the highest German civil court, the Federal Court of Justice (Bundesgerichtshof, or BGH), placed an important restriction on the use of genetic fingerprints. In a decision in 1992, extending its analysis in an opinion from 1990, the BGH found that although genetic fingerprints could be introduced in criminal trials, the judiciary had an "obligation for critical assessment." Courts were required to hear expert testimony establishing "the basis for scientific conclusions." As part of this testimony, courts were obliged to consider "the informational basis" upon which "the expert witness derived the frequency of the examined characteristics from the population." To be sure, judges could view positive results of DNA fingerprinting as offering evidence capable of strongly incriminating a defendant. This evidence was, however, generally not "binding, rather merely one indication—if also an important one." Courts were also to consider other evidence and the testimony of witnesses.[77]

The German legislature has now spent more than six years preparing and debating different drafts of bills to provide detailed regulation of the use of genetic evidence through amendment of the Criminal Procedure Code. One of the most critical issues treated in these bills is how "genetic fingerprints" will be used for purposes beyond mere comparisons with evidence found at a crime scene.[78] Most bills have restricted any analysis that would reveal health information about the suspect. Federal Data Protection Commissioner Jacob has criticized a number of aspects of existing legislative proposals. He has stressed the need to test DNA not under the suspect's name but through an assigned number. In addition, Jacob has objected to one bill's simple statement that testing results might also generally be introduced in civil trials. At a minimum, he wishes to see a clear set of legal norms that regulate the conditions of such further use of these tests.[79]

Another set of regulatory issues in Germany concerns the use of genetic information in the administration of public social insurance and private insurance policies. The German system of social insurance includes statutory health care insurance, accident reimbursement, and retirement funds. Genetic information is *not* used within this system as an underwriting mechanism; eligibility for social insurance depends on objective, statutorily fixed criteria rather than one's personal characteristics.[80] Someone who is receiving certain public social insurance benefits may, however, agree to genetic testing. For example, a health care consumer can seek genetic counseling before or during a pregnancy. Like other personal medical data, this information is subject to the confidentiality provisions of Section 35, Book I, of the Social Welfare Law.

The German private insurance system currently does not make use of personal genetic information. However, one legal scholar has called for a statute that would foreclose any such application. Günther Wiese argues that private insurers might be tempted to practice adverse selection techniques to increase their profits and lower the premiums of their remaining clients: "An exclusion of genetically encumbered persons from private insurance would be unsatisfactory for the society as a whole; the state and the general public of taxpayers would be responsible for these individuals, after all, and the system of private insurance would end by being discredited. This exclusion would be especially problematic if, due to demographic trends, public social insurance benefits could only be set at a low level."[81] Profit maximizing by private companies that use personal genetic data does not increase social wealth. Rather, it inefficiently shifts costs to taxpayers and, to a lesser extent, back onto health care providers who may be forced to provide uncompensated or undercompensated care.

The European approach to the establishment of fair information practices has led to a generally high level of legal protection. And yet the European method of data protection serves as more than a positive example of comparison. Both European-wide law and domestic law contain provisions that allow the embargoing of data exports to countries with insufficient data protection. The United States is thus obliged to consider international norms in this area.

On the European-wide level, the European Union's directive and the Council of Europe's convention set rules not only for the processing of personal data *within* Europe but also for the transfer of these data to any "third country," including the United States. The directive and convention permit the prohibition of data transfers, including those involving medical information, to countries with insufficient data protection.

The European Union's Directive gives responsibility to each member government to oversee the conditions of transfers to nonmember nations. Its critical requirement is that data transfers be permitted "only if the third country in question ensures an adequate level of protection." The adequacy of protection is to be "assessed in the light of all the circumstances surrounding a data transfer operation or set of data transfer operations." Among the circumstances to be assessed are "the legislative provisions . . . in force in the third country in question." The adequacy of protection can also depend on "professional rules," such as a given company's business practices or code of conduct.[82]

According to the Council of Europe's convention, a signatory nation may prohibit data transfers to third countries that occur "through the intermediary of the territory of another party." Such *indirect* transfers can be prevented when they would cause the circumvention of specific heightened regulations for certain categories of data.[83] Although the Convention does not discuss the treatment of *direct* transfers to third countries, it has generally been held to require an equivalent level of protection in third countries. The council's Draft Recommendation on the Protection of Medical Data is more explicit in this regard. It requires domestic legal provisions that are "in conformity" with the convention before a transfer of personal information to a state which has not ratified this treaty.[84]

Data exports can also be limited under the national law of various European nations. For example, the French omnibus data protection law allows the French data protection agency, the CNIL, to oversee the conditions of the transfer of information from France to foreign nations "to ensure compliance with the principles laid down in this Act."[85] The French law of 1994 that regulates the use of personal data in health care research has a section that governs international transfers of personal data. International transmission of non-anonymous health care data for use in research projects is permissible only when "the legislation of the destination state contains an equivalent protection to French law."[86]

In Europe, planned transfers have been modified because of concerns regarding privacy protection. The French data protection commission has permitted international transfers of personal information in two instances only after the foreign parties involved agreed to set up contracts that would increase protection of the data.[87] One of these transfers concerned personal medical information that a French medical center wished to send to Belgium. The transfer was to take place as part of the establishment of a European electronic network of cancer information named EUROCODE. At the time of the planned transfer, Belgium did not have a national data protection law. The CNIL permitted the transfer only after discussions with all concerned parties and modifications of the original agreement. The Belgian data center agreed to receive only anonymous data from France. The keys that revealed the identify of patients listed in these data were to be kept at all times in France. The French medical institute was also required to negotiate a contract with EUROCODE. In this contract, the Belgian data center pledged to observe all the protections of French law and European-wide data protection. Specifically, the Belgian institution was obliged to specify limitations on the release to third parties of information in the electronic data bank. In addition, it had to set restrictions on any further application of the data.[88]

What do these provisions for blocking data exports mean for the United States? They indicate that transfers of personal data from Europe to America will depend upon the adequacy of protection that such data will receive once transferred. This decision is likely to be made first through an examination of the nature of the data and the specific processing context and then by an evaluation of legal safeguards and prevailing business practices.[89]

The idea of permitting transfers of personal data only to nations with sufficient data protection has appeal even beyond Europe. An American bill that seeks to improve the protection of health care information has adopted this technique. The Fair Health Information Practices Act, which Representative Gary Condit (D-California) introduced in the 103d and 104th Congresses, permits access to health information outside the United States only if certain statutory standards are met. One such standard is that the foreign country provide "fair information practices . . . that are equivalent to the fair information practices provided for by this Act."[90]

The weaknesses in U.S. data protection law could lead to blockage of international transfers of data to the United States.[91] Even when such transfers are not forbidden, the transactions in which they are involved will be subject to heightened scrutiny. The inevitable result will be dramatically increased expenditures by American businesses and litigants with interest in personal genetic information from Europe.

CONCLUSION

Modern genetics permits the creation of a powerful flood of information about individuals. Computers can make this information instantly accessible to a range of institutions and individuals. The legal order should structure the social application of this information.

The European approach to data protection is based on shared agreements regarding both the appropriate process for regulation and a core group of fair information practices. The European process of regulation foresees an active state role in protecting individual interests and the enactment of both general data protection statutes and sectoral regulations. Another essential element of this process is involvement by data protection commissions in the creation of a regulation of personal information use. As to the core group of fair information practices, European laws center around four principles: the creation of a statutory fabric that defines obligations with respect to the use of personal information; the maintenance of "transparent" processing of personal information; the assignment of special protection for sensitive data; and the establishment of enforcement rights for the individual and effective oversight of the treatment of personal information. These principles have been expressed in legal standards that control the allocation and application of personal medical information.

In the area of medical privacy, European regulation of medical information occurs through the interplay of different kinds of measures. European-wide law and domestic statutes have combined to create a legal standard that is higher than that found in the United States. One area of concern in the United States is the lack of knowledge about how personal data are currently used; there is widespread ignorance, for example, about the marketing of lists of people with specific medical conditions. Yet the European approach is currently being challenged by such new technological developments as the introduction of chip cards in Germany. European data protection commissioners are playing a significant and positive role in the social debate concerning the use of medical information.

With general data protection laws and medical privacy statutes already in place, the European response to genetic privacy has generally been through highly targeted regulations rather than broad genetic privacy laws. One example of this approach is the draft bill in Germany that amends the Criminal Procedure Code to regulate the use of "genetic fingerprints." This law and additional statutes are likely to be enacted in Germany and elsewhere in Europe to structure the use of personal genetic information. Finally, European transnational and domestic law allow embargoes to be placed on data exports to nations with insufficient data protection. These laws indicate a need for ongoing attempts in the United States to improve the protection of the privacy of personal health care information.

NOTES

Author's note: I am grateful for the insightful comments on drafts by David Dow, Martin Flaherty, Robert Gellman, Jutta Körbel, Joel Reidenberg, Mark Rothstein, Spiros Simitis, and William Treanor. Terri Yeakley helped in countless ways with her administrative skills. My warm thanks also go to Anne Arendt, David Gay, and Sally Kelley for their bibliographical assistance. Unless otherwise noted, translations are my own.

1. In the words of the astronomer and cybersleuth Clifford Stoll, "lots of little computers have taken over where once giant mainframes roamed." Stoll, *Silicon Snake Oil: Second Thoughts on the Information Highway* (New York: Doubleday, 1995), 94.
2. Paul M. Schwartz and Joel R. Reidenberg, *Data Privacy Law: A Study of United States Data Protection* (Charlottesville, Va.: Michie, 1996), 12–16.
3. Ibid.
4. U.S. Congress, Office of Technology Assessment, *Protecting Privacy in Computerized Information* (Washington, D.C.: Government Printing Office, 1993), 13; Institute of Medicine, *The Computer-Based Patient Record: An Essential Technology for Health Care* (Washington, D.C.: National Academy Press, 1991), 156.
5. See John Riley, "Know and Tell: Sharing Medical Data Becomes Prescription for Profit," *Newsday,* Apr. 2, 1996, A17.
6. Joel R. Reidenberg, "Setting Standards for Fair Information Practice in the U.S. Private Sector," *Iowa Law Review* 80 (1995): 497, 523. For a fairly comprehensive catalogue offering marketing lists for sale, see Standard Rate and Data Service, *Direct Marketing List Source* (Wilmette, Ill.: SRDS, 1996).
7. Reidenberg, "Setting Standards for Fair Information Practice," 515–23, quotations on 517, 521. Robert Gellman, "Confidentiality and Telemedicine," *Telemedicine Journal* 1 (1995): 191.
8. Paul M. Schwartz, "Privacy and Participation: Personal Information and Public Sector Regulation in the United States," *Iowa Law Review* 80 (1995): 565–66.
9. Paul M. Schwartz, "The Protection of Health Privacy in Health Care Reform." *Vanderbilt Law Review* 48 (1995): 295, 314–20.
10. 429 U.S. 589 (1977).
11. Ibid., 599–604.
12. See, e.g., Doe v. Attorney General, 941 F.2d 780, 795 (9th Cir. 1991); American Civil Liberties Union v. Mississippi, 911 F.2d 1066, 1069–70 (5th Cir. 1990); Walls v. City of Petersburg, 895 F.2d 188, 192–94 (4th Cir. 1990); Gutierrez v. Lynch, 826 F.2d 1534, 1539 (6th Cir. 1987); Mann v. University of Cincinnati, 824 F.Supp. 1190, 1198–99 (S.D. Ohio 1993); Doe v. Borough of Barrington, 729 F.Supp. 376, 382 (D.N.J. 1990).

13. For example, the Privacy Act fails to control the use of personal information for purposes beyond the original one for which the data was collected. For a discussion of the shortcomings of the Privacy Act, see Schwartz, *Privacy and Participation,* 582–87.

14. Cal. Const. art. I, § 1. For cases interpreting this right, see Urbaniak v. Newtown, 277 Cal. Rptr.2d 354, 357–58 (Ct. App. 1991); Division of Med. Quality v. Gherardini, 156 Cal. Rptr.2d 55, 61–62 (Ct. App. 1979).

15. See, e.g., Cal. Civ. Code § 56; Wis. Stat. Ann. § 146.82; R.I. Gen. Laws § 5–37–9. For cases interpreting the duty of confidentiality, see Horne v. Patton, 287 So.2d 824, 827–30 (Ala. 1974); Hague v. Williams, 181 A.2d 345, 347–49 (N.J. 1962). See also Robert Gellman, "Prescribing Privacy: The Uncertain Role of the Physician in the Protection of Patient Privacy," *North Carolina Law Review* 62 (1984): 255, 274–78.

16. For an overview and excellent analysis, see Karen H. Rothenberg, "Genetic Information and Health Insurance: State Legislative Approaches," *Journal of Law, Medicine and Ethics* 23 (1995): 312.

17. The weaknesses of these state solutions become clear when one considers the common law right of privacy. One branch of this interest has been found to prevent public disclosure of private fact; *Restatement (Second) of Torts,* § 652D (1977). Most courts have, however, found that such a tort claim requires widespread disclosure to the public, which will not occur in most cases involving the release of medical information; Porten v. University of San Francisco, 134 Cal. Rptr. 839, 841 (Ct. App. 1976). Another restrictive element of the public disclosure tort is the requirement found by many courts that disclosure be to someone without a "legitimate interest" in the information. Some courts have found employers to have a legitimate interest in their workers' medical information; W. Page Keeton et al., *Prosser and Keeton on the Law of Torts,* 5th ed. (St. Paul, Minn.: West, 1984), 857–58.

    A second branch of the tort right of privacy prevents intentional intrusions upon the private affairs or concerns of an individual; *Restatement Second of Torts,* § 652B. Such intrusion must be "highly offensive"; moreover, something in the nature of "prying or intrusion" must occur. Keeton et al., *Prosser and Keeton on the Law of Torts,* 855. Courts have failed to find that disclosure of sensitive medical information by an employer to an individual's coworkers create such an "intrusion"; the employee had, after all, "voluntarily" provided the information to her employer. Miller v. Motorola, 560 N.E.2d 900, 903 (Ill. App. 1990).

18. Rothenberg, "Genetic Information and Health Insurance," 317.

19. See generally Joseph White, *Competing Solutions: American Health Care Proposals and International Experiences* (Washington, D.C.: Brookings Institution, 1995), 61–162.

20. Schwartz and Reidenberg, *Data Privacy Law,* 39–41; Herbert Auernhammer, *Bundesdatenschutzgesetz,* 3d ed. (Cologne: Carl Heymanns Verlag, 1993), 22.

21. Directive on the Protection of Individuals with Regard to the Processing of Personal Data and on the Free Movement of Such Data, J.O., L 281/31 (Nov. 23, 1995) (hereinafter cited as Directive on Data Protection).

22. Sacha Prechal, *Directives in European Community Law: A Study of Directives and Their Enforcement in National Courts* (New York: Oxford University Press, 1995), 18–43; Stephen Weatherill and Paul Beaumont, *EC Law* (New York: Penguin, 1993), 116.

23. Directive on Data Protection, Preamble (1), Arts. 8, 6–25.

24. Convention for the Protection of Individuals with Regard to Automatic Processing of Personal Data, opened for signature Jan. 28, 1981, No. 108 (hereinafter cited as Convention for the Protection of Individuals). Regarding the lack of binding power of the Convention, see Reinhard Ellger, *Der Datenschutz im grenzüberschreitenden Datenverkehr* (Baden-Baden: Nomos, 1990), 463; and A. C. M. Nugter, *Transborder Flow of Personal Data Within the E.C.* (Amsterdam: Kluwer, 1990), 26.

25. Convention for the Protection of Individuals, Art. 6

26. Ibid., Arts. 5–11.

27. Council of Europe, Regulations for Automated Medical Data Banks, Recommendation no. R(81)1, Jan. 23, 1981. The Explanatory Memorandum to the Recommendation states: "the operation of every automated medical data bank [should be] subject to a specific set of regulations. The general purpose of these regulations should be to guarantee that medical data are used not only to ensure optimal medical care and services but also in such a way that the data subject's dignity and physical and mental integrity are fully respected" (13).

28. See Project Group on Data Protection, Report, CJ–PD (93) 37 (Strasbourg, Sept. 17, 1993) (hereinafter cited as Draft Recommendation).

29. This right was first identified in an important decision of the German Constitutional Court, 65 Entscheidung des Bundesverfassungsgerichts [hereinafter cited as BVerfGE] 1 (1983). An English translation of this case with commentary is found in Donald P. Kommers, *The Constitutional Jurisprudence of the Federal Republic of Germany* (Durham, N.C.: Duke University Press, 1989), 332–36. Since this initial decision, the Federal Court of Justice (Bundesgerichtshof, or BGH) has further developed this important right; see, e.g., Neue Juristische Wochenschrift (hereinafter NJW) 707 (1989), NJW 2805 (1987).

30. 65 BVerfGE at 43–52. For a discussion of this decision, see Paul M. Schwartz, "The Computer in German and American Constitutional Law: Towards an American Right of Informational Self-Determination," *American Journal of Comparative Law* 37 (1989): 675, 689–92.

31. The Federal Constitution of the Swiss Confederation, Amendments, Art. 24novies (adopted 17 May 1992), in Albert P. Blaustein and Gisbert H. Flanz, eds., *Constitutions of the World* (New York: Oceana Press, 1995) (hereinafter cited as Swiss Constitution).

32. English translations of these laws are found in Spiros Simitis, Ulrich Dammann, and Marita Körner, eds., *Data Protection in the European Union* (Baden-Baden: Nomos, 1995). See generally Colin J. Bennett, *Regulating Privacy: Data Protection and Public Policy in Europe and the United States* (Ithaca, N.Y.: Cornell University Press, 1992), 153–92.

33. Gesetz zur Fortentwicklung der Datenverarbeitung und des Datenschutzes, vom 20.12.1990 (BGBl I, S. 2954) (hereinafter cited as German Data Protection Law); Loi no. 78–17 relative à l'informatique, aux fichiers et aux libertés (hereinafter French Data Protection Law), reprinted in Simitis, Dammann, and Körner, eds., *Data Protection in the European Union.*

34. Sozialgesetzbuch, Allgemeiner Teil, Vom 11.Dezember 1975 (BGBl I, S. 3015); SGB V,

Vom 20.Dezember 1988 (BGBl I, S. 2477); SGB X, vom 18.August 1980 (BGBl I, S. 1469) (hereinafter cited as German Social Welfare Code). Strafgesetzbuch, § 203 I, Nr. 3 (hereinafter cited as German Criminal Code). Krebsregistergesetz vom 1994, BGBl I, S. 3351; for a discussion of this law, see *Berliner Datenschutzbeauftragter, Jahresbericht 1994*, 89–90.

35. German Data Protection Law, § 28(2)(b). See Auernhammer, *Bundesdatenschutzgesetz*, 375.

36. German Social Welfare Code, Book X, §§ 67–78.

37. BGH, Judgment of July 10, 1991, NJW 2995–56 (1991).

38. Ibid., 2956–57. See Bürgerliches Gesetzbuch, § 134 (hereinafter cited as Civil Code); German Criminal Code, § 203 I Nr. 1.

39. BGH, Judgment of July 10, 1991, NJW, 2957. For a discussion of this important decision, see Marita Körner-Dammann, *Weitergabe von Patientdaten an ärztliche Verrechnungsstellen*, NJW 729 (1992); and Herbert Auernhammer, "Zum Honorareinzug durch ärztliche Verrechnungsstellen," *Datenschutz und Datensicherung* 16 (1992): 182.

40. For an explanation of Germany's provision of medical services, see John K. Iglehart, "Germany's Health Care System," *New England Journal of Medicine* 324 (1991): 503; and Uwe E. Reinhardt, "Reforming the Health Care System: The Universal Dilemma," *American Journal of Law and Medicine* 19 (1993): 21. For a discussion of the reform of this system in the 1980s, see Iglehart, "Germany's Health Care System," 1750, 1751–55; and Jan Kuhlmann, "Die Verarbeitung von Patientendaten nach dem SGB V. und das recht auf selbstbestimmte medizinische Behandlung," *Datenschutz und Datensicherung* 17 (1993): 198, 199–200.

41. White, *Competing Solutions*, 75–77.

42. German Social Welfare Code, Book V, §§ 284–305. Among the most important uses of the information gathered with the use of these cards is to place a global cap on the cost of medical services that any given physician may furnish. A physician who exceeds the average costs of services in a given time by more than 20% is to be refused additional insurance compensation for this work. Kuhlmann, "Verarbeitung von Patientendaten," 204.

43. German Social Welfare Code, Book V, §§ 284–305.

44. Ibid., § 291.

45. See generally "Die Lunte Brennt," *Der Spiegel* 47 (1994): 62–79; Rita Wellbrock, "Chancen und Risiken des Einsatzes maschinenlesbarer Patientenkarten," *Datenschutz und Datensicherung* 18 (1994): 70, 74; and Der Hessische Datenschutzbeauftragte, 22. Tätigkeitsbericht (1993), 59–61 (hereinafter cited as Hessian Data Protection Commissioner, Twenty-Second Activity Report).

46. Der Hessische Datenschutzbeauftragte, 23.Tätigkeitsbericht (1994), 47–50 (hereinafter cited as Hessian Data Protection Commissioner, Twenty-Third Activity Report).

47. See Landesbeauftragte für den Datenschutz, Bremen, 16. Jahresbericht (1994), 63–66; Landesdatenschutzbeauftragte für den Datenschutz, Bremen, "Ärztliche Behandlung und Abrechnung der Leistungen demnächst nur noch mit Chipkarte," *Datenschutz und Datensicherung* 16 (1992): 276; Hessen Data Protection Commissioner, Twenty-Second Activity Report, 58–93.

48. See generally David Flaherty, *Protecting Privacy in Surveillance Societies: The Federal Republic of Germany, Sweden, France, Canada, and the United States* (Chapel Hill: University of North Carolina Press, 1989), 21–90.

49. Beschluβ der 47. Konferenz der Datenschutzbeauftragten des Bundes und der Länder vom 09./10. März 1994 zu Chipkarten im Gesundheitswesen (hereinafter cited as Potsdam Resolution), reprinted in Hessen Data Protection Commissioner, Twenty-Third Activities Report, 194–98.

50. Ibid., 194–95.

51. For an insightful discussion of the complexities of this doctrine, see Peter Schuck, "Rethinking Informed Consent," *Yale Law Journal* 103 (1994): 899, 902–4.

52. Potsdam Resolution, 195.

53. Ibid.

54. Hessen Data Protection Commissioner, Twenty-Third Report, 48.

55. Potsdam Resolution, 195–96.

56. "Neue Ära," *Der Spiegel* 10 (1996): 68.

57. Hessen Data Protection Commissioner, Twenty-Second Report, 65; 14. Tätigkeitsbericht des Bundesbeauftragten für den Datenschutz (1993), 159.

58. Loi no. 94–548 du 1er juillet 1994 relative au traitement de données nominatives ayant pour fin la recherche dans le domaine de la santé, J.O., 9559 (July 2, 1994) (hereinafter cited as French Health Research Law).

59. Ibid., Art. 40–2.

60. The CNIL is organized as a miniparliament; its 17 members come from the government and important social groups. This form reflects a desire for a diversity of opinion and a broad basis of support for decisions once reached. A staff, which is organized in three different bureaus, assists the commissioners and has a large role in handling routine matters. Flaherty, *Protecting Privacy in Surveillance Societies*, 165–242.

61. French Data Protection Law, Arts. 15–21.

62. French Health Research Law, Art. 40–2.

63. Ibid., Arts. 40–3, 40–4, 40–5.

64. Loi no. 93–8 du 4 janvier 1993, Art. 15.

65. Decret no. 95–564 du 6 mai 1995, J.O. 7371 (May 7, 1995).

66. CNIL, Deliberation no. 95–035 du 21 mars 1995 relatif au projet du décret portant application de l'article L161–29 du Code de la sécurité sociale (copy on file with author).

67. Ibid., quotations on 3, 5, 5–6.

68. See Olivier Guillod, "Réglementation de l'analyse génétique humaine: quelques remarques de droit comparé" in *Human Genetic Analysis and the Protection of Personality and Privacy* (Lausanne: Swiss Institute of Comparative Law, 1994), 167; and Noëlle Lenoir, "Aspects juridiques et éthiques du diagnostic prénatal: le droit et les pratiques en vigueur en France et dans divers autres pays," in ibid., 29.

69. Swiss Constitution, Art. 24novies(1), (2)(f).

70. Gentechnikgesetz, BGBl S. 4111 (July 12, 1994), §§ 5–79.

71. Ibid., § 71.

72. Ibid., § 71(1).

73. Ibid., § 71(4).

74. Spiros Simitis, "Allgemeine Aspekte des Schutzes genetischer Daten," in *Human Genetic Analysis,* 126.

75. LG Heilbronn, Judgment of Jan. 19, 1990, NJW 784 (1990); LG Berlin, Judgment of Dec. 12, 1988, ibid. 787 (1989).

76. Strafprozeβordnung, republished Sept. 12, 1950, BGBl I, S. 455.

77. BGH, Judgment of Aug. 12, 1992, NJW 2977 (1992). See also BGH, Judgment of Aug. 8, 1990, ibid. 2944 (1990).

78. For a discussion, see Alexander Dix, "Der genetische Fingerabdruck vor Gericht," *Datenschutz und Datensicherung* 17 (1993): 281.

79. Der Bundesbeauftragte für den Datenschutz, 15. Tätigkeitsbericht, 1993–1994 (1995), 69–71.

80. Günther Wiese, *Genetische Analysen und Rechtsordnung* (Berlin: Luchterhand, 1994), 69–73.

81. Wiese, *Genetische Analysen und Rechtsordnung,* 82.

82. Directive on Data Protection, Art. 26(1).

83. Convention for the Protection of Individuals , Art. 12(3)(a). For analysis of this provision of the convention, see Joel R. Reidenberg, "The Privacy Obstacle Course," *Fordham Law Review* 60 (1992): 161–62.

84. Draft Recommendation, 11.4. The Draft Recommendation adds that such transfers may occur even in the absence of such conformity if "a. necessary measures, including of a contractual nature, to respect the principles of the Convention and this Recommendation have been taken and the data subject has the possibility to object to the transfer, or b. the data subject has given his consent." Ibid.

85. French Data Protection Law, Art. 24.

86. French Health Research Law, Art. 40–9.

87. CNIL, *Dixième rapport d'activité* (1991), 32–34.

88. Ibid., 34–37.

89. See Directive on Data Protection, § 26(2). For a discussion of the necessary analysis, see Spiros Simitis, "Datenschutz und Europäische Gemeinschaft," *Recht der Datenverarbeitung* 6 (1990): 3, 20.

90. H.R. 435, Sec. 152.

91. Paul M. Schwartz, "European Data Protection Law and Restrictions on International Data Flows," *Iowa Law Review* 80 (1995): 471; Priscilla Regan, "The Globalization of Privacy," *American Journal of Economy and Society* 52 (1993): 257, 264–65.

Chapter 22 International and Comparative Concepts of Privacy

Sonia Le Bris and Bartha Maria Knoppers

It is important that the respect for privacy imposes the protection of real values—liberty, responsibility, loyalty—and does not become an alibi for hypocritical behaviors.
Daniel Becourt

Privacy is a fluid concept without consensual definition. It "comes within the scope of institutions that history has crafted in order to ensure the equilibrium of social relations between not only its members but also with the public or private authorities."[1] Traditionally defined as the right to be left alone, privacy cannot in fact be dissociated from society; indeed, privacy, rather than the staking out of a sphere of solitude, constitutes one of the modalities of life in society.[2] A "constellation of values, claims and interests in a universe of concurring and competing values, of supporting and antagonistic claims, of allied and adverse interests"—privacy "is more felt than defined."[3] Illustrative of the balance within a given culture at a specific time, privacy as a legal concept, then, reflects the "image of an indistinct nebula" with many legal sources and differing legal status.[4]

The accession of privacy to legal status in Europe can be explained by four factors. First, technological advances in fixing image and sound and in intercepting and recording speech (notably phone conversations), as well as the progress of statistical methods, have enhanced the capacity of intrusion into the private life of individuals. Second, a mass culture has gradually replaced that of cloistered societies of the past. With the development of the media, it became necessary to counterbalance the liberty of an increasingly sophisticated and intrusive press by protecting the privacy of individuals. In this way, two rights—privacy and the right to information—have had a parallel, though often conflictual, development. Third, beginning in the nineteenth century, such attributes of personality as "honor" and one's "image" acquired pecuniary value. Last, as a result of the disappearance of shared traditional values and the emergence of pluralistic societies, the private domain has gradually been extended and state control has gradually diminished.[5]

The notion of privacy now ranks among the fundamental rights. It is based on two concepts: human dignity and respect for individual freedom as understood in light of the Kantian notion of self-determination.[6] Human dignity is the most fundamental and absolute principle of human rights. Although it is the fount of all other human rights and is found in the majority of international texts, human dignity has never been specifically defined.[7] Freedom constitutes an important element of human dignity, notably the liberty to make decisions, from whence issues an obligation on the state to respect individual choice. According to Robert Hallborg, the right to privacy can be derived from the respect due to individual freedom as found in Kant.[8] Kant defined freedom as "the only original right belonging to every man by virtue of his humanity."[9] This right allows each person to claim the protection of personal choice in so far as it is now acknowledged that the right to liberty includes "the right to make fundamental personal decisions without the intervention of the State."[10]

In fact, the notion of privacy is founded on "the exaltation of individuality," which stems from the impossibility of individual expression in a totally public environment.[11] Therefore, the need to be left alone not only is part of personal development but also underlies autonomy, which becomes possible only in the context of freedom. From this private-public sphere of personal expression stems the narrow correlation between privacy and liberty.[12] In fact, as mentioned, privacy is not a fundamental value in itself, around which other values gravitate; rather, it integrates itself with other values and increases their impact.[13]

In addition to these historical and philosophical considerations, the concept of privacy is often accorded differing interpretations and definitions in various countries and under various laws. An international and comparative study of these positions as well as of the variability of the ambit of privacy is therefore justified. After a brief overview of the concept of privacy in Europe, we will examine, albeit succinctly, its interpretation at the national level.

RECOGNITION OF PRIVACY IN EUROPEAN INSTRUMENTS AND CASE LAW

In the aftermath of World War II, different international texts seeking to proclaim human rights were adopted. They recognized certain fundamental rights as being inherent to the person, that is, "those rights and faculties without which a human being cannot fully develop his personality."[14] In the spirit of the Universal Declaration of Human Rights,[15] official European bodies have specifically recognized the existence of the right to privacy. The Council of Europe reiterated this right in the European Convention for the Protection of Human Rights and Fundamental Freedoms, as did the European Community through the decisions of its Court of Justice.

On the international level, the right to privacy is recognized as an inherent individual right. Nevertheless, it is not framed in the same terms in the Universal Declaration of Human Rights, the International Covenant on Civil and Political Rights,[16] and the European Convention for the Protection of Human Rights and Fundamental Freedoms. Although the right to privacy was seen initially as a right to be left alone, the interpretation of the European Convention has transformed it into a positive obligation on public authorities not to interfere and has extended its ambit of protection even further to private parties.

First enunciated in the Universal Declaration,[17] the right to respect for privacy was reaffirmed in the European Convention[18] as well as in the International Covenant[19] (to cite only the most important international instruments). However, a comparative textual analysis of these articles relating to the right to privacy reveals important differences in wording and content. Although both Article 12 of the Universal Declaration and Article 17, § 1, of the International Covenant recognize a right to privacy, they do so only indirectly. The European Convention, though inspired by the Universal Declaration, specifically recognizes this right while also distinguishing between privacy and reputation.[20]

The Universal Declaration and the International Covenant affirm the right to privacy only as "a consequence of the duty of every person not to intrude in the private life of another."[21] The European Convention, by contrast, affirms that "every person has a right to the respect for his familial and private life, for his home and correspondence."[22] These different formulations are significant. Indeed, in the Universal Declaration and the International Covenant, privacy is a derivative right, a protection by default, as attested to by the term *consequence*. Under this formulation, the recognition of a right to privacy results in an obligation of nonintrusion, whether arbitrary or illegal; it is this obligation of noninterference that is directly enunciated. Moreover, in the Universal Declaration and in the International Covenant, the right to privacy is expressed, on one hand, in terms of banning attacks or interference and, on the other, in terms of a right to legal protection against such interferences. In contrast, respect for privacy is directly recognized in the European Convention. Under this approach, the respect for privacy is the principle, and the limits are the exception. It seems, therefore, that under the Universal Declaration and the International Covenant, protection is against an attack on the right to privacy, the protection resting essentially on the duty not to intrude; under the European Convention, it is really the right to a private sphere that is envisaged, that sphere which contains private and familial life, home, and correspondence.

Second, whereas the Universal Declaration and the International Covenant envisage interference only within the ambit of arbitrariness[23] and illegality,[24] the European Convention innovates in enumerating possible legal interference with privacy if three requirements are met.[25] The interference must be provided for under law; the interference must be legitimate in a democratic society; and it must meet certain predetermined goals (goals that include health protection).[26] This apparent distinction between the texts of the Universal Declaration and the European Convention, however, should be seen in context. Article 29, § 2, of the Universal Declaration lists legitimate limitations that apply to all the rights stated in the declaration, and not just to the right to privacy.[27]

This direct recognition of a right to privacy per se in Article 8 of the European Convention is complemented, moreover, by the evolving interpretation of this right to respect for privacy by the European Commission of Human Rights and the European Court of Human Rights.

If we refer to the spirit in which the European Convention was drafted, human rights were limited "to those fundamental individual rights which imply on the part of obligated states only abstentions, obligations of not doing and of not violating such rights."[28] In the case of privacy, this means a ban on the involvement of public authorities in the exercise of this right by individuals.[29] This negative obligation of abstention—that is, the obligation of not doing—included the protection of the secrecy of privacy against investigation and disclosure by the state as well as the protection of the liberty of privacy.[30] The only reservations are those intrusions specifically allowed by the law within the context of a democratic society and within the limited objectives of Article 8, § 2. This interpretation of the respect of privacy in terms of a negative obligation "reflects a liberal view of right, according to which human rights pertain to an area of freedom enjoyed by the individual, an area upon which the State may impinge only in defined circumstances and upon showing just cause."[31]

Nevertheless, the European Commission of Human Rights and the European Court of Human Rights, referring to the principles of interpretation set out in the Vienna Convention on the Law of Treaties of 1969, in particular that of the interpretation "in good faith, in accordance with the ordinary meaning to be given to the terms of the treaty in their context and in the light of its objects and purpose,"[32] have gradually come to consider that this right to privacy in the same way as other rights imposes positive obligations on the state.[33]

Moreover, it is interesting to note that the European Court of Human Rights has for the interpretation of Article 8 in particular extended its role "to controlling the substantial content of the norms of the States." Every time a state takes advantage of Article 8, § 2, to justify interference in the privacy of a person under its jurisdiction, the court has not hesitated to verify if the "proportionality principle" has been respected. In so doing, the court ensures that the legislature did not have at its disposal other means more respectful of the right of privacy as recognized in Article 8, § 1, in order to meet the legitimate objective it was seeking.[34]

Such a positive interpretation results in part from the fact that, contrary to other articles of the European Convention that explicitly foresee procedural guarantees and recourses, the content of the right to privacy, as stated in the first paragraph of Article 8, is not limited, leaving the article open to an "evolving and extensive interpretation."[35] This interpretation charges the state with the obligation to create mechanisms for the protection of both the secrecy and the liberty of privacy. Thus, under this interpretation, there is a positive obligation on the state to protect and promote the right to privacy, while paragraph 2 specifies the negative obligations incumbent on the public authorities. This recognition of a positive obligation conveys the social concept of human rights under which states must take all necessary measures in order to promote human dignity.[36]

A recent case has thus held that there are "positive obligations inherent in an effective respect for private or family life [which] may involve the adoption of measures designed to secure respect for private life even in the sphere of the relations of individuals between themselves."[37] This brings us to examine a third evolution, that concerning the opposability of the right to privacy under the European Convention.

In the absence of precise indicators in the European Convention itself or in the preparatory texts that preceded its adoption, Article 8, § 1, has inspired extensive doctrinal debate. Two schools of thought govern the question of whether the right to privacy applies only to the actions of public authorities or also to the actions of individuals.[38] The origin of this debate resides no doubt in the originality of the European Convention itself. Indeed, according to certain authors, the convention resembles not a classical treaty between states but a federal constitution.[39]

Even beyond these particularities of its elaboration, an examination sensu stricto of Articles 2 to 12—guaranteeing fundamental rights—provides no clarification on the question of the *erga omnes* (with regard to all) applicability of the convention. In support of a liberal interpretation, some have asserted that the very general wording of each of the fundamental rights stated would obligate not only states but also individuals. Certain provisions in using such phrases as "Nobody can . . . " and "Every person has a right . . . " could be interpreted as aiming to set a general and absolute range to the rights cited and in this way to make them opposable to each other.[40] For example, Article 8, § 1, of the European Convention enunciates the right to respect of private life without specifying to whom this right may apply. Some commentators have argued that paragraphs 1 and 2 are inseparable, the second limiting the principle enunciated in the first to relations between the state and private citizens.[41] This restrictive interpretation seemed to have been accepted to a certain extent during the discussion of Article 17 on respect for privacy under the International Covenant.[42] Others have defended the idea that the first paragraph of Article 8 aimed at both private-public and private-private relations, while paragraph 2 imposed certain limitations on the public authorities, state interference being an important source of discrimination.

Finally, the application erga omnes of Article 8, § 1, is largely the result of the evolution of the case law of the European Commission and Court of Human Rights.[43] For a long time, it was uncertain whether the case law of the European Commission and Court was in favor of either the absolute or relative effect of the rights guaranteed by the European Convention. On the basis of its interpretation of Articles 19[44] and 25,[45] the commission seemed to have as its function the respect of the obligations taken by the contracting parties—that is, of the member states of the Council of Europe who had signed the European Convention.[46] The court has always expressly maintained that it has the right to find a state responsible with regard to the rights in the European Convention and to acts between individuals. This position has slowly evolved toward a more explicit recognition of the opposability erga omnes of the European Convention[47] and, in particular, in the decisions rendered under Article 8 of the European Convention concerning the relations between public authorities and private persons.[48] This approach admits that human rights (and the right to privacy in particular) should be recognized not only in the relations between public authorities and individuals but also in the relations between individuals—the "horizontal or reflex effect."[49] Such an extension of the obligations arising from human rights translates a social concept of those rights, an extension maintained by some authors and particularly developed in Belgian law.[50]

The case law of the European Commission and Court of Human Rights includes within the freedom of privacy "to a certain degree, the right to establish and to develop relationships with other human beings, especially in the emotional field for the development and fulfillment of one's own personality."[51] Such a recognition of a right to personal fulfillment can be effective only if the right to privacy includes relationships between individuals.[52]

This case law does not signify, however, that an individual has direct recourse to the courts; only contracting states do. Any legal action directed against an individual on the basis of the violation of one of the rights found in the European Convention would be declared unacceptable *ratione personae* (by reason of the person concerned).[53] A contracting state engages its responsibility insofar as it can be proven that it did not protect the victim as required by the convention. It is the abstention of the state that is at fault, and this applies even when the case originates between individuals over a right found in the European Convention.[54]

The broader interpretation of privacy also raises the question whether the private sphere is identical for each individual or whether the circumstances specific to each case and the characteristics specific to each individual must be considered in determining privacy. The case law of the European Commission and Court of Human Rights seems to favor the subjective test—that is, an *in concreto* (a contextual approach) interpretation of the notion of privacy as stated in Article 8. Moreover, privacy is further circumscribed in opposition to the notions of both public life and public interest. If the notion of public life is a classical reference in matters of privacy, such is not the case for that of public interest, the extent and content of which remain undetermined.[55]

The European Commission of Human Rights and the European Court of Human Rights, therefore, have extended the protection of the right to privacy in their case law.[56] This same approach can be found to a certain extent within the European Community.

Even if the European Community has an economic objective, the Court of Justice of the European Community (not to be mistaken with the European Court for Human Rights) has clarified that "fundamental rights are an integral part of the general principles of law the observance of which the Court ensures." It also considered that "international treaties for the protection of human rights, on which the Member States have collaborated or of which they are signatories, can supply guidelines which should be followed within the framework of Community law."[57] This is particularly true of the European Convention.[58] Moreover, the preamble of the European Act of Union, signed on February 17, 1986, states that the member states have "decided to promote democracy together as founded on fundamental rights recognized in the Constitutions of member States, in the *European Convention for the safeguard of human rights and fundamental liberties* and in the *European Social Charter*."[59]

There is no doubt, then, privacy has become a fundamental right in the European Community. Although privacy is protected differently in all the member states, all the members of the European Union have ratified the European Convention, of which Article 8 expressly recognizes a right to the respect of private and family life.

Nevertheless, because each member state has its own internal law and is thus only partially affected by community law, the impact of decisions of the Court of Justice differ depending on whether the litigation falls under community law or under domestic law of a member state.[60] In recent years, however, the Court of Justice has attempted to reinforce the integration of its case law in relation to fundamental rights into the law of the member states.[61] In contrast to the case law of the European Court of Human Rights, the cases of the Court of Justice have no direct effect on national laws.[62]

Last, although the European Court of Human Rights and the Court of Justice of the European Community protect the secrecy of privacy in the same way, the protection of the liberty aspects of privacy is more elaborated upon in the case law of the European Court of Human Rights.[63] It is important to point out that the case law of the Court of Justice should be consolidated with the introduction of Article F, § 2, of the Treaty on European Union.[64] The Court of Justice could in future extend its protection of privacy to elements other than those it has thus far recognized.[65]

Yet even if the case law of the European Court of Human Rights and the Court of Justice of the European Community has allowed us to draw general conclusions about the extent of the right to privacy and its domain of application, the sources of this right remain controversial at the level of national legislation.

THE CONTROVERSIAL NATURE OF PRIVACY IN COMPARATIVE LAW

The need to protect the sphere of privacy appeared at approximately the same time in both the common law tradition and the Romano-Germanic law tradition. There is heterogeneity of both terminology and interpretation of the concept of privacy in most European countries. Furthermore, if privacy is generally recognized in all European countries and in Canada, its legal basis differs between the two legal systems—common law and Romano-Germanic law—as well as within the same legal system, where the understanding of privacy under public law can differ from that of private law.[66] Nevertheless, these antinomic conceptions of privacy seem to be moving toward greater harmony due to a common tendency to erase the public-private dichotomy in favor of the acceptance of the notion of privacy as a fundamental freedom.[67]

Pluralistic Sources of Privacy in Romano-Germanic Law

It is important to note at the outset that for many years under civil law the only category of rights covering personal interests or such personality rights as privacy was that of delict (an offense against the law).[68] Delict under civil law permitted recovery in the case of an act that was illicit and considered to be a fault. It was this requirement of proof of an illicit character that in the past seriously limited the field of protection of privacy. A more recent comparative study of countries with a civilian tradition reveals the emergence of additional sources for the concept of privacy. Linked to temporal and cultural contingencies, the dominant doctrinal approach in most European countries that operate under civil law today is to consider privacy as a subjective right and nonproprietary in nature.[69] Subjective rights are actionable per se and do not require proof of fault. Furthermore, in most civilian countries, the right of privacy is protected not only by the Civil Code but also through the notion of human freedoms and fundamental rights as laid down in the Universal Declaration and in the European Convention. By way of illustration, we discuss the notion of privacy in Belgium, France, Germany, Italy, the Canadian province of Quebec, the nations of Scandinavia, Spain, and Switzerland.

Privacy in Belgium. In Belgium, the notion of privacy in the internal legal system is recognized through ratification of the European Convention.[70] No article in either the Civil Code or a specific statute defines privacy, in spite of the recent adoption of a statute regarding the use of personal automated data.[71] This statute simply declares that every human being has the right to respect for privacy when personal data are processed.[72] The refusal of the Belgian legislature to define privacy is due, in part, to the complex nature of the concept.[73] In the absence of specific legal provisions, rules on civil liability apply. This means that the illicit character of the interference must be proven.

Privacy in France. It is now generally admitted in France that the right to private life constitutes a right of personality, a subjective right, found under Article 9 of the Civil Code.[74] This qualification creates certain problems, the category of personality rights being itself subject to controversy as to its legal nature.[75]

Although the debate on the legal qualification of the right of privacy may seem purely theoretical, it has a significant impact. Indeed, the legal qualification of a right determines the regime of protection. Subjective rights have as their goal both the protection of material interests and of moral interests. When the law accords an attribute to a person to assure the protection principally of moral interests (the main goal of personality rights), it then becomes a subjective right and not a legal situation governed only by the traditional rules of civil liability.[76] This distinction is important because the rules of civil liability offer only limited protection.[77] Indeed, the rules of civil liability foresee compensation for harm rather than protection and therefore are insufficient to prevent breach of privacy. Moreover, Article 1382 of the Civil Code, which states the rule of civil liability, requires proof of damage.[78] In most cases, proof of harm in the realm of privacy is difficult to establish, leaving the victim without recourse. The qualification as a subjective right then has a certain advantage in that, as we have mentioned, the breach of a subjective right does not require proof of damage, the breach itself constituting harm.

In France, as elsewhere in Europe, the right to privacy is not protected solely via personality rights. It is also protected through the notion of public liberties and fundamental rights as laid down in the Universal Declaration, International Covenant, and European Convention, which apply to France.[79] A public liberty is thereby grafted to any subjective right of a civil nature, rights whose preeminence is increasingly affirmed in the context of the internationalization of norms.

Finally, in France, the most serious invasions of privacy, such as those of medical secrecy, are sanctioned by penal law.[80] At the same time, a number of administrative measures have been implemented to ensure the secrecy of private life.[81]

The protection provided by civil, administrative, or penal French texts aims more at the secrecy of privacy than the liberty of privacy. Essentially, a material and physical approach prevails, a protection against interference by others. The notions of personal fulfillment and autonomy are absent. This state of events results no doubt from the circumstances surrounding the inclusion of the notion of privacy in the Civil Code of France. Indeed, it was in reaction against systemic abuses of information that the right to the respect for the intimacy of private life was inserted in both the Civil and Penal Codes.[82]

Privacy in Germany. To determine the legal status of the right to privacy in Germany, it is necessary to understand the general right of personality that is found in Germany's civil and constitutional law.

German scholars of private law were the first to develop the notion of personality rights (*das allgemeine Persönlichkeitsrecht*) in order to include certain situations inherent to the individual that lacked satisfactory recourse outside the legal system.[83] Rights of personality were defined as "the right of the person to be his own end, to affirm himself, and to develop as an end unto himself."[84] The German right of personality includes "the control of bodily and intellectual faculties, of all fundamental liberties, and, notably, the freedom to move and to choose one's domicile or religion."[85] This notion gained prominence in the late nineteenth century through the work of Kohler and Gierke, who viewed the rights of personality as subjective rights.[86]

Parallel to this reflection on personality rights as defined by the private law doctrine, the German public law scholars of the nineteenth century began their own analysis of the rights of personality. They maintained that personality rights found their protection in the laws of the state and were therefore of a purely public nature.[87]

With the enactment of the Civil Code in 1900, the general notion of personality rights was abandoned.[88] It was revitalized, however, in the light of the Basic Law of the Federal Republic of Germany of May 23, 1949, and then again by the Federal Court of Civil Justice (Bundesgerichtshof) in the Schacht case of 1954.[89]

The contemporary German doctrine of personality rights centers around three approaches. The first approach, found in the Böll case, establishes a distinction between the principal attributes of personality rights (intimacy, privacy, and secrecy), which are well protected by the general rights of personality (*die Persönlichkeit*), and other attributes for which the textual basis in German civil law is weak because of their origin in the general rules of civil liability, notably in cases of harm to life, physical integrity, health, and liberty (BGB § 823 al.1). The second approach, that of German doctrine, regroups different personality rights around certain concepts by either a bipartite division into the spheres of intimacy (*Individualsphäre*) and secrecy (*Geheimsphäre*) or a tripartite division, adding the sphere of personal development (*Persönliche Entfaltung*).[90]

The third approach comes from the interpretation by the Federal Constitutional Court of Articles 2 al.1 and 1 al.1 of the Basic Law of 1949.[91] On the basis of these introductory provisions, the Federal Constitutional Court recognized a general personality right. This personality right has been inspired by the Basic Law, which is a constitutional document, but it still belongs to the domain of private law. It has been qualified as the civil version of the constitutional liberty (*das allgemeine Persönlichkeitsrecht*), which carries the same name. This has been defined as "the right of a person vis-à-vis another to respect for dignity and for the development of individual personality" as long as "its expression did not violate the rights of others or the constitutional order and morality."[92] This interpretation of the Basic Law provides for a right to informational self-determination, which, while not absolute, imposes an obligation on the state to organize information collection, conservation, and communication in such a way as to respect this personal autonomy. This general right of personality includes the right to privacy.[93]

The duality between constitutional and civil law personality rights in Germany has prompted certain authors to affirm that in addition to those rights of personality expressly enunciated by statute, there exists in the name of civil public order a general right of personality that, though constitutional in its essence, belongs to civil law.[94] This recognition of a general right of personality has as its consequence the possibility of compensation for moral damages. Thus, the Federal Constitutional Court considered that Articles 1 and 2 of the Basic Law, in recognizing the existence of a general right of personality, constituted exceptions to the civil rule (BGB § 253), which limits the conditions under which moral damages can be claimed.[95]

In conclusion, under German constitutional law, fundamental rights constitute "a real system of values infiltrating all of objective law." At the same time, the Basic Law protects individuals not only from the state but also from other individuals.[96]

Privacy in Italy. In a decision of April 12, 1973, the Italian Constitutional Court held that the right to privacy (*riservatezza diritto*) and to intimacy were inviolable human rights under Articles 2; 3, § 2; and 13, § 1, of the Constitution. Furthermore, these rights merited protection under civil laws.[97]

As in Germany, Italian legislators have implemented extensive legal controls, in particular a control of the constitutionality of the laws, in order "to prevent the destruction of a State of law" as happened under the Fascists. Thus, the control of the constitutionality of Italian laws is entrusted to specialized jurisdiction, the Constitutional Court (Corte Costituzionale), and not to civil judges.[98]

Taking into account the similar historical contingencies (fascism and the reaction against this type of political power), Italian law has been greatly influenced by German law and is similar in two respects with regards to the legal nature of the right to privacy. First, as in Germany, the Italian Civil Code and several statutes protect certain attributes of personality without containing provisions of a general nature. Second, Italian constitutional case law has tied certain personality rights to fundamental rights, notably to Article 2 of the Italian constitution. According to some Italian authors, one could interpret the riservatezza diritto as including a right to self-determination under Article 3 of the Italian constitution instead of Article 2. Whatever the textual foundation, personality rights and, more specifically, the right to privacy in Italy have a constitutional base reinforced by Article 8 of the European Convention.[99]

Privacy in Quebec. Influenced by a civil law tradition, Quebec is the Canadian province that offers the most extensive protection of privacy. This comprehensive protection stems from three sources: the civil code, the general notion of personality rights, and the Quebec Charter of Human Rights and Freedoms.[100] Since 1975 the Quebec Charter has stipulated in Article 5 that "every one has a right to respect for his private life." Although Article 5 may appear innovative, it is in fact a codification of case law. Yet it is an important provision in that every person has a direct action in the case of violation of a right or a freedom enunciated in the Quebec Charter—that is, a right to require that any illicit attack on an individual's privacy cease and to obtain compensation for any resulting material or moral damage. This is because Article 49 of the Quebec Charter specifically provides such a remedy.[101] Such a direct recourse allows the Quebec debate on privacy to concentrate on the elaboration of a coherent, continuous, and evolving definition of the concept of privacy rather than on the issue of harm. However, although the Quebec Charter was adopted in 1975, only after it was amended in 1982 did privacy dispositions, like others, prevail over provincial legislation unless the statute in question expressly stated that it applied despite the charter.[102] The Quebec Charter constitutes an important step in the evolution of the theory of personality rights in Quebec in that it shifts them from the domain of private law to that of fundamental human rights.[103]

Privacy has always been protected in Quebec under the concept of personality rights through an action in civil liability.[104] This action permitted compensation of the victim, albeit indirectly by proving fault, contrary to subjective rights which allow an action for breach per se.[105] The adoption of the new Civil Code, in effect since January 1, 1994, has put an end to any recourse under civil liability because privacy is now directly protected under Article 35.[106]

The concept of privacy introduced in Article 35 and following of the new Civil Code, however, has been weakened by the fact that its wording introduces what is essentially a criminal law approach. The article describes physical and material interference in privacy without introducing the concept of psychological or informational interference (although informational interference was recognized by the Supreme Court of Canada in the Dyment case of 1989).[107] Recent statutes on privacy, however, have expanded its ambit to personal information in both the public and private sectors.[108]

Privacy in Scandinavia. Norway, Denmark, and Sweden have neither elevated the respect of privacy to the level of a subjective right as in France nor admitted the existence of a general right of personality as in Germany. Protection of privacy is offered through penal provisions concerning private life and any intrusion on it. Under civil law in these nations, the only sanction that seems to have been admitted by the doctrine is a right to demand the prohibition or cessation of any attack on privacy with a limited compensation for moral damages. Yet the Scandinavian countries, in particular Sweden, have an original approach toward the protection of privacy. They assure this protection by two different means: the principle of "governmental publicity" and the more contemporary approach of data protection.[109]

Privacy in Spain. As with many other countries of the civil law tradition, the recognition and protection of personality rights under Spanish case law and doctrine rely on the general principles of civil liability (Art. 1.902 of the Spanish Civil Code). Contrary to the French and Swiss Civil Codes, however, there is no explicit recognition, either enumerative or global, of any personality rights in Spain's Civil Code. This absence is compensated by the affirmation of fundamental rights in the Spanish constitution of 1978. The Article 10.1 proclaims, albeit in very general terms, the right to respect for dignity as well as for the fundamental rights derived therefrom within the respect of law and public order. In addition, the interpretation of these rights under case law refers to the international texts ratified by Spain, such as the Universal Declaration or the European Convention. This has often resulted in an extensive interpretation of these fundamental rights, including the right to privacy.[110]

Article 18.1 of the constitution guarantees the rights to honor, to personal and familial private life, and to one's image. Article 3.1 of the Organic Law of 1982 reaffirms these rights in civil law.[111] It is worth noting that these three rights are handled in a unitary fashion in Spain. Considering the close links among them, it seems obvious that a violation of any of these rights may harm the other two.

These rights are not absolute. Article 2, § 1, of the Organic Law maintains that they may be limited by law, social customs, or previous conduct of the individual. Moreover, Article 7 enumerates the illegitimate invasions of privacy, while Article 8 describes legitimate invasions,—that is, those in conformity with the law or those that conform to a superior interest (historical, scientific, or cultural).[112]

Privacy in Switzerland. In Switzerland, the right of privacy is recognized in Article 28 of the Civil Code as amended in 1983. It provides recourse against "all illicit attacks on personality," which includes the right to privacy.[113] Still, the wording of Article 28 remains vague, and several Swiss authors have interpreted it to include a special category of subjective law, personality rights.[114] Sometimes qualified as "innate rights" in Swiss doctrine, these personality rights in Switzerland as elsewhere are nevertheless linked to the social climate and thus capable of evolving.[115] All authors admit the need for more specific legal protection of the essential attributes of the person, including the right to privacy.[116]

More contentious has been the controversy on the issue of the unity or plurality of personality rights. Torn between the French example of a plurality of personality rights—an enumerative approach—and the German example of a general right to personality with manifold aspects—a global approach—the Swiss legislature opted for a general formula of "personal interests" that are not explicitly enunciated. This approach permits creative legal interpretation. Thus, today, under Article 28 of the Civil Code, privacy is viewed as a legal precept that covers the personal interests inherent in the notions of both secrecy (*geheimsphäre*) and privacy (*privatsphäre*).[117]

As with other personality rights under civil law, however, compensation under Article 28 requires proof of fault and of the illicit character of the intrusion of privacy. This may not be so difficult a requirement since paragraph 2 of Article 28 establishes a rebuttable presumption of the illicit character, thus granting civil judges a wide power of appreciation.[118]

In Switzerland, then, these personality rights, including privacy, lack the protection accorded to the essential attributes of the individual. Protection is ensured by the general rules of civil liability and by the increasingly important role allotted to individual freedoms as explicitly named or implicitly recognized in the constitution. It should be noted that in Switzerland (according to the predominant opinion reinforced by numerous decisions of the federal court), these individual freedoms can be invoked only with regards to the state or one of its organs, not in relation to private relations. This restriction does not apply, however, to the freedoms enunciated in the European Convention, which is exactly the case as regards the respect of privacy as stated in Article 8 of the constitution.[119]

The Notion of Privacy in English and Canadian Common Law

In contrast to Romano-Germanic countries, the notion of privacy as such is not specifically recognized under British and Canadian common law. This does not mean that there is no protection of privacy. It means that privacy is governed by the classical causes of action. At the same time, there is also a gradual emergence of a general right of privacy via the avenue of fundamental rights.

Privacy in Great Britain. Parliament has repeatedly refused to legislate a right to privacy. The courts also have been reluctant to determine a certain number of constitutional or common law principles underlying the concept of privacy. The British government has refused to recognize through legislation a fundamental right to privacy as enunciated in the Universal Declaration and the International Covenant even though it has ratified these texts. Great Britain has always denied the necessity of a legislative intervention in the matter, putting forward the multiple forms of existing protection without direct links to the International Covenant but nevertheless always in conformity with it. With regard to Article 8 of the European Convention, the British government declared in a report submitted to the secretary general of the Council of Europe in 1967: "Any power a public authority may have to interfere with a person's right to respect for private life and family life, his home and correspondence must be provided by Law."[120]

One reason why, in spite of ratification, international texts have little impact on English common law comes from the English constitutional principles. These principles do not recognize the direct application of international texts in internal law. Moreover, even if the English courts have had occasion to interpret some international texts in a broad and flexible way, they have been timorous in their interpretation of the European Convention, presuming that their existing laws provided sufficient protection of all the rights contained in the European Convention, including the right to privacy.[121]

Last, although Great Britain has signed the option under the European Convention that permits every citizen to start proceedings directly before the European Court of Human Rights, this has had no direct effect on the government's position.[122]

In the absence of legislative intervention and of the direct importation of international texts, case law has alluded "to a legally protectable interest in privacy" and even to the "right to privacy in limited contexts" through three approaches: the protection of property; the confidentiality of communications; and the protection of personal information.[123] Rejecting a generic concept of privacy, English doctrine and case law treat different situations affecting privacy enumeratively and sanction them as such.[124] This refusal of a concept of privacy per se is due to the reluctance of common law to recognize the notion of moral damages, fearing an onslaught of claims. Change has occurred in the past twenty-five years, however, the notion of a fundamental right to privacy being more frequent in the decisions of British courts.[125] Recent decisions of the House of Lords have explicitly referred to the notion of privacy in each of three spheres: protection of property, confidentiality of communication, and protection of personal information.[126] There seems to be a tendency to recognize this emerging tort of invasion of privacy even if there is no "new legal right of action in tort."[127]

Privacy in Canada. The protection of privacy in Canadian common law, which applies in all provinces but Quebec, is multifaceted. This is due in part to the confusion between confidentiality and privacy and in part to the complexity of the divisions of power within a federal state. Privacy protection derives from a multitude of sources in Canada, and the division of the state's powers can make it difficult to sort out the the mechanisms in place for the protection of individual rights.

There is no a priori constitutional recognition of a right to privacy at the federal level in Canada because the Canadian Charter of Rights and Freedoms does not explicitly enunciate such a right.[128] Yet, in fact, in a number of dispositions of the charter, the Supreme Court of Canada has asserted such a right. At the provincial level the right of privacy is not explicitly recognized, but an action in tort remains possible. Four provinces have adopted privacy acts. These legislative interventions have nevertheless been perceived as fragmentary in that they are limited to private parties.

Failing a specific provision regarding the right to privacy, Canadian courts, following the Supreme Court of Canada, have deemed privacy to be a fundamental right recognized by the Canadian charter but having limited scope when conflicting with other fundamental rights: "First the court must recognize the privacy component of a specific right or freedom. Once the court determines that a privacy right has been infringed, the court must ask under section one of the Charter whether the limits imposed on privacy are 'reasonable' and can be 'demonstrably' justified in a free and democratic society."[129]

The first decision to recognize a right to privacy on the basis of section 8 of the Canadian Charter was the case of Hunter v. Southam.[130] The Supreme Court declared that section 8 concerns an aspect of privacy—the right of citizens to be protected in matters of private life in a free and democratic society. The court stated that this section "guarantees a broad and general right to be secure from unreasonable search and seizure" and that its finality is "to protect individuals from unjustified state intrusion upon their privacy."[131]

Following this decision, Canadian courts have begun to apply its principles in various situations in order to better delineate the frontiers of the concept.[132] In 1989, in the case of The Queen v. Dyment, the court pushed its reasoning further and declared through Justice Gérard V. Laforest that the "seriousness of a violation of the sanctity of a person's body constitutes an affront to human dignity." Under Article 8, which protects against unreasonable search or seizure, the court maintained: "Like other Charter rights, [the privacy of individuals] must be interpreted in a broad and liberal manner . . . . Its spirit must not be constrained by a narrow legalistic classification based on notions of property and the like which served to protect this fundamental human value in earlier times."[133]

Thus, in Dyment, the Supreme Court explicitly rejected the formalistic and narrow approach of the right to property in matters of privacy in order to extend it even beyond the integrity of the person. It reaffirmed the physiological dimension of the notion of privacy—that is, integrity of the person—but also clearly recognized that the right to privacy is informational. The court stated, "There is privacy in relation to information. This too is based on the notion of dignity and integrity of the individual." Moreover, it specified that "the use of a person's body without his consent to obtain information about him, invades an area of personal privacy essential to the maintenance of his human dignity."[134]

Relying on a teleological analysis of the protections guaranteed by the Canadian Charter, the Supreme Court attempted to determine other potential foundations of the right to privacy. In this respect, the minority opinion of Justice Bertha Wilson in the case of Morgentaler v. The Queen suggests that the right to liberty, such as stated in section 7 of the charter, guarantees the right to privacy or at the least "a decisional autonomy with regards to important decisions affecting in an intimate manner the private life."[135]

Finally, certain authors reasoning by analogy consider that the American thesis of "penumbral rights" created by the First, Fourth, Fifth, and Ninth Amendments of the U.S. Constitution (implicit sources of the right to privacy) have their corollaries in the Canadian Charter. Some Canadian authors, drawing an analogy between Article 26 of the Canadian Charter and its twin, the Ninth Amendment, maintain that it is possible to consider "privacy in its widest acceptation [as] a fundamental right worthy of appearing side by side with the rights and liberties enumerated in the Canadian Charter." In order to justify that the protection of privacy falls under section 26, these authors assert that "to attribute to this value a constitutional qualification contributes to its development and to ensuring this liberty, necessary for allowing the exercise of other named rights."[136]

In conclusion, privacy though not explicitly mentioned, is covered by the Canadian Charter. Nevertheless, one can deplore the fact that although this notion of privacy has been interpreted widely, no amendment to the charter has been put forward so as to institute an explicit constitutional right to privacy.[137] Moreover, even though this emerging recognition of a right to privacy is important, the Canadian Charter protects individuals only against public authorities, not against the acts of private organizations or other individuals. The recognition of a general right to privacy in common law is thus of interest.

Even though the right to privacy is not recognized as such in Canadian common law, its violation constitutes a tort.[138] As Peter Burns wrote in 1976, "At a superficial level, the common law of privacy is simple to summarize: There is no protection for personal privacy *per se*. . . . There is no general right, instead where that term is used, it is taken to be a statement of principle in support of some other already recognized right or a cause of action."[139]

This absence of a general right to privacy in no way, however, obviates the fact that certain levels of privacy are in concrete terms protected by more classical means: among them trespass to land, trespass to the person, nuisance, defamation, injurious falsehood, and breach of confidence. The most efficient (though fragmentary) protection remains the actions for defamation and for breach of confidence.[140] In order to counter this absence of a general right to privacy, some provincial parliaments have adopted laws to establish such a right. Saskatchewan, British Columbia, Manitoba, and Newfoundland have adopted legislation to create a "tort actionable without proof of damage."[141] Yet these laws are sketchy in many regards. First, their application is restricted to private relations between individuals and private organizations without including the relationship between the individual and the state. Second, they do not define the notion of privacy, instead enumerating such factors as the fact that the nature or degree of privacy one can envisage depends on the circumstances and the interests of others, which must be considered. Determining a violation of privacy, then, depends, on one hand, on the nature and consequences of the action at fault and, on the other, on the nature of the relationships between the involved parties. These laws, therefore, have not had the impact that was expected.

In this regard, Burns has been very critical. Not only does he refer to these laws as "nondevelopment," but he affirms that "it can be argued . . . that these *Acts* do not grant real protection to the privacy interests they were set up to safeguard, at least, at the most visible levels," the right to privacy in reality being pronounced half-heartedly.[142] Finally, some provisions of criminal law indirectly protect the right to privacy in Canada, notably in Part VI of the Criminal Code, entitled "Violations of Privacy."[143] The criminal approach to the protection of privacy is essentially material and physical since it is organized chiefly around the protection against interception of written and spoken communications.[144]

Whether in English or Canadian common law, the tendency thus seems to be to reject a common law tort of invasion of privacy. It will be interesting to follow developments on both sides of the Atlantic because of the continued opposition to this tort in Great Britain and the time needed to study the scope of provincial privacy legislation with regard to new scientific challenges. Finally, it will be interesting to follow developments in the other common law provinces. As mentioned, however, Canada seems to have gone further than Great Britain to the extent that, through the interpretation of the Canadian Charter, the right to privacy has achieved some legitimacy, even though, contrary to the United States, the specific recognition of such a right is still lacking.

CONCLUSION

This comparative study on the nature of the right to privacy at both the European and national levels demonstrates that although privacy is a commonly used and frequently invoked concept, it is multifaceted, fluid, and evolving. Any attempt to circumscribe the concept in a uniform and monolithic manner is inappropriate. Indeed, such an approach would undermine the very richness, fluidity, and malleability of the concept, which, as we have seen, can include both liberty, secrecy, and intimacy within its ambit. Its translation as an actionable subjective right and as a fundamental constitutional or civil right, along with its more limited interpretation under the rules of ordinary civil liability, also attest to its multifaceted nature. The varying legal traditions of Canada, the European countries examined here, and indeed of Europe itself as a political entity eschew any common approach or definition. There is no doubt, however, that the German concept of informational self-determination and the French notion of an actionable subjective right have great potential. Furthermore, should the tendency to expand the application of Article 8, § 1, of the European Convention to encompass not only the relationship between the state and the individual but also that between private parties continue, its acceptance as a judicial principle distinct from and yet integrating within itself other fundamental rights may be ensured.

In short, privacy should be considered as a legal principle since a principle has more flexibility. A principled response in the formulation of a generic formula is more susceptible to influence and can shape and foster the evolution of the law. It is the flexibility of the wording and the fluidity of the content that confer an intrinsically judicial value to the principle. Moreover, a principle, unlike a statutory disposition, can adapt to social transformations to ensure a more just appreciation of the surrounding reality. This concept of privacy, besides its ability to adapt to different legal systems, becomes particularly interesting in light of fundamental transformations generated through scientific progress, especially in the domain of genetics. Future legal developments will determine whether it can protect such highly personal data as well as personal freedom in "genetic" decision making—the dual components of privacy.

NOTES

Authors' note: All translations are by the authors.

Note to epigraph: Daniel Becourt, "La protection de la vie privée, nécessité et limites," in *Vie privée et droits de l'homme, Actes du troisième colloque international sur la Convention européenne des droits de l'homme, Bruxelles, 30 septembre–3 octobre 1970* (Brussels: Bruylant, 1973), 140.

1. Ibid., 139.
2. François Rigaux, *La protection de la vie privée et des autres biens de la personnalité* (Brussels: Bruylant, 1990), 694.
3. Task Force Established Jointly by Department of Communications and Department of Justice, *Privacy and Computers* (Ottawa: Information Canada, 1972), 11. Jacques Velu, *Répertoire pratique de droit belge.* See European Convention for the Protection of Human Rights and Fundamental Freedoms, adopted November 4, 1950, Council of Europe, entered into force September 3, 1953, hereinafter European Convention), no. 652.
4. Task Force Established Jointly by Department of Communications and Department of Justice, *Privacy and Computers,* 11; quotation from Marie-Thérèse Meulders-Klein, "Vie privée, vie familiale et droits de l'homme," *Revue internationale de droit comparé* 4 (1992): 769.
5. François Rigaux, "La liberté de la vie privée," *Revue internationale de droit comparé* 3 (1991): 546–47.
6. Meulders-Klein, "Vie privée, vie familiale et droits de l'homme," 771.
7. Mureille Delmas-Marty, "L'homme des droits de l'homme n'est pas celui du biologiste," *Esprit* 11 (1987): 121.
8. Robert B. Hallborg, "Principles of Liberty and the Right of Privacy," *Law and Philosophy* 5 (1986): 175.
9. Immanuel Kant, *The Metaphysics of Morals* (Cambridge: Cambridge University Press, 1991), 63.
10. R. V. Morgentaler [1988], 1 S.C.R. 30 at 166.
11. Rigaux, "La liberté de la vie privée," 10.
12. Jean Velu, as cited by A. Vitalis, *Informatique, pouvoir et libertés,* 2d ed. (Paris: Economica, 1988), 152.
13. Arnold Simmel, "Privacy Is Not an Isolated Freedom," *Nomos* 13 (1971): 71.
14. René Cassin, "Droits de l'homme et méthode comparative," *Revue internationale de droit comparé* 3 (1968): 476.
15. U.N. General Assembly, Dec. 10, 1948, U.N. Doc. A/810 (1948), 71. Universal Declaration of Human Rights, G.A. Res. 217A (III) (hereinafter Universal Declaration).
16. U.N. General Assembly, Dec. 16, 1966, International Covenant on Civil and Political Rights, G.A. Res. 2200A (XXI). 21 U.N. GAOR Supp. (No. 16) 52, U.N. Doc. A/6316 (1966), 999 U.N.T.S. 171, entered into force Mar. 23, 1976 (hereinafter International Covenant).
17. International Covenant, Art. 12: "*No one shall be subjected to arbitrary interference* with his privacy, family, home or correspondence, nor to attacks upon his honour and reputation. Everyone has the right to the protection of the law against such interference or attacks" (emphasis added).
18. Ibid., Art. 8, § 1: "*Everyone has the right to respect* for his private and family life, his home and his correspondence" (emphasis added). Art. 8, § 2: "There shall be no interference by a public authority with the exercice of this right except such as is in accordance with the

law and is necessary in a democratic society in the interests of national security, public safety or the economic well-being of the country, for the prevention of disorder or crime, for the protection of health or morals, or for the protection of the rights and freedoms of others."

19. Ibid., Art. 17, § 1: "*No one shall be subjected to arbitrary or unlawful interference* with his privacy, family, home or correspondence, nor to unlawful attacks on his honour and reputation" (emphasis added).

20. Alpha M. Connelly, "Problems of Interpretation of Article 8 of the European Convention on Human Rights," *International and Comparative Law Quarterly* 35 (1986): 569; Pierre Kayser, *La protection de la vie privée*, 3d ed. (Paris: Economica, 1995), 20.

21. Kayser, *La protection de la vie privée*, 20.

22. International Covenant, Art. 8, § 2.

23. Universal Declaration, Art. 12.

24. International Covenant, Art. 17, § 1.

25. International Covenant, Art. 8, § 2.

26. Kayser, *La protection de la vie privée*, 20; International Covenant, Art. 8, § 2: "for the protection of health and . . . ."

27. International Covenant, Art. 29, § 2: "In the exercise of his rights and freedoms, everyone shall be subject only to such limitations as are determined by law solely for the purpose of securing due recognition and respect for the rights and freedoms of others and of meeting the just requirements of morality, public order and the general welfare in a democratic society."

28. Pierre-Henri Teitgen, "Introduction à la Convention européenne des droits de l'homme," *Journées d'information sur la Convention européenne, Annales de l'Université des sciences sociales de Toulouse*, vol. 29, Dec. 4–5, 1980, 14.

29. Kayser, *La protection de la vie privée*, 17.

30. Indeed, the commission considers that the right to privacy "comprises . . . to a certain degree, the right to establish and to develop relationships with other human beings, especially in the emotional field for the development and fulfilment of one's own personality." X. v. Iceland, Decision of May 18, 1976, *Decisions and Reports* 5 (1976): 87; Meulders-Klein, "Vie privée, vie familiale et droits de l'homme," 771, 773; Kayser, *La protection de la vie privée*, 28.

31. Connelly, "Interpretation of Article 8," 571.

32. Vienna Convention on the Law of Treaties, Art. 31, § 1: "A treaty shall be interpreted in good faith in accordance with the ordinary meaning to be given to the terms of the treaty in their context and in the light of its object and purpose"; Golder, Feb. 21, 1975, Ser. A, no. 18, 2 Eur. H.R. Rep. 524, 532, cited by Connelly, "Interpretation of Article 8," 568.

33. This position was defended in the Marckx decision in particular, and then reaffirmed in the Airey decision. Marckx v. Belgium, June 13, 1979, Ser. A, no. 31, 2 Eur. H.R. Rep. 330, 342: "[Article 8] does not merely compel the State to abstain from . . . interference"; in addition to this primarily negative undertaking, there may be positive obligations inherent in an effective "respect" for private life. Airey v. Ireland, Oct. 9, 1979, Ser. A, no. 32, 2 Eur. H.R. Rep. 305, 319: "Effective respect for private or family life obliges Ireland to

make this means of protection effectively accessible, when appropriate, to anyone who may wish to have recourse thereto."

34. Rigaux, *La protection de la vie privée*, 142.

35. Kayser, *La protection de la vie privée*, 27.

36. Connelly, "Interpretation of Article 8," 575, where with regards to this social conception of human rights he states: "it attributes a much greater role to the State in the promotion of human welfare than does the liberal view. In the latter, the individual is to be protected from the State; in the social view, the individual achieves freedoms and dignity through the State. The positive approach clearly bears the imprint of socialist philosophy, and in the West, is associated with the development of the welfare State."

37. X. and Y. v. Netherlands, Mar. 26, 1985, Ser. A, no. 91, 8 Eur. H.R. Rep. 235, 239–40.

38. Of those who have given an opinion against an extensive interpretation of Art. 8, § 1, of the European Convention see H. C. Guradze, *Die Europäische Menschenrechts Konvention* (Berlin, 1968), 187; and E. Ehrun, "La convention européenne des droits de l'homme" (Thesis, 1953), 240, cited by Jean De Meyer, "Le droit au respect de la vie privée et familiale, du domicile et des communications dans les relations entre personnes privées et les obligations qui en résultent pour les états parties à la Convention," in *Vie privée et droits de l'homme,* 373. Rigaux himself denies this extensive interpretation which he considers concerns only the relation between individuals and the state, in Rigaux, *La protection de la vie privée*, 676ff. For an opposing view, see Leisner, cited by De Meyer, "Le droit au respect de la vie privée et familiale," 373; Marc-Andre Eissen, "La convention et les devoirs de l'individu," in *La protection internationale des droits de l'homme dans le cadre européen* (Paris: Dalloz, 1967), 184, as cited by De Meyer, "Le droit au respect de la vie privée et familiale," 373; Kayser, *La protection de la vie privée,* 77–78; Meulders-Klein, "Vie privée, vie familiale et droits de l'homme," 776.

39. "As with any constitutional or legislative act, it [the European Convention] has acquired an existence independent of the will of its authors, and seems to be subjected to an objective and evolving interpretation. It is not excluded that its application could, in certain cases, move away from this will, especially insofar as this will no longer corresponds to the evolution of judicial conscience or to social needs. . . . Thus, it could be argued that the particular problem of an eventual validity erga omnes of the fundamental rights guaranteed by the Convention must not necessarily be resolved in a manner other than would be the case of an identical problem arising with regard to the fundamental rights guaranteed by the constitutions of various countries." De Meyer, "Le droit au respect de la vie privée et familiale," 366–67.

40. Marc-Henri Eissen, "La cour européenne des droits de l'homme," *Revue de droit public* (1986): 1586.

41. Guradze, *Die Europäische Menschenrechts Konvention,* 22; Ehrun, "La convention européenne des droits de l'homme," 373.

42. Doc. A/4625, cited by De Meyer, "Le droit au respect de la vie privée et familiale," 372.

43. X. and Y. v. Netherlands, 235.

44. Article 19: "To ensure the observance of the engagements undertaken by the High Contracting Parties in the present Convention, there shall be set up: (a) A European

Commission of Human Rights, hereinafter referred to as 'the Commission'; (b) A European Court of Human Rights, hereinafter referred to as 'the Court.'"

45. Article 25: "(1) The Commission may receive petitions addressed to the Secretary-General of the Council of Europe from any person, non-governmental organisation or group of individuals claiming to be victim of a violation by one of the High Contracting Parties of the rights set forth in this Convention, provided that the High Contracting Party against which the complaint has been lodged has declared that it recognises the competence of the Commission to receive such petitions. Those of the High Contracting Parties who have made such a declaration undertake not to hinder in any way the effective exercise of this right. (2) Such declarations may be made for a specific period. (3) The declarations shall be deposited with the Secretary-General of the Council of Europe who shall transmit copies thereof to the High Contracting Parties and publish them. (4) The Commission shall only exercise the powers provided for in this Article when at least six High Contracting Parties are bound by declarations made in accordance with the preceding paragraphs."

46. De Meyer, "Le droit au respect de la vie privée et familiale," 374.

47. Ibid., 375.

48. Connelly, "Interpretation of Article 8," 567.

49. Kayser, *La protection de la vie privée*, 76; Connelly, "Interpretation of Article 8," 595; Meulders-Klein, "Vie privée, vie familiale et droits de l'homme," 776, 793; Rigaux, *La protection de la vie privée*, 639 (quotation).

50. See, in particular, Connelly, "Interpretation of Article 8," 575. Jacques Velu and Rusen Ergec, *La convention européenne des droits de l'homme* (Brussels: Bruylant, 1990), 78.

51. X. v. Iceland, Decision of May 18, 1976, *Decisions and Reports* 5 (1976): 87. This approach has been confirmed by the commission: see, e.g., Van Oosterwijck v. Belgium, Report, Mar. 1, 1979, 3 Eur. H.R. Rep. 581, 583–84.

52. Kayser, *La protection de la vie privée*, 79. The European Court has had the chance to clarify its position in the Marckx decision and especially in its decision in X. and Y. v. Netherlands. See Marckx v. Belgium, 411; and X. and Y. v. Netherlands, 239–40: "Although the object of Article 8 is essentially that of protecting the individual against arbitrary interference by the public authorities, it does not merely compel the State to abstain from such interference: in addition to this primarily negative undertaking, there may be positive obligations inherent in an effective respect for private or family life. These obligations may involve the adoption of measures designed to secure respect for private life even in the sphere of the relations of individuals between themselves."

53. Velu and Ergec, *La convention européenne*, 77; De Meyer, "Le droit au respect de la vie privée et familiale," 375.

54. Everta Alkema, "The Third Party Applicability or 'Drittwirkung' of the European Convention on Human Rights," in *Protection des droits de l'homme: la dimension européenne; mélanges offerts en l'honneur de G. J. Wiarda* (Cologne, 1988), 38; Connelly, "Problems of Interpretation of Article 8," 593; De Meyer, "Le droit au respect de la vie privée et familiale," 375.

55. Connelly, "Problems of Interpretation of Article 8," 579, 583.

56. Such as it results from a wide conception of privacy which includes the right to establish

and maintain relationships with other human beings so as to develop and accomplish his own personality. Kayser, *La protection de la vie privée*, 16–17, 45–63.

57. Nold v. Commission, May 14, 1974, case 4/73, E.C.J.; J. Rideau, *Droit institutionnel de l'Union des Communautés européennes* (Paris: L.G.D.J., 1994), 135–36; Kayser, *La protection de la vie privée*, 83.

58. Déclaration commune des représentants de l'Assemblée, du Conseil et de la Commission des communautés européennes, en date du 5 avril 1977, in which they recognize "the primary importance [of] the respect of fundamental rights as they result amongst other things for the Constitutions of the member States as well as for the European Convention." *Official Journal of the European Community*, C 103, Apr. 27, 1977, 1; Rideau, *Droit institutionnel de l'Union des Communautés européennes*, 136.

59. Single European Act (SEA), *Official Journal of the European Community*, L 169/87, entered into force July 1, 1987. "[This] attachment to the principles of liberty, democracy and respect for human rights and fundamental freedoms and of the rule of law has been confirmed in the preamble to the Maastricht Treaty, which was signed on February 7, 1992."

60. Ibid.; Cinéthèque SA and Others v. Fédération nationale des cinémas français, joined cases 60/84 and 61/84, July 11, 1985, E.C.J., 2605: the Court of Justice of the European Community considers that "although it is the duty of the Court to ensure observance of fundamental rights in the field of Community law, it has no power to examine the compatibility with the European Convention for the Protection of Human Rights and Fundamental freedoms of national legislation which concers an area within the remit of the national legislator"; Demirel v. Stadt Schwäbisch Gmünd, Sept. 30, 1987, case 12/86, E.C.J., 3719.

61. See ERT AE v. Dimotiki Etairia Plioroforissis and others, case E–260/89, June 18, 1991, E.C.J., I–2925; The Society for the Protection of the Unborn Children v. Grogan, case C–159/90, Oct. 4, 1991, ibid., I–4685; Commission v. Germany, case C–62/90, Apr. 8, 1992, ibid., I–2575.

62. Kayser, *La protection de la vie privée*, 84.

63. Ibid.

64. Rideau, *Droit institutionnel de l'Union des Communautés européennes*, 139. Article F, § 2: "The Union shall respect fundamental rights, as guaranteed by the European Convention for the Protection of Human Rights and Fundamental Freedoms signed in Rome on 4 November 1950 and as they result from the constitutional traditions common to the Member States, as general principles of Community law."

65. Kayser, *La protection de la vie privée*, 84.

66. Rigaux, *La protection de la vie privée*, 7.

67. Rigaux, "La liberté de la vie privée," 559.

68. Rigaux, *La protection de la vie privée*, 7.

69. The fundamental distinction between a subjective right and a liberty interest resides in the fact that a subjective right is, by necessity, circumscribed. It also has defined characteristics and is actionable per se. A liberty interest is, by necessity, undetermined and is a principle, accompanied by a power of self-determination. For a discussion on this question, see Rigaux, "La liberté de la vie privée," 557–59.

70. Velu, *Répertoire pratique de droit belge.*

71. Law of Dec. 8, 1992, relative to the protection of privacy in relation to personal auto-mated data. Article 7 of the statute regulates medical data of a personal nature; *Moniteur belge,* Mar. 18, 1993.

72. Ibid., Art. 2.

73. Commentaires de documents, Ministère de la Justice, Documentation interne, *Projet de loi relatif à la protection de la vie privée à l égard des traitements de données à caractère personnel,* 6.

74. Civil Code, Art. 9: "Each has a right to respect for his private life . . . ."

75. For a review of this controversy, see Pierre Kayser, "Les droits de la personnalité," *Revue trimestrielle du droit civil* 70 (1971): 445–509.

76. Gerard Cornu, *Droit civil: introduction, les personnes, les biens,* 7th ed. (Paris: Montchres-tien, 1994), 191–93.

77. Kayser, "Les droits de la personnalité," 454.

78. "Every act of a person causing damage to another obliges that person to repair the damage."

79. Jean Morange, *Libertés publiques* (Paris: PUF, 1982), 148; Kayser, *La protection de la vie privée,* 19.

80. Article 368 of the old Penal Code, now Art. 226–1, provides: "The fact of infringing voluntarily someone's privacy, by whatever means, is punishable with one year of imprisonment and 300,000 francs. For example: (1) by receiving, registering or copying, without consent, personal and private declarations, without consent; (2) by fixing, registering or copying, without consent, the portrait of a person who is in a private place, without consent . . . ."

81. For example, law no. 78–17 of Jan. 6, 1978, "relative à l'informatique, aux fichiers et aux libertés," *Journal officiel,* Jan. 7, 1978, 227–31.

82. Article 9 of the Civil Code and old Art. 368 of the Penal Code were introduced by law no. 70–643 of July 17, 1970. This law reinforced the individual rights of citizens. *Journal officiel,* July 19, 1970, 6751–61.

83. G. F. Putcha, *Geschichte des Rechts bei dem römischen Volk* (Leipzig: Breitkoff und Härtel, 1881), 50. Putcha was the first author to use this notion in 1832, according to Rigaux, *La protection de la vie privée,* 612.

84. C. Neuner, *Wesen und Arten der Privatrechtsverhsltnisse* (Kiel: Schwers'sche Buchhandlung, 1866), 16, cited by Rigaux, *La protection de la vie privée,* 612.

85. Rigaux, *La protection de la vie privée,* 612.

86. Josef Kohler, "Das Autorrecht," *Jherings Jahrbücher* 18 (1880): 254–59; Otto Friederich Von Gierke, "Deutsches Privatrecht," in K. Binging and Friederich Oetker, *System-atisches Handbuch der Deutscher Rechswissenschaft* (Leipzig: Verlag von Dunker und Humblot, 1895). See Kayser, *La protection de la vie privée,* 104; and Rigaux, *La protection de la vie privée,* 613–14.

87. Rigaux, *La protection de la vie privée,* 615–16. Rigaux indicates that according to Thon, civilists could speak of a private right of personality but that they should be conscious of the fact that such a right depends on the will of the state and is public in nature. Georg Jellinek (*System der Subjektiven öffentlichen Rechte* [Tübingen: Mohr, 1905]) defined

personality rights as the totality of faculties afforded by law (*die Rechtsordnung*) to an individual. Jellinek considered that life, health, liberty, and honor are not objects possessed by humans, but rather constitutive qualities of their concrete being (*Eigenschaften die sein konkretes Wesen ausmachen*). Therefore, these rights fall not within the domain of rights that one has but rather among those of "being," hence, the notion of liberty rights, *Freiheitsrechten.*

88. Kayser, *La protection de la vie privée*, 104, refers to the decision of the Reichsgericht of May 22, 1902 (RGZ 51, 369) according to which "the recognition of a general subjective right of personality does not have its place in the positive system of our civil code" (373).

89. The Basic Law for the Federal Republic of Germany (Grundgesetz) of May 23, 1949, *Federal Law Gazette*, May 23, 1949. Schacht, Federal Court of Civil Justice (Bundesgerichtshof), May 25, 1954, BGHZ 13, 334.

90. Heinrich Böll, June 3, 1980, BVerwGe, 54, 208. Rigaux, *La protection de la vie privée*, 15, 621.

91. Article 2 al. 1 recognizes that "every one shall have the right to the free development of his personality insofar as he does not violate the rights of others or offend against the constitutional order or the moral code." Article 1 al. 1: "The dignity of man shall be inviolable. To respect and protect it is the duty of all state authority." See David Flaherty, "On the Utility of Constitutional Rights to Privacy and Data Protection," *Case Western Reserve Law Review* 41 (1991): 841; Rigaux, *La protection de la vie privée*, 621; Kayser, *La protection de la vie privée*, 105; and Meulders-Klein, "Vie privée, vie familiale et droits de l'homme," 791–92.

92. Kayser, *La protection de la vie privée*, 105; Meulders-Klein, "Vie privée, vie familiale et droits de l'homme," 791.

93. Walther C. Zimmerli, "Ethical Aspects of the Legal Problem of Confidentiality," in International Workshop, *The Human Genome Project: Legal Aspects* (Bilbao: Fundacion BBV, 1995). Flaherty, "Utility of Constitutional Rights to Privacy," 842, 841.

94. Meulders-Klein, "Vie privée, vie familiale et droits de l'homme," 791; Rigaux, *La protection de la vie privée*, 621–22.

95. Kayser, *La protection de la vie privée*, 487.

96. Meulders-Klein, "Vie privée, vie familiale et droits de l'homme," 792.

97. C. Cast., Apr. 12, 1973, n. 38, Giur. Cost., 1973, I, 354–362, cited by Rigaux, *La protection de la vie privée*, 651. S. Rials, *Textes constitutionnels étrangers* (Paris: PUF, 1991), 88–89: "Article 2: The republic recognises and guarantees the fundamental human rights of a person, as much in his capacity of individual as in the social groups in which his personality is exercised. Article 3 al.2: The republic has the duty to smooth out the economic and social obstacles which . . . hinder the full development of the human person. . . . Article 13 al.1: The liberty of a person is inviolable."

98. Rigaux, *La protection de la vie privée*, 149. In Germany, constitutional control of legislation is exercised by the Bundesverfassungsgericht, which limits the possibility for appeal in civil matters, in order not to take over the role of the Bundesgericht (the federal Civil Court).

99. Rigaux, *La protection de la vie privée*, 149, 627. The Italian Supreme Court, in a famous decision on privacy of May 27, 1975, implicitly recognized the existence of a general right

of personality. Cass. Civ. I, May 25, 1975, n. 2629, Principessa Soraya Esfandari, Giust. Civ. I, 1975, 1686, as cited in ibid., 628.

100. Charter of Human Rights and Freedoms, S.Q. 1975, c. 6; R.S.Q., c. C–12.

101. Article 49: "Any unlawful interference with any right or freedom recognized by the Charter entitles the victim to obtain the cessation of such interference and compensation for the moral or material prejudice resulting therefrom. In case of unlawful and intentional interference, the tribunal may, in addition, condemn the person guilty of it to exemplary damages."

102. Karim Benyekhlef, *La protection de la vie privée dans les échanges internationaux d'informations* (Montreal: Themis, 1992), 24. Even if the Supreme Court of Canada has constantly reaffirmed the fundamental character of the Quebec Charter and its quasi-constitutional status, doctrinal discussions still surface about its obligatory nature.

103. Ibid.; Patrick A. Molinari, "Les nouveaux moyens de reproduction et les droits de la pérsonalité," *Revue du barreau* 46 (1986): 721.

104. H. Patrick Glenn, "Le droit au respect de la vie privée," *Revue du barreau* 39 (1979): 881.

105. Benyekhlef, *La protection de la vie privée*, 22.

106. Article 35: "Every person has a right to the respect of his reputation and privacy. No one may invade the privacy of a person without the consent of the person or his heirs unless authorized by law." This means that privacy is now a substantive, subjective right. This codification of the principle of respect for privacy is then only the confirmation of case law, which for many years already considered privacy as "a rampart against illicit invasions of the fundamental rights of the person."

107. The Queen v. Dyment [1988], 2 S.C.R. 417. For example, Art. 36, C.c.Q., in its description of acts considered as invasions, includes inter alia interception of communication, observance of others, and use of name, image, etc., of another.

108. An Act Respecting the Protection of Personal Information in the Private Sector, L.Q. 1993, c. 17; An Act Respecting Access to Documents Held by Public Bodies and the Protection of Personal Information, R.S.Q., c. A–2.1.

109. Kayser, *La protection de la vie privée*, 111. For example, Art. 390, al.1, of the Norwegian Penal Code and Art. 263, al.1, of the Danish Penal Code; "Norway has, since 1899, had a criminal statute forbidding violations of 'the peace of private life,' and there has been case law which is remarkably similar to that in USA," James Michael, *Privacy and Human Rights* (Paris: UNESCO, 1994), 181.

   "[The principle of governmental publicity] provides a general right of public access to government documents. Although this does not seem to have been intended originally as a privacy protection measure, many of those who exercise the right do so, in order to inspect records that relate to them personally." Ibid., 14. The principle of governmental publicity has been introduced in Sweden, by its constitution, in 1766. It has existed in Finland since 1951 and in Denmark and Norway since 1971.

110. J. Lete Del Rio, *Derecho de la persona* (Madrid: Tecnos, 1986), 173, 175. Article 10.1 of the Spanish constitution expressly proclaims: "La dignidad de la persona, los derechos inviolables que le son inherentes, el libre desarrollo de la personalidad, el respecto a la ley y a los derechos de los demas son fundamento del orden politico y de la paz social."

111. Lete Del Rio, *Derecho de la persona*, 187.

112. Article 7: "Recoge en terminos de razonable amplitud diversos supuestos de intromision o injerencia que pueden darse en la vida real." Article 8(1): "Con carácter general, las actuaciones autorizadas o acordadas por la autoridad competente de acuerdo con la ley, ni cuando predomine un intérés histórico, científico o cultural relevante." Lete Del Rio, *Derecho de la persona,* 187.

113. Article 28 as modified by the law of Dec. 16, 1983, entered into force July 1, 1985.

114. Until 1983, the term *personal interest* was used instead of *personality right* even though it had a similar content. The modification, in 1983, of the Code of Obligations and the introduction of the term *personality* in Art. 28 have established the new terminology in Swiss law. Pierre Engel, "La protection des données personnelles: Etat de la législation et tendance de la jurisprudence en Suisse," *Revue internationale de droit comparé* 3 (1987): 628.

115. Rigaux, *La protection de la vie privée,* 626.

116. Henri Deschenaux and Paul-Henri Steinauer, *Personnes physiques et tutelle* (Bern: Stäntsli, 1980), 130. "The inviolability of privacy is not only a moral principle; it is a rule of law, an attribute of the person that is protected by law"; Engel, "La protection des données personnelles," 629.

117. Deschenaux and Steinauer, *Personnes physiques et tutelle,* 134, 138; Engel, "La protection des données personnelles," 633.

118. Deschenaux and Steinauer, *Personnes physiques et tutelle,* 140. Article 28 al. 2: "Any intrusion is illicit, unless justified by the consent of the victim, by a superior public or private interest, or by the law." Rigaux, *La protection de la vie privée,* 337.

119. Deschenaux and Steiner, *Personnes physiques et tutelle,* 132, 131. The European Convention was ratified by Switzerland on Nov. 28, 1974.

120. David J. Seipp, "English Judicial Recognition of a Right to Privacy," *Oxford Journal of Legal Studies* 3 (1983): 326, 350. Doc. H (67) 2, published Jan. 10, 1967, cited in ibid., 351.

121. Ibid., 351, 352.

122. Ibid., 353.

123. Ibid., 331, 334–37. "The principle stated in a dissenting judgement in 1769 had become the rule, that every man has a right to keep his own sentiments, and a right to judge whether he will make them public, or commit them only to the sight of his friends"; Millar v. Taylor (1769), 98 Eng. Rep. 201, 242 (Yates, J. dissenting), cited in ibid., 338. "Nineteenth-century English courts afforded only a precarious protection to intangible personal information but showed some of their greatest legal inventiveness when they did act to protect this privacy interest" (341).

124. Rigaux, *La protection de la vie privée,* 636.

125. Bernstein v. Skyviews and General, Ltd. [1978] Q.B. 479; Miller v. Jackson [1977] Q.B. 966.

126. Inland Revenue Commissioners v. Rossminster, Ltd. [1980] A.C. 952 (property). Riddick v. Thames Board Mills [1977] Q.B. 881; Harman v. Sec'y of State for the Home Dep't [1982] 2 W.L.R. 338 (communication). British Steel Corp. v. Granada Television, Ltd. [1981] A.C. 1096 (personal information).

127. Seipp, "English Judicial Recognition," 362. But "this judicial recognition of a right to privacy in a broad range of contexts, the culmination of a decade or more of decisions

focusing explicitly on privacy interests, delineates the present scope of a healthy, exuberant new branch of English common law. Privacy law, no longer the interstitial and incidental by-product of other doctrines, is about to come on its own" (363).

128. Canada Act 1982, Schedule B, 1982 (U.K.), c. 11.

129. Regina v. Oakes [1986] 1 S.C.R. 104.

130. Article 8: "Every one has the right to be secure against unreasonable search or seizure." Hunter v. Southam [1984] 2 S.C.R. 145.

131. Ibid., 159, 158, 160.

132. Flaherty, "Utility of Constitutional Rights to Privacy," 847.

133. Queen v. Dyment, 429, 426.

134. Ibid., 429.

135. Article 7: " Every one has the right to life, liberty and security of the person and the right not to be deprived thereof except in accordance with the principles of fundamental justice."

136. Benyekhlef, *La protection de la vie privée*, 32, 34, 36. Article 26: "The guarantee in this Charter of certain rights and freedoms shall not be construed as denying the existence of any other rights or freedoms that exist in Canada." The particular attention afforded by some American judges to the Ninth Amendment is not without interest since this provision could constitutionally protect certain fundamental rights not explicitly enunciated in the text of the amendment.

137. Flaherty, "Utility of Constitutional Rights to Privacy," 849.

138. Benyekhlef, *La protection de la vie privée*, 13.

139. Peter Burns, "The Law and Privacy: The Canadian Experience," *Revue du barreau canadien* 54 (1976): 12.

140. Ibid., 14–23.

141. Privacy Act, R.S.S., 1979, c. P–24 (Sask.); Privacy Act, R.S.B.C., 1979, c. 336 (B.C.); Privacy Act, S.M., 1970, c. 74 (Man.); An Act Respecting The Protection of Personal Privacy, S.N., 1981, c. 6 (Nfld.). Burns, "The Law and Privacy," 32.

142. Burns, "The Law and Privacy," 33.

143. Criminal Code, R.S.C. (1985), c. C–46, mod. by R.S.C. (1985), c. 2 (1st supp.)

144. Article 184 (1): "Everyone who, by means of any electro-magnetic, acoustic, mechanical or other device, wilfully intercepts a private communication is guilty of an indictable offence and liable to imprisonment for a term not exceeding five years."

Part Six **Recommendations**

Chapter 23 Genetic Secrets:

A Policy Framework

Mark A. Rothstein

Before the last half of the twentieth century, human genetic secrets belonged exclusively to nature. They were locked securely within the genes. Except for the most rudimentary associations of phenotypes in families, genetic secrets were unknown and unknowable to human-kind. Genetic afflictions were seemingly caused by the indecipherable and unpredictable hand of fate. Gene expression was the only mean-ingful endpoint. There were no genetic secrets involving individuals who were presymptomatic or predisposed to late-onset disorders or unaffected carriers of recessive or X-linked disorders.

Today concern has shifted to a different type of genetic secret. The secrets no longer belong solely to nature. Some belong to humans as well. As we learn many of nature's genetic secrets, we must consider whether, when, and how individuals should have access to their ge-netic legacy, and when this information must be shared with other individuals and entities. An expanding array of genetic secrets about individuals is now ascertainable before or in the absence of gene expression. In the future, an even wider range of genetic information will be discoverable about an individual virtually from the first moments after conception.[1]

The previous chapters of this book have explored some of the many ways genetic information may be obtained and used. In the face of serious concerns about psychological harm, stigmatization, and discrimination, policy makers have been tempted to advocate or even to enact legislation to protect genetic privacy and confidentiality. In some instances, however, these efforts have not been preceded by a searching inquiry into the theoretical underpinnings, practical limitations, and future implications of such legislative actions.

Although the avowed purpose of many of these laws is to protect privacy and confidentiality, it is essential to identify the public policy interests to be served by any new legislation or other policy initiatives. Some of the key policy goals underlying any effort to protect privacy and confidentiality of genetic information include the following: (1) preventing at-risk individuals who want to undergo genetic testing from being dissuaded from doing so because of a fear that the information generated by the tests may be used to their detriment; (2) preventing individuals from being coerced into genetic testing; (3) preventing individuals untrained in genetics, both laypeople and health professionals, from making decisions based on genetic information, which they may misinterpret; (4) conserving medical resources by preventing genetics professionals and medical technologies from being used for inappropriate nonmedical purposes; (5) preserving the quality of genetic testing and counseling by limiting their use in nonclinical settings, where testing may not be of the best quality and counseling may not be provided; (6) conserving human resources by not disqualifying individuals from current activities (such as employment) because of a fear of future illness; (7) preventing discrimination based on genetic information; and (8) preventing genetic reductionism and determinism, in which genetic explanations for health and behavior are the predominant factor in evaluating various aspects of human affairs.

In this chapter, drawing on the contributions of the preceding chapter authors as well as other sources, I present the rationale and strategy for regulating genetic information. In so doing, I address a range of difficult but essential questions. These include the following: What is genetic information? Does it differ from other types of medical information? Why is it important to protect genetic secrets? Why is genetic information important to third parties? When do the benefits of protecting genetic privacy outweigh the costs? Is it possible to protect the confidentiality of genetic information? What legal and political approaches are most likely to be successful?

PRIVACY AND CONFIDENTIALITY

In common parlance, privacy and confidentiality are often used interchangeably. As Anita Allen observes, however, there are four important classes of privacy: informational privacy, physical privacy, decisional privacy, and proprietary privacy.[2] Although each of these aspects is explored in this volume, Allen notes that many of today's privacy claims refer to informational privacy. The essence of informational privacy is controlling access to personal information.

Sonia Le Bris and Bartha Maria Knoppers explore the "richness, fluidity, and malleability" of the concept of privacy in the international and comparative law field.[3] They note that privacy is more of an evolving legal principle than a static legal rule. Privacy includes, for example, the German concept of informational self-determination and the French notion of an actionable subjective right.

Confidentiality may be considered, along with secrecy and anonymity, as branches of informational privacy. Confidentiality often refers to an individual's right to prohibit the redisclosure of sensitive information originally disclosed within a confidential relationship (e.g., patient-physician) or otherwise released on assurances that the information will not be redisclosed without consent. Thus defined, issues of the confidentiality of genetic information need to be resolved only after other privacy issues, especially physical privacy (e.g., issues of bodily integrity surrounding genetic testing) and decisional privacy (e.g., issues of the right to make autonomous health choices based on genetic information) are decided. Nevertheless, when the possible uses of new genetic information have been raised, concern has frequently focused on confidentiality and informational privacy rather than on physical or decisional privacy.

Some genome scientists, entrepreneurs, and members of the public feel that politicians and lawyers need to "fix" the confidentiality problem immediately. In essence, they assert that if at-risk individuals and the public were free of worries about discrimination in insurance and employment, then no remaining obstacles would exist to the widespread introduction of genetic testing. Yet the purpose of laws related to genetics, including antidiscrimination laws, is not to make the world safe for the unfettered pursuit of genomic research or mass genetic screening programs of unproven need or efficacy.

Confidentiality is an important concern not merely because of the structure of the U.S. health care system but also because of broader societal interests in how individuals view themselves, individuals' right to autonomy in health care decision making, and the need to preserve the trust essential to patient-physician relations. If concerns about the confidentiality of genetic information would be obviated by adoption of a health care system in which preexisting conditions or predispositions did not adversely affect access to health care, then one might assume that in Western Europe and Canada there would be less concern by the public about the confidentiality of medical records and relatively less legal regulation of medical records than in the United States. As Paul Schwartz points out, however, the opposite is true, with laws in several European countries, such as France and Germany, containing stringent limitations on and even criminal sanctions for the disclosure of health information.[4] Obviously, privacy and confidentiality are considered important social values in themselves, regardless of the possible use of the information by the health care system. By contrast, in the United States, widespread public sentiment exists in favor of privacy and confidentiality in the abstract, yet we tolerate a political and social structure in which privacy and confidentiality are poorly protected.

Many issues of genetic privacy and confidentiality revolve around the proper use of personal genetic information developed in the clinical setting. As more genetic tests are available for and used in the clinical setting, more genetic information will be generated. Therefore, determining when it is appropriate to introduce a new genetic test beyond the research setting is the first step in controlling the flow of genetic information. Before introducing any new medical test into clinical practice or as a screening device, there should be careful consideration of the test's analytic validity, clinical validity, and clinical utility, the cost-effectiveness of medical interventions, and other traditional criteria for health care technology assessment.

Once these technical criteria are satisfied, the focus can turn to the social and legal consequences of the testing. There is much more to consider than discrimination. Indeed, the discrimination model deals only with one aspect of the consequences of genetic information; it fails to address such threshold issues as autonomy, liberty, and justice. For example, what rights do individuals have to obtain genetic information, decide with whom to share the information, receive appropriate medical services based on the information, and manage their own health affairs as a result of the information?

Even if a decision were reached to promote widespread genetic testing of any particular type, it is certainly not clear that "fixing" confidentiality holds the key to encouraging testing. Two threshold questions are whether confidentiality will encourage more genetic testing and whether more genetic testing is good. As Scott Burris and Lawrence O. Gostin point out, HIV confidentiality was similarly considered an integral part of the public health strategy of encouraging HIV testing. Yet they observe that the broader strategy of encouraging HIV testing has produced questionable public health benefits in reducing the spread of HIV.[5] There is far less of a compelling public health rationale for genetic testing, and thus we should have far less confidence that the "problem" will be "fixed" by confidentiality legislation.

DEVELOPING A LEGISLATIVE FRAMEWORK

Although many of the problems posed by new genetic information can be lessened through education and voluntary approaches, new legislative initiatives must be an integral part of any comprehensive scheme of protecting genetic privacy and confidentiality. Devising appropriate legislative strategies is extremely difficult. Indeed, as I argue below, most of the legislative enactments and proposals to date have been ineffective or ill-advised. As in other areas of public policy, well-meaning but imprudent legislation to protect genetic secrets may have serious unintended consequences.

In the pages that follow, I suggest a number of possible legislative initiatives in specific subject areas. Before reaching these specifics, however, more basic questions of the nature and structure of such legislation need to be addressed. In particular, I discuss whether new legislative initiatives should: (1) be comprehensive or incremental, (2) be national or state, (3) be genetic or generic, (4) regulate access to information or use of information, and (5) regulate unauthorized or authorized disclosures. Several of these considerations are interrelated.

Comprehensive versus Incremental Approaches

Issues of genetic privacy and confidentiality have many ramifications, but at the core they are primarily issues of health—personal, familial, and societal. In suggesting approaches to remedy some of the problems, it is tempting to propose a sweeping revision of the U.S. health care system. As noted earlier, it has been asserted that if the United States adopted a universal access, single-payer health care system, then the issue of genetic discrimination in health insurance would be irrelevant, the way it is in Canada or many Western European countries.[6] Because all individuals are assured of access to health care under such a system, a genetic predisposition will be solely an individual concern that does not affect insurance coverage or health care allocation decisions. As Madison Powers has written, "A health care finance policy that eliminates the market incentives for gaining access to genetic information can be as effective as an instrument of genetic privacy protection policy as legal prohibitions."[7]

The merits of fundamentally restructuring the U.S. health care system have been debated many times and in many places, and there is minimal value in restating the arguments here. There can be little dispute, however, that the likelihood of a drastic change occurring soon in the United States is exceedingly small. As I have previously noted, genetic privacy and confidentiality are important under any health care system. Nevertheless, I will address the potential risks of invasion of genetic privacy and breach of genetic confidentiality within the general framework of the current, mostly private, voluntary health insurance system in effect in the United States.

Genetic privacy and confidentiality cannot be protected adequately by a single piece of legislation. Instead, in this chapter I propose a series of laws, each dealing with a particular subject area in which privacy and confidentiality are threatened. In a sense, this approach is neither comprehensive nor incremental; it is context-specific.

National or State Laws

Almost every law specifically directed at an aspect of genetic information since 1990 has been enacted at the state level. Thus, by 1997, at least 12 state laws prohibit genetic discrimination in employment, at least 16 state laws prohibit genetic discrimination in health insurance, and more than 40 state laws authorize the establishment of DNA data banks for law enforcement purposes. There are several explanations for this phenomenon. First, some issues, such as regulation of insurance, are matters traditionally left to the states. Second, under our system of federalism, to paraphrase Justice Louis Brandeis, the states are the "laboratories of democracy," often taking the lead in initiating experimental approaches to solve the problems of the day.[8] Third, Congress has been slow to enact federal legislation in this area.

It is difficult to say, in the abstract, whether state or federal action is preferable. To a great extent, it depends on the particular subject being regulated. The need for uniformity and the ability of computers to transfer entire medical files across the country in an instant militate in favor of federal regulation to protect the security of medical records. And yet certain institutions, such as schools, are traditionally regulated at the state and local levels. Regulation of genetic information obtained by schools, therefore, would be best achieved through state school records laws.

In allocating regulatory responsibility between federal and state governments, policy makers need to consider the possible effect of the law of federal preemption. Basically, unless Congress indicates otherwise, federal law preempts state laws as to matters that the federal government has chosen to regulate. Sometimes, federal preemption results in gaps in protection for individuals. For example, the federal Employee Retirement Income Security Act (ERISA) preempts states from regulating employer-provided pension and welfare plans. As to pension plans, Congress has detailed the requirements for pension plan reporting, vesting, solvency, portability, and other matters. As to welfare plans (including employee health benefits), Congress has not enacted substantive limitations on the ERISA-qualified plans of self-insured employers. The result is that states are prohibited from regulating the health plans of self-insured employers but there are no substantive federal provisions.[9]

Many of the federal antidiscrimination laws, such as the Americans with Disabilities Act (ADA), permit states to enforce their own laws so long as they are consistent with federal law and provide protection at least as stringent. In the area of genetics, it may be valuable to enact a combination of laws: preemptive federal laws, nonpreemptive federal laws, and state laws. These alternatives, however, should be carefully weighed to avoid gaps, overlaps, and unintended consequences.

Genetic versus Generic Legislation

The most difficult legislative strategy question is whether new enactments should focus specifically and exclusively on genetics or whether genetics should be merely one part of a broader statute. I believe, as a practical matter, that it is impossible to separate genetic conditions, tests, and information from other medical conditions, tests, and information. I also believe that it is possible to craft effective, general legislation and that this approach is preferable to legislation focusing specifically on genetics.

To begin with, as a medical and scientific matter, it is extremely difficult to develop a satisfactory definition of *genetic, genetic information, genetic testing,* or any other essential term. Even as to monogenic disorders, in which the condition is caused by a single gene, although it is clear that the condition is "genetic," it is not clear whether a non-DNA-based test is a "genetic test." For example, is a sweat chloride test, a common diagnostic measure of cystic fibrosis, a "genetic test"? Moreover, as the emphasis of genetic research turns increasingly to complex disorders, scientists will identify a genetic component of numerous common health conditions. Scientists have already demonstrated a genetic role in some forms of diabetes, hypertension, hypercholesterolemia, epilepsy, osteoporosis, and various cancers. Because these and similar complex or multifactorial disorders are likely to be the main focus of future genetic inquiries in both the clinical and nonclinical settings, a DNA-based definition of *genetic* would be demonstrably underinclusive. Yet, a more comprehensive definition would include virtually all medical conditions.

The second practical problem in enacting "genetic" legislation involves medical records. If genetic information is to be treated differently from non-genetic information, some easy way must be found to separate the information so that only nongenetic information can be reported to third parties, such as employers and insurers. Unfortunately, this would be extremely difficult to accomplish. Most medical records are interspersed with information about family health histories and similar matters. Editing or otherwise expunging genetic information from reportable medical records would be burdensome and impractical. It might also compromise the quality of patient care.

Another possibility is to use anonymous genetic testing, as some have suggested,[10] but this approach is unlikely to be effective. Because an insurer will not pay for an anonymous test, the use of anonymous testing would be restricted to those who could afford to pay for genetic services in cash. Moreover, if genetic testing were inexpensive and anonymous testing were common, insurers and other similarly interested parties, to avoid adverse selection, would soon begin their own mandatory genetic testing programs, thus defeating the purpose for which anonymous testing was started.[11] Health care providers may need to develop policies on how to respond to occasional patient requests for anonymous genetic testing, but this practice should not be promoted as the solution to the problems of genetic privacy and confidentiality.

In his chapter, Thomas Murray closely examines what he calls "genetic exceptionalism" and concludes that there is essentially no difference between ordinary medical information and genetic information, and thus both types of information should be subject to the same protections.[12] I reach the same conclusion; genetic information should not be protected separately. We both recognize, however, the significance of the distinction between genetic and other medical information. Genes reveal information about the health of family members (e.g., parents, siblings, children), parentage, reproductive options, and future health risks. In addition, genetic information is transgenerational; as a result, it goes to the essence of humanity, self-identity, and individuality. Finally, genetic information often carries a great degree of stigma and not long ago was used as the "scientific" justification for racism, eugenics, and geno-cide.[13]

The preceding reasons for distinguishing genetic information from other medical information, however, are overwhelmingly social rather than scientific phenomena. Genetic information is unique because it is regarded as unique. This fact supports the need for legislation to protect genetic privacy and confidentiality, but not separately from other medical information. Enacting special legislation to deal with genetic information could well have the effect of reinforcing the stigma of genetic conditions, creating a self-fulfilling prophecy.

Because of the special public concerns raised by the specter of widespread disclosure of genetic information, it may be easier politically to gain popular support for legislation that limits the uses of genetic information. Coalitions of consumers of genetic services can make a persuasive case for statutory protection. Indeed, at least at the state level, the trend thus far has been to enact specific laws prohibiting genetic discrimination in health insurance and employment. As further described below, however, these laws offer little protection to affected individuals, and they may create even more problems in the long run.

The enactment of specific HIV-AIDS laws in the 1980s does not support the passage of genetic-specific legislation. Unlike the thousands of genetic disorders and traits, HIV-AIDS is a single condition (although variably manifested) with a largely predictable course and outcome. Seropositivity for HIV is relatively easy to establish with a simple and cheap test, which generates a result that, by itself, is relatively easy to isolate in a medical record. By contrast, genetic information is so extensive and pervasive that a law limited to genetics would not succeed. Carefully crafted generic—rather than reflexively genetic—laws hold the greatest promise for protecting genetic secrets.

Regulate Access to Information or Use of Information

If the goal is to protect genetic privacy and confidentiality, is it more likely to be achieved by a law that bans access to the information by third parties, use of the information by third parties, or both? Federal employment discrimination laws are instructive. Title VII of the Civil Rights Act of 1964 prohibits discrimination in employment on the basis of race, color, religion, sex, or national origin. Title VII bans using the information in a discriminatory manner rather than collecting the information. Technically, it is lawful for an employer to ask an applicant to reveal information such as race or sex, although hardly any employers do so because there are few circumstances under which such information can be used lawfully. Thus, by prohibiting the *use* of certain information, Title VII also works to limit collection of the information.

By contrast, Title I of the Americans with Disabilities Act, which prohibits discrimination in employment on the basis of disability, also restricts access to information. For example, by limiting an employer's preemployment inquiries about disabilities, the law attempts to exclude irrelevant health criteria from the employer's decision-making process. Unfortunately, the ADA also permits complete access to an individual's medical records after a conditional offer of employment, thereby compromising genetic privacy and facilitating surreptitious disability discrimination.[14] This latter issue is addressed below.

In the genetics context, if privacy and confidentiality are the goals, then access to the information should be prohibited to the extent possible. As a practical matter, however, access by third parties to some information may be unpreventable or may even serve a positive function. In those instances, the use of the information must be carefully circumscribed, thereby protecting individuals from the adverse consequences of disclosure.[15]

Regulate Unauthorized or Authorized Disclosures

Some proposals to protect genetic privacy and confidentiality, notably the Genetic Privacy Act drafted by George Annas, Leonard Glantz, and Patricia Roche, use procedural mechanisms in an attempt to prevent the unauthorized disclosure of genetic information.[16] The proposed act contains detailed oral and written notice provisions, written informed consent provisions, a right to view and correct genetic records, a right to order the destruction of genetic samples, and numerous other procedural rights. Although these provisions, if enacted, would afford some protections to individuals, as Philip Reilly observes, complying with these myriad procedures will be onerous and expensive for health care providers to implement.[17]

This approach has an even more fundamental problem, as Wendy Parmet notes. "Procedural laws may not prevent what substantive laws permit."[18] The proposed legislation seeks to prevent unlawful, inadvertent, and unauthorized disclosures of genetic information. This is a laudable goal, but the more significant problem is the *authorized* disclosure of genetic information. The issue of authorized disclosure is not addressed by this or other procedural proposals. Thus, as a condition of employment, insurance, or other opportunities, an individual lawfully may be required to execute a release authorizing the disclosure of medical (including genetic) information. All the procedural measures in the world will not protect the confidentiality of the information under these circumstances. As a result, it is clear that substantive provisions need to be enacted to prevent the compelled, authorized disclosure of health records. According to Madison Powers, "the best vehicle for protecting the interests underlying our concerns about genetic privacy may require changes in the economic and social institutions themselves."[19]

As discussed in Chapter 20, several bills introduced in Congress in the mid-1990s have sought to preserve the privacy and confidentiality of medical records. The bills have sparked a considerable debate among health care providers, insurance companies, privacy advocates, and other interested groups and individuals. The fundamental problem with these proposals has been not that they were too restrictive or too lax in permitting the disclosure of medical information. The problem is that these bills have been largely irrelevant.

Medical records privacy bills thus far have been procedural proposals, which seek to regulate *unauthorized* disclosure of medical information through fair information practices. In this respect, they are similar to the proposed Genetic Privacy Act. Regulation of medical records disclosure practices is necessary but not sufficient to provide meaningful and effective protection for privacy and confidentiality. Substantive laws regulating the *authorized* disclosure of information are far more important, yet they will be considerably more difficult to enact. It simply will not be possible to enact a single new law to protect the diverse substantive rights implicated by disclosure of genetic and other medical information.

The dilemma for policy makers is easy to summarize but difficult to resolve. Procedural protections are likely to be complicated, expensive, and ineffective. Genetic-specific laws are likely to be limited in scope and afford inadequate protection. Without a doubt, substantive changes in several laws must be made. Among other things, laws must be enacted to eliminate the incentives for commercial entities to gain access to various types of health-related information about individuals. Nevertheless, fundamental or radical changes, such as replacing our current private health finance system with a universal access public system, are unlikely to be forthcoming. Thus, legislative and policy proposals to protect genetic privacy and confidentiality must go beyond empty procedural reforms and walk a fine line between effective substantive changes and unrealistic radical proposals.

GENES AND FAMILIES

Before exploring the complex issues of competing claims to genetic information asserted by various individuals, institutions, and commercial entities, it is important to focus on the individual and the family. In the first instance, genetic information is information about families. Do individuals have a duty to share genetic information with members of their family? According to Lori Andrews, there may be a moral duty to share genetic information within families, but there is no corresponding legal duty.[20] This assertion is in accord with the position taken by the Committee on Assessing Genetic Risks of the Institute of Medicine.[21]

Families are not monolithic. Some are in close contact; others are dispersed and out of touch. Some families have a warm, loving relationship; others are abusive and openly hostile. Some individuals would be extremely uncomfortable in disclosing personal genetic information even to first-degree relatives. In families where one member is affected and another one is unaffected, genetic information could severely strain relationships, perhaps even evoking "genetic resentment" in an affected individual or "survivor guilt" in an unaffected individual. No public policy therefore ought to require individuals to notify family members about genetic risks. The only realistic public policy is to provide individuals with sufficient genetic education and appropriate client-centered genetic counseling to enable them to make informed decisions about whether to share this information.

A similar set of issues pertains to whether health care providers have a duty to notify the relatives of their patients regarding genetic risks when the patient has refused to do so. According to the Committee on Assessing Genetic Risks: "The committee recommends that confidentiality be breached and relatives informed about genetic risks only when attempts to elicit voluntary disclosure fail, there is a high probability of irreversible or fatal harm to the relative, the disclosure of the information will prevent harm, the disclosure is limited to the information necessary for diagnosis or treatment of the relative, and there is no other reasonable way to avert the harm."[22] These instances are likely to be extremely rare.

Notwithstanding these guidelines, it is still possible that a lawsuit could be brought in which the plaintiff asserts a claim for failure to warn against a health care provider. For example, in a Florida case decided in 1995, a woman received medical treatment for medullary thyroid carcinoma, an autosomal dominant disorder, in 1987.[23] In 1990, the woman's adult daughter also was diagnosed with medullary thyroid carcinoma. The daughter later brought a medical malpractice action against her mother's physician, alleging that her mother's physician had a duty to warn her mother that medullary thyroid carcinoma was a genetic condition and that her children should be tested. According to the daughter's legal complaint, if she had been tested in 1987, her condition, more likely than not, would have been curable. The Florida Supreme Court held that under the state's medical malpractice statute, the mother's physician had a duty to inform the mother that her condition was genetic and that her children were at risk. Nevertheless, the court expressly stated that the physician had no duty to warn the patient's children.

The opposite result was reached in a New Jersey case in 1996.[24] The plaintiff's father was diagnosed with adenomatous polyposis coli, an autosomal dominant disorder, and died at age 45. Twenty-six years later, after the plaintiff, then age 36, was also diagnosed with adenomatous polyposis coli, she sued the estate of her father's physician. The lawsuit alleged that the physician's negligent failure to warn the daughter prevented her from undergoing prophylactic treatment. The trial court dismissed the action, but the appellate court reversed. In specifically refusing to follow the Florida case, the New Jersey court said that "the duty to warn of avertible risk from genetic causes, by definition a matter of familial concern, is sufficiently narrow to serve the interests of justice."[25]

Although the purpose of establishing a duty to warn relatives about genetic risks is to promote public health, it is also arguable that the absence of a duty to warn promotes public health. Preserving the confidentiality of genetic information may be seen as encouraging individuals to avail themselves of genetic services without fear that their genetic secrets will be disclosed. The proliferation of lawsuits alleging failure to warn about genetic risks could lead to legislative action either establishing specific statutory disclosure duties or immunities for health care providers who fail to disclose.

GENETIC INFORMATION AND HEALTH PROFESSIONALS

Several surveys have revealed that many clinical geneticists do not consider maintaining the confidentiality of genetic information to be a high priority.[26] These geneticists indicated a willingness to make disclosures to relatives over the objections of their patient, as well as to disclose the information to third parties (e.g., employers, insurers) even in the absence of consent by their patient. This lack of concern for confidentiality does not bode well for the future.

With fewer than 800 board-certified clinical geneticists in the United States, the vast majority of future genetic testing in the clinical setting will be performed in the offices of family practice physicians, internists, obstetricians and gynecologists, and pediatricians. If substantial numbers of clinical geneticists, who should be the most knowledgeable about the consequences of disclosure of genetic information, fail to make confidentiality a priority, then it is questionable whether nongeneticist physicians will be more vigilant. All health care providers must be cognizant of the psychosocial consequences of disclosing genetic information. In particular, health care providers must be diligent in obtaining informed consent for all tests, and they should tell patients in advance of providing any genetic services how the confidentiality of their genetic secrets will be protected.[27] The failure to preserve the confidentiality of genetic information is already considered unethical practice and may lead to a range of professional sanctions and legal liability.[28]

A related issue is the quality of genetic counseling services that will be provided in primary care settings. With only 1,200 master's-level trained members of the National Society of Genetic Counselors, responsibility for much of the future of genetic counseling is likely to be assigned to the nurses, physician assistants, or other nonphysicians working with primary care providers. Yet there are only 120 clinical nurse specialists in the International Society of Nurses in Genetics. Major new educational initiatives are needed to train primary care providers and their professional staffs about both the substantive issues in genetic testing and in the psychosocial issues of genetic counseling. An increased used of videotapes, computer-assisted learning programs, Internet, and other information sources will also be needed to supplement face-to-face counseling of patients.

Professional education programs for physicians and nurses must occur before or concurrently with the introduction of large-scale genetic testing in the clinical setting.[29] In the absence of professional and public education, misunderstanding of test results and inappropriate disclosures could cause a loss of confidence in the health care professions' ability to provide appropriate genetic services. One response could be for state legislatures and licensing agencies to restrict the ability to offer DNA-based genetic testing to medical professionals who have been certified to provide genetic services.

The confidentiality of genetic information is also likely to be affected by two trends in health care, managed care and computerization. With regard to managed care, increased utilization review means that more people, including administrators, will be reviewing medical records and patient information to decide whether to preapprove medical care and to determine whether medical services have been rendered appropriately. Entire charts, rather than simply billing information, may be shared with nonclinical personnel at remote sites. The sensitivity of genetic information dictates that these disclosures should be limited. Some specific proposals in this regard appear below.

Computerization also threatens medical record confidentiality.[30] Even before computerized medical records, hospital charts were subject to insufficient limitations on access. Greater restrictions on access, through passwords, encryption, or other means, are necessary to ensure that every hospital computer terminal is not an open portal to genetic and other sensitive information. Similarly, optical memory computer cards ("smart cards"), which can contain a patient's entire medical record since birth on what looks like a standard credit card, should not be introduced unless confidentiality concerns have been satisfactorily resolved.[31]

MEDICAL RESEARCH

Both publicly and privately funded genetic research raise important questions of privacy and confidentiality. Informed consent is often considered the starting point in evaluating research ethics. Under this doctrine, consent to participate in biomedical research must be competent, voluntary, and informed. In obtaining informed consent, researchers often overestimate the value of their assertions to research subjects that information disclosed in the research will be kept confidential. Even if information is not disclosed by the researchers, subjects may be asked by third parties whether they have ever participated in genetic research, and an inference may be drawn that if they participated in genetic research the individuals may be at risk of a genetic disorder.[32] The records of genetic research also may be deliberately or inadvertently placed in an individual's medical records, thereby raising many of the same issues as medical records generated in the clinical setting.

Informed consent has traditionally been regarded as an individual right, and this right is usually considered adequately protected if research data are not available in individually identifiable form. In the genetics context, as well as other medical contexts, even information that is not in individually identifiable form may be harmful to individuals and groups. Although the family members of a subject do not consent to research, information learned about one family member may have serious consequences for other members. Genetic research also may indicate the propensity of certain genetic traits to be expressed in particular ethnic or racial groups. Thus, the individual subject as well as other group members may be harmed by the accumulation of group data, such as the prevalence of a specific mutation in the breast cancer 1 (BRCA1) gene in Ashkenazic Jewish women.[33]

Informed consent for research, including anonymous research, should disclose the possibility of individual and group harms that result from the research. Among other things, investigators should disclose what steps have been and will be taken to preserve the confidentiality of research information and the situations (e.g., legal process) when the confidentiality of research information will not be protected.

A similar issue is raised with regard to the reanalysis of stored samples. Investigators have recognized that millions of samples of blood, tissue, and other specimens already are available for DNA analysis. These samples were probably collected for one purpose, such as clinical care or legally mandated newborn screening, and consent was given, if at all, only for that purpose. Subsequently, the researchers may seek to use the samples for another purpose without obtaining additional consent. If information will be used in individually identifiable form, express consent should be obtained. Even if the results of the research will not be disclosed in an individually identifiable form, institutional review board (IRB) procedures should be used to ensure that in any new research undertaken without obtaining additional consent the researchers have taken steps to eliminate or reduce the risks to subjects from group data.

It has been suggested that the use of certificates of confidentiality, issued pursuant to the Public Health Service Act,[34] is an effective way to preserve the confidentiality of research records.[35] Certificates of confidentiality prevent the compelled disclosure of research data pursuant to legal process. By regulation, these certificates are issued "sparingly,"[36] although in fiscal 1994, 258 certificates of confidentiality were granted by the assistant secretary for health and the Office of Protection from Research Risks of the National Institutes of Health.[37] The right to apply for the certificate belongs exclusively to the researchers; the subjects have no assurance that the researchers will exercise the right; and there is no private right of action. Thus, as currently authorized and used, certificates of confidentiality do not adequately protect subjects of research.

The use of genetic information during and as a consequence of commercial research raises additional concerns. Undoubtedly, one effect of commercialization is to increase demand for genetic testing, which can lead to greater threats to individual privacy and confidentiality.[38] In addition, during commercial research, detailed pedigree information may be shared by many laboratories, thereby raising issues of the confidentiality of the information.[39] Commercial research is not directly funded by the federal government, and therefore traditional IRB procedures are not required. Nevertheless, because commercial genome research is often undertaken in collaboration with government-funded researchers, it may be subject to IRB review. Additional protections for research subjects may be needed, either through the professional licensure process or through new legislation mandating more stringent IRB procedures in the public and private sectors.

MEDICAL RECORDS

Protecting the security of medical records in the hospital setting is essential in the age of computers. As mentioned earlier in this chapter, restrictions on remote access to medical records, such as from physicians' offices and from multiple locations within a hospital, can be controlled through password entry, encryption of sensitive data, and "electronic audit trails," which record all computer entries to medical files.[40] In addition to increased security measures, unauthorized access to medical records as well as the sale of medical records in any setting should be prohibited by law.

Perhaps the most difficult problem in medical record confidentiality arises from billing records. Numerous public and private payers need specific medical information about the health care received by specific individuals. In general, however, they do not need individual identifiers. Each individual in a government program, managed care organization, employee benefits program, or other health plan should be assigned a separate medical record number. This should not be the individual's Social Security number, which is widely used in numerous contexts and is easily obtained by third parties. All billing to third-party payers, including self-insured employers, should include only the number of the patient treated. A conversion table (or encryption access) with the names and numbers should be accessible only to approved personnel and only on a need-to-know basis, such as to correct erroneous records. Computer programs can be developed to provide such protection, and their use should be statutorily mandated.[41]

As discussed below, the Health Insurance Portability and Accountability Act of 1996 provides some modest measures for preventing genetic discrimination in health insurance. Significantly, the law serves as the first federal regulation of both self-insured employee welfare plans under ERISA and of commercial health insurers. Therefore, it is well suited for a provision to protect the confidentiality of billing records processed by group health insurers. The law could be amended to provide that all billing records submitted pursuant to self-insured and commercially insured plans must be submitted in a coded format. At the least, Congress could mandate the use of pilot programs to test the efficacy of such systems.

INSURANCE

Concerns about insurance—especially health insurance—dominate any discussion about the possible adverse consequences of disclosure of genetic information. It is extremely difficult to achieve meaningful protection for medical, including genetic, privacy and confidentiality without restructuring the current U.S. health care system. There are, however, a number of measures, some modest and others more sweeping, that will strengthen protections for genetic secrets within the confines of our largely private, voluntary health insurance system.

Insurance is a mechanism for the pooling of resources against unknown risks. To the extent that the health claims of individuals become predictable or are believed to be predictable, then the entire concept of insurance must be reconsidered. Medical underwriting in health insurance is sometimes cast as a struggle between actuarial fairness (treating similar risks in a similar way) and moral fairness (safeguarding equal access to the essential good of health care).[42] With regard to genetic information, framing the debate in such a manner may give "actuarial fairness" more credit than it deserves. There is little evidence that the state of the art in genetics is sufficiently developed or that medical directors of insurance companies have the expertise in genetics to base medical underwriting on predictive genetic information. For example, among the results of a 1992 questionnaire survey of the medical directors of life insurance companies, "more than one in four indicated that they believed that genes are composed of chromosomes rather than the other way around, and . . . [o]nly half knew that DNA is composed of four nucleotides."[43] Thus, even if no changes were made to current laws that permit the acquisition and use of genetic information, it is still essential that the information be used correctly.

There are several possible ways of improving the level of genetic knowledge among the medical directors of insurance companies. The simplest way would be for the medical directors and their organization, the American Academy of Insurance Medicine, to sponsor a series of educational programs on the actuarial significance of new genetic discoveries. One problem, of course, is that there is often inadequate information from which to assess the actuarial significance of genetic discoveries, although merely reaffirming this notion may be an important achievement in itself. More likely, it will be necessary for regulatory or statutory intervention to ensure that genetic medical underwriting is based on good science.

One way to institutionalize the review of genetic developments for the insurance industry would be to establish a panel comprising members from the American Academy of Insurance Medicine, American Academy of Actuaries, American College of Medical Genetics, National Association of Insurance Commissioners, consumer representatives, epidemiologists, and other interested parties to evaluate the predictive significance of genetic information. The panel would determine, among other things, which carrier states are benign and should not be the basis of underwriting, which disorders have such variable penetrance or expressivity that prediction is too speculative, which genetic disorders are treatable, and what effect health status has on the cost of care. With current and sound data, the policy debate on whether genetic information ought to be used and, if so, how, at least can be better informed. Even without more fundamental reforms, consumers will be less subject to erroneous or irrational discrimination in insurance.

A second relatively modest reform would be to enact legislation prohibiting the redisclosure or sale to third parties of information submitted for medical underwriting. At present, it is unclear how medical underwriting information may be used. Individuals are forced to take at face value the claims by the Medical Information Bureau and insurance companies that medical information is not made available to third parties or put to unapproved uses.[44] With sensitive genetic information being added to medical files, legislation should expressly prohibit insurance companies and their agents from using information beyond its stated and immediate purpose.

Some people fear that insurance companies will begin wholesale discrimination against individuals based on their genotypes. If insurance companies adopt the practice of using substantial amounts of genetic information in underwriting, however, they are more likely to do so as a defensive matter. The issue of adverse selection, in which individuals at risk are more likely to seek insurance, has been addressed widely.[45] Another way that insurers could be "forced" to use genetic information is as follows: Suppose Insurance Company A begins offering a "good gene" discount of 50% on its individual health, disability, or life insurance policies to any applicant who voluntarily takes 10 selected genetic tests and is found not to carry any of the specific mutations. Low-risk individuals will flock to Company A for the discount. Company B will lose some of its low-risk insureds. It would then either have to raise its rates to reflect the greater risk of its pool of policyholders or also use genetic tests (perhaps requiring the tests, instead of making them optional as Company A did) to further limit its risk. The actions of Companies A and B will put pressure on Company C, and the other companies, with the result that even reluctant companies will have no choice but to use genetic information. This is what actuaries generally refer to as an "assessment spiral."

To prevent this from occurring, legislation should be enacted to prohibit insurance companies from using genetic information to sell any insurance product *below* standard rates. At present, some insurers permit at-risk individuals (such as an individual known to be at risk of Huntington disease) to obtain coverage by submitting genetic test data showing that the individual did not inherit the mutation. These practices would still be permitted under the proposed legislation, because the policy will not be written at substandard rates.

Some existing laws would have to be amended. For example, an Ohio law enacted in 1993 prohibits insurers from requiring genetic testing or using genetic information to "make a decision adverse to the applicant."[46] It also provides that "an insurer may consider the results of genetic screening or testing if the results are voluntarily submitted by an applicant for coverage and the results are favorable to the applicant."[47] The law fails to address the issue of substandard rates and therefore would not prevent an assessment spiral.

The Ohio statute is typical of the laws enacted in 16 states, largely between 1991 and 1997, which attempt to prohibit genetic discrimination in health insurance.[48] Although these laws have been praised and additional legislation has been advocated,[49] these laws in fact afford little protection against the adverse use of genetic information in health insurance. To begin with, the laws prohibit the use of genetic test information, and the definition of a genetic test is often narrow. For example, the Colorado law, enacted in 1994, defines "genetic testing" as "any laboratory test of human DNA, RNA, or chromosomes that is used to identify the presence or absence of alterations in genetic material which are associated with disease or illness . . . [and] includes only such tests as are direct measures of such alterations rather than indirect manifestations thereof."[50]

The first problem with Colorado's law, as with most other state laws, is that it does not prohibit the use of genetic information derived from family histories or other similar sources. As Deborah Stone has written, "The problem with all these proposals is that genetic information is too deeply embedded in the structure of general medical underwriting to be effectively regulated separately."[51] Even in states that prohibit the use of genetic information derived from family histories, insurers would have an incentive to use other, less precise measures of future genetic risks.

During the early years of the HIV epidemic, some health insurers attempted to require HIV testing as a precondition of insurance. When this was prohibited by state insurance laws, some insurers used T-cell counts; when this was prohibited, some used sexual orientation; when this was prohibited, some used zip code or occupation as surrogates for identifying supposedly at-risk, gay male applicants.[52] There is a legitimate concern that similar, surrogate measures for genetic traits could be adopted by one or more insurers if genetic testing were prohibited. For example, nonspecific diagnostic criteria could be used to predict the onset of a genetic disorder. Less likely, but more troubling, an insurer might refuse to insure members of a certain ethnic group because the group has a higher prevalence of a particular genetic disorder, regardless of legal prohibitions on such conduct.

The second problem with current state antidiscrimination laws is their lack of coverage. About half of the nonelderly insured population in the United States receives its health insurance coverage through a self-insured employer plan. Most large companies in the United States are self-insured. The federal Employee Retirement Income Security Act preempts state insurance laws from regulating ERISA-qualified plans.[53] Thus, state insurance laws fail to reach most of the individuals covered by plans sponsored by the nation's largest companies.

The third problem with the approach of these state laws is the most serious. The laws only prohibit the refusal to insure individuals who are asymptomatic. The laws do not prohibit insurers from refusing to insure individuals who are symptomatic with a genetic disorder, nor do they prohibit insurers from canceling the policy or raising the rates significantly of an individual once the individual becomes symptomatic. For example, under a typical state law, an individual with a mutation of the BRCA1 gene cannot be denied coverage until the individual begins to have symptoms of breast cancer, but then the insurer may lawfully decide not to renew the policy or may increase the rates to levels where the individual may not be able to afford to continue the policy. Thus, the individual will not have health insurance at the precise time and for the precise condition that she needs it the most.[54]

Despite serious drawbacks, these state laws still have some value. Some individuals with a genetically increased risk of cancer or other health problems will never get the condition for which they were at increased risk. These individuals will have coverage for all of their other illnesses. Even individuals who develop the condition for which they were at increased risk (and are eventually dropped from coverage) will be insured for their other illnesses in the interim.

For advocacy groups that succeed in obtaining enactment of these types of state laws, however, exultation should not be the order of the day. At best, this genre of state insurance reform should be viewed as "fallback" or "default" legislation. The laws can be improved, such as by more broadly defining genetic information and prohibiting discrimination based on other surrogate measures, but so long as they permit the cancellation of coverage after illness or rate increases that have the same effect, they will have limited utility. Of equal concern is that policy makers and legislatures will regard this type of legislation as adequate to resolve the problem.

The federal Health Insurance Portability and Accountability Act of 1996 provides some protection against discrimination based on genetic factors.[55] The law permits group health plans and group health insurers to exclude from coverage for only a limited time a covered individual's preexisting health conditions. Because "genetic information" is not a preexisting condition, there can be no exclusion at all based on genetic predisposition. Also, genetic information may not be used to limit coverage or benefits. Thus, genetic information may not be used to deny coverage or limit the portability of health benefits to individuals changing employment.

As widely noted, the new law does not address many of the pressing needs for health care reform. It does not require employers to offer health benefits, and it does not prohibit an employer from dropping or limiting coverage. It does not deal with individuals who are uninsured nor with those who have individual health insurance policies. It does not limit the rates that commercial insurers may charge employer groups based on their claims experience. Although the law guarantees a right of access to health insurance for individuals converting from group to individual coverage, it does not guarantee that premiums will not be at levels where insurance is no longer affordable.

Finally, the "administrative simplification" provisions of the new law, designed to lower costs and improve delivery through electronic data interchange, raise serious threats to individual privacy and confidentiality. By mandating the creation of a unique health identifier for every patient, vast databases of individually identifiable health records will be connected. Rather than confronting the substantial privacy issues before enacting the legislation, Congress simply delegated to the secretary of Health and Human Services the task of resolving the issues.

Having demonstrated the ineffectiveness of the current reforms (both enacted and proposed), I return to the dilemma raised at the beginning of this chapter. Is it possible to enact effective health insurance reform without totally dismantling the current system? The problems are easier to list than they are to solve. They involve the following five interrelated challenges: (1) the current health insurance system is largely a for-profit business and not a social entitlement and therefore the premium structure must be adequate for the expected claims; (2) the only way that high-cost or high-risk individuals can participate in the system is if their premium contributions are subsidized by low-cost or low-risk individuals; (3) because the system is voluntary, community rating or other forms of risk spreading will raise the rates for low-risk individuals, such as younger, healthier individuals, and encourage them to opt out of the system, creating an assessment spiral of rising rates and declining numbers of enrollees, a problem that threatens the individual and small group market; (4) increasing employer mandates within the structure of a voluntary group insurance system will cause more employers to drop health insurance coverage altogether, thereby putting increased pressure on the public health insurance system; and (5) using the government as insurer of last resort could help save the rate structure of the private market, but it would require substantial new revenues, it also might cause individuals and groups to drop their coverage and opt for the public system, thereby requiring additional public revenues, and it has the potential to create a two-tiered health system in which individuals with genetic conditions and other health problems will be in the least desirable tier.

Regrettably, it is not possible to fix the problem of genetic discrimination in insurance without addressing the broader issue of health care financing. Devising an effective strategy is ultimately a matter of determining what reforms are politically feasible. Any proposal must deal with the five problems noted above and must move toward some combination of mandatory participation by low-risk individuals and increased governmental participation or subsidies. Once the basic structure is in place, the role of genetic information is easier to discern. In my view, no medical information regarding preexisting conditions or predispositions should be used to deny coverage for a basic health insurance package (however defined), but that for premium coverage (however defined) an insurer should be free to consider any actuarially sound medical data, so long as the information is kept confidential and not redisclosed. The basic health insurance package must provide coverage for all reasonable and necessary medical services.

I have previously suggested this same basic approach to life insurance.[56] Unlike health insurance, life insurance is generally not regarded as a necessity. Nevertheless, the use of genetic information in life insurance underwriting implicates important issues of privacy, confidentiality, and fairness. To protect these interests while not creating irresistible pressure for adverse selection, all individuals should be permitted to purchase life insurance up to a specified amount using standard mortality tables but without using any predictive medical underwriting. The amount could be a specific dollar amount or a percentage of the individual's income. To prevent individuals from applying for coverage at the end of life, insurers should be permitted to require a relatively long waiting period (e.g., one year from application) until the policy is in force for nonaccidental death. In the United States, small life insurance policies already are sold without medical underwriting. Thus it is merely a matter of determining what level of coverage strikes a fair balance between affording a decent level of income replacement without undermining the rate structure of insurance.

In the Netherlands, a five-year moratorium trial period, in which no genetic information may be used in underwriting policies below 200,000 guilders (about $100,000), has been extended indefinitely while proposed legislation is debated in Parliament.[57] Any limit should apply to the total of all life insurance policies to prevent an individual from "stacking" a series of small policies. No doubt the insurance industry easily could determine the total amount of an individual's life insurance policies in force. For policies in excess of the cutoff limit, insurers should be permitted to engage in any form of medical underwriting, so long as it is actuarially based and the information is kept confidential and not redisclosed.

The issues surrounding disability insurance are similar to those involved in life insurance, where the principal concern is balancing the risk of adverse selection against the desire to make available an important but not essential insurance product on an equitable basis. Long-term insurance is another area that may be of increasing importance, because of the impending retirement of the "baby boomers" and expected cutbacks in Medicaid's contribution to nursing home expenses. Widespread genetic testing for predisposition to Alzheimer's disease, although scientifically unwarranted at present, must be viewed as a growing social threat.[58] In terms of political response to this threat, I would consider the issue to be governed by the principles discussed for health insurance, where no predictive testing for a basic package of care should be permitted.

EMPLOYMENT

New genetic discoveries may be used in assessing whether individuals are at risk of developing occupational diseases and, through the use of biomarkers, predicting the course of future occupational illness.[59] The paramount concern with genetic discrimination in employment, however, is that employers will use genetic predictions of future illness to exclude from the work force individuals who are thought to be at risk of nonoccupational illness, thereby eliminating individuals who are perceived as likely to increase the employer's health benefits costs.

There is no question that health care costs will continue to affect employee selection and retention decisions. In any given year, the top 5% of health care claimants use 50% of health care resources, and the top 10% use 75% of resources. For employers, average annual health care costs in 1996 were about $4,000 per employee; they were over $6,000 at companies with the most generous benefits. Although the shift to managed care in the mid-1990s halted the double-digit annual growth in employer costs, most analysts believe that the pause in cost increases is temporary. Employers therefore will continue to have tremendous incentives to take steps to exclude from the workforce and benefits rolls employees and their dependents who are believed to be high-cost consumers of health care dollars.

Although legal measures to prohibit discrimination based on presumed health care utilization already exist and could be strengthened, it is questionable whether traditional antidiscrimination laws will be effective. After all, since the mid-1960s there have been laws enacted prohibiting discrimination based on race, color, religion, sex, national origin, and age. Nobody would seriously contend that discrimination on the basis of these factors has been eliminated, and discrimination on the basis of these criteria do not have the actual or perceived economic incentives that discrimination on the basis of future health status do. Effective legislation therefore must prevent employers from gaining access to the medical information from which such future health projections can be made.

For the near term, employers are unlikely to perform their own genetic tests because they are too expensive and there is no reason for them to do so. So long as it is lawful for employers to require individuals to sign a release authorizing the disclosure of their medical records, employers will have access to vast amounts of genetic information and at-risk individuals will be discouraged from having genetic testing.

The primary legislative response to the problem of genetic discrimination in employment has paralleled the response to the problem of genetic discrimination in health insurance. Twelve states have enacted laws specifically prohibiting genetic discrimination in employment. As with state health insurance discrimination laws, state employment discrimination laws are woefully inadequate. Their first problem is how they define their protection. Three of the 12 states enacted their laws in the 1970s and apply only to sickle-cell trait, where the concern is that employers will erroneously consider the individuals to be ill or at risk of illness. Even in states with broader definitions, except in New Jersey, the laws do not extend to information obtained from medical records or family histories (as opposed to DNA-based tests), and no state law affords adequate protection against employer access to sensitive genetic information.[60]

As previously discussed, the most promising avenue for protecting genetic privacy in employment is through the general laws prohibiting discrimination in employment on the basis of disability. As of 1997, no cases have yet been decided under either the ADA or its state law analogs involving alleged discrimination against an asymptomatic individual based on genotype.[61] Even the much-heralded interpretation of the ADA by the Equal Employment Opportunity Commission (EEOC) in 1995, that when individuals are subject to discrimination because they are predisposed to genetic disorders they are "regarded as" individuals with disabilities,[62] fails to afford adequate protection. The current interpretation does not necessarily apply to the unaffected carriers of recessive or X-linked disorders. Employers may also require, as a condition of employment, that individuals release all their medical records to the employer and consent to *any* medical tests.

The ADA can serve as an example of how to structure a general statute to protect against third parties unnecessarily obtaining access to and discriminatorily using genetic information. Although as a political matter amending the ADA may not be possible at present, the same basic approach can be used in amending state laws that prohibit discrimination in employment based on disability. In the pages that follow, I set out two proposed amendments to the ADA as well as other suggested reforms. Although they are designed to prohibit genetic discrimination in employment, to avoid the definitional problems previously noted, none of the amendments uses the word *genetic*. The amendments prohibit discrimination in employment based on future health risks and prohibit employers from gaining access to non-job-related medical information.

The major concern regarding genetic discrimination in employment is that employers might exclude currently capable individuals because of a belief that the individuals will be unable to work in the future or may cause increased health insurance costs. This concern is addressed directly by amending the definitional section of the ADA, section 3(2), as follows:

(2) DISABILITY.—The term "disability" means, with respect to an individual—
(A) a physical or mental impairment that substantially limits one or more of the major life activities of such individual;
(B) a record of such an impairment;
(C) being regarded as having such an impairment; *or*
(D) having a risk of a future physical or mental impairment that would substantially limit one or more of the major life activities of such individual, having a record of such a risk, or being regarded as having such a risk.

Either by statute or regulation, the ADA also should include within the definition of "disability" the carrier state for recessive and X-linked disorders that, if manifested, would substantially limit one or more of the major life activities of an individual.

The other proposed amendment prohibits employers from gaining access to an employee's medical records containing non-job-related genetic information (by requiring the signing of a general release of medical records) as well as performing their own genetic tests. The proposal would amend the relevant section of the ADA, section 102(d)(3), which prescribes the conditions under which medical examinations may be performed after a conditional offer of employment.

(3) EMPLOYMENT ENTRANCE EXAMINATION.—A covered entity may require a medical examination after an offer of employment has been made to a job applicant and prior to the commencement of the employment duties of such applicant, and may condition an offer of employment on the results of such examination, if—
(A) all entering employees are subject to such an examination regardless of disability;
(B) information obtained regarding the medical condition or history of the applicant is collected and maintained on separate forms and in separate medical files and is treated as a confidential medical record . . . ;

(C) the results of such examination are used only in accordance with this title; *and (D) a covered entity shall not require a medical examination, shall not undertake a review of medical records, and shall not make inquiries of an applicant as to whether such applicant is an individual with a disability or as to the nature or severity of the disability, unless such examination, medical records review, or inquiry is shown to be job-related and consistent with business necessity.*

Under the ADA, preemployment medical inquiries of applicants are prohibited altogether, and postemployment inquiries of current employees must be either voluntary or job-related and consistent with business necessity. By requiring that post-offer examinations and inquiries of conditional offerees also have to be job-related and consistent with business necessity, employers will not be permitted to perform their own genetic tests nor will they be able to mandate that individuals sign blanket releases of personal medical records.

Most of the current proposals to prohibit genetic discrimination in employment merely prohibit employer use of genetic information. Those that also attempt to prohibit employers from gaining access to genetic information still permit access to all nongenetic medical information through comprehensive post-offer medical examinations or general releases. If genetic information is defined too narrowly (e.g., DNA-based test results), then the employer can still get access to much genetic information. If it is defined too broadly (e.g., including health information from relatives and that related to any illness with a genetic component), then employers will be precluded from access to essential medical information indicating whether the individual will be able to perform the job safely.

A better way of structuring the law is to prohibit employers from access to all non-job-related medical information while permitting access to all job-related information. It is not necessary to focus on "genetic information" at all. Such a strategy already has been effective in Minnesota since 1983. This approach eliminates the problem of defining "genetic" and does not single out any condition for special treatment. It also leaves open the possibility that, in the future, employers might be able to get access to job-related genetic information if the employer could show that such information were medically recognized as valid; it was essential to prevent the risk of a possible imminent, serious, threat to public safety; and there was no other way to avert the risk.

The ADA does not change the common law rule that no patient-physician relationship exists in the occupational setting. In the absence of this relationship, individuals subjected to workplace medical examinations lack the right to receive information about the nature of the test being performed and the uses to which the information may be put. As I have previously urged, as an "Examinee's Bill of Rights," each individual subjected to a medical examination at his or her employer's direction should have a right to: (1) be told the purpose and scope of the examination; (2) be told for whom the physician works; (3) provide informed consent for all procedures; (4) be told how examination results will be conveyed to management; (5) be told about confidentiality protections; (6) be told how to obtain access to medical information in the employee's file; and (7) be referred for medical follow-up if necessary.[63] These modest suggestions are already standard practices at some progressive companies.

The final area of the employment relationship that needs reform involves the employer's role in health insurance. I have suggested earlier in this chapter that all health insurance claims information should be submitted by number rather than in a personally identifiable form. This measure would help to preserve the medical confidentiality of individuals working for both self-insured and commercially insured companies. The ADA provides that medical information may not be stored in personnel files. The law also should provide that health insurance claims information may not be stored in personnel files.

COURTS

Genetic information has the potential to be of increasing significance in three types of legal matters: criminal law, personal injury litigation, and domestic relations. As the use of genetic information in court becomes more widespread, there is a growing risk that genetic privacy and confidentiality may be compromised. Although the range of cases in which genetic information may be sought to be introduced varies tremendously, there is one common element. In an adversarial system, lawyers are the advocates of their clients. They are retained to urge any plausible theories that advance the interests of their clients. Courts will inevitably be besieged with requests to introduce genetic evidence well before the scientific community would support the theories, associations, or conclusions that are urged in court. The legal system must be careful not to give inappropriate weight to genetic explanations of behavior and genetic predictions of future health.

Criminal Law

As noted by Franklin Zweig, Joseph Walsh, and Daniel Freeman, genetic information may be used in criminal cases on three likely occasions.[64] First, at trial, a defendant might seek to introduce evidence of a genetic defect in an attempt to prove that he or she lacked the mental capacity to commit the crime. Although the jurisdictions vary on the substantive law applied to the issue of insanity or diminished capacity, biological explanations, such as organic brain syndrome, have long been considered to be relevant and admissible evidence by criminal courts. The practical concern is that juries might be persuaded that genes are destiny and therefore that they might give undue weight to genetic exculpatory evidence.

The second possible use of genetic information is at the sentencing stage. Having failed to convince the jury that a genetic predisposition precludes a finding of guilt, the defendant might seek to introduce the same or similar evidence as a mitigating factor in the penalty phase of the trial. If genetic factors could explain (even though not excusing) the defendant's behavior, this might result in a lesser sentence.

The third possible use of genetic information in criminal justice is at a parole hearing. Unlike the prior two examples, in which the defendant would seek to introduce the genetic evidence, at the parole hearing the government might attempt to show that a genetic predisposition to violence or other antisocial behavior makes the individual likely to be a recidivist who should not be granted parole. Any attempt to use biological information to deny an individual liberty would raise serious issues of constitutional law.

In the 1942 case of Skinner v. Oklahoma, the Supreme Court struck down an Oklahoma law that authorized the sterilization of a "habitual criminal," defined as someone convicted two or more times of a crime of moral turpitude.[65] The majority based its decision on equal protection, because some crimes, such as larceny, could lead to sterilization, but other similar crimes, such as embezzlement, could not. Chief Justice Harlan Fiske Stone's concurring opinion asserted that the statute violated due process because it did not provide for an individual hearing to determine whether the offender had inherited criminal tendencies. Justice Robert H. Jackson's concurring opinion raised an even broader issue, and one certain to be raised if eligibility for parole were to be affected by genotype.

> I also think the present plan to sterilize the individual in pursuit of a eugenic plan to eliminate from the race characteristics that are only vaguely identified and which in our present state of knowledge are uncertain as to transmissibility presents other constitutional questions of gravity. . . . There are limits to the extent to which a legislatively represented majority may conduct biological experiments at the expense

of the dignity and personality of a minority—even those who have been found guilty of what the majority define as crimes.[66]

More recently, Kansas v. Hendricks involved a pedophile convicted five times of molesting at least 10 children over a period of 40 years.[67] In 1994, after Hendricks had served nearly 10 years in prison for his most recent crime, Kansas sought to have him civilly committed to a mental institution for an indeterminate period under its Sexually Violent Predator Act, which it had enacted only months earlier. Although the Kansas Supreme Court held that the statute violated due process, the U.S. Supreme Court reversed and upheld the law by a vote of five to four. According to Justice Clarence Thomas's majority opinion, the law did not violate either the double jeopardy or the ex post facto clauses of the Constitution.

It is hard to have sympathy for Hendricks, and the state has a substantial interest in keeping him off the streets, but the method chosen by the state raises serious concerns. Rather than impose longer sentences for the crime of child molestation, and after making no effort to treat Hendricks during his confinement, the state sought to commit him indefinitely because of its admittedly well-founded fear that he might commit another crime. This approach, however, is perilous because it merges incarceration for crimes with civil commitment. The latter procedure is supposed to be used only for individuals whose severe mental illness creates a serious danger to themselves or others, and it was conceded by the state that Hendricks did not meet this definition. Under a law similar to the one upheld in this case, what is to prevent the civil commitment of individuals based on behavioral genetic profiles that suggest they would be or might be dangerous to society?

The introduction of genetic information into the criminal justice system may demand a reassessment of society's view of individuals as responsible agents.[68] The effects on the criminal law of new genetic discoveries could be similar to the changes caused by advances in our understanding of psychiatry, which necessitated a new paradigm for dealing with insanity.

Personal Injury Litigation

Each year nearly one million personal injury lawsuits are filed in the federal and state courts of the United States. The cases are based on, among other things, products liability, premises liability, vehicular accidents, and medical malpractice. In a substantial but unknown number of these cases the plaintiffs seek damages for permanent injury. In assessing these damages, the courts and juries make an initial determination of the individual's life expectancy and work-life expectancy. Traditionally, this calculation is based on standard mortality tables, but specific evidence of the plaintiff's health is admissible. Thus, if a defendant were able to prove that the plaintiff's preinjury life expectancy was shorter than the mortality tables provide, the defendant could save thousands or millions of dollars in damages. Defendants in personal injury cases therefore have a tremendous economic incentive to obtain and introduce in court evidence of a plaintiff's reduced life expectancy. The results of genetic tests, both those performed in the clinical setting and obtained through the lawsuit discovery process and those conducted pursuant to a court order, could become standard sources of predictive medical information.

Although there are, as yet, few reported incidents in which defendants have sought to compel genetic testing of plaintiffs in personal injury actions, and although none of these tests have been sought solely to estimate damages, there is some evidence that courts would permit such examinations. For example, in a lawsuit brought in state court in Minnesota in 1996, the plaintiff attempted to recover for injuries sustained in a two-car auto accident. After obtaining the plaintiff's medical records through discovery, the defendant suspected that the plaintiff might have Huntington disease and requested a court order requiring the plaintiff to submit to DNA tests and a neurological examination. Over the objection of the plaintiff (who had not been tested before and did not want to know the results), the court ordered the DNA testing. The defendant was attempting to prove that the accident was not caused by the fault of the defendant but by the effect of Huntington disease on the plaintiff's driving ability.[69]

I have written in some detail about the threat to genetic privacy and confidentiality posed by defendants seeking to discover the genetic profiles of plaintiffs in personal injury cases that do not otherwise concern genetics.[70] The simplest way to prevent defendants from embarking on "genetic fishing expeditions" is to have the trial judge issue a protective order to limit the discovery of genetic information and bar physical examinations. Because of the problem of defining what is "genetic," a problem identified in this chapter on more than one occasion, it may be difficult to isolate some genetic information, such as family histories, in a routinely discoverable, general medical record. Nevertheless, if all the medical information were subject to confidentiality protections, DNA-based test results were not discoverable, and predictive genetic information (broadly defined) were inadmissible, then genetic privacy and confidentiality would be greatly enhanced.

There are at least two other possible approaches to limit access to and use of genetic information in personal injury litigation. First, a specific statute could be enacted to limit the discoverability and admissibility of predictive medical and genetic information. Second, the jurisdictions could adopt a variable period payment of damages statute. In effect, if damages were due in installments for as long as the plaintiff lives, it would be unnecessary to predict life expectancy. Predictive genetic information would thus be irrelevant.

Under any of these approaches, to protect the rights of defendants, plaintiffs should be prohibited from introducing evidence of their genetic predisposition to longevity. It is important to remember that without a consideration of genetic information in any cases, in the aggregate all defendants will be liable to all plaintiffs for the appropriate amount of damages based on standard mortality tables. The fairness to individual defendants of using presumably more accurate predictions of life expectancy in individual cases is offset by a variety of public policy considerations. These include not requiring plaintiffs and their families to learn genetic information that they do not want to know, not compromising individual privacy and confidentiality in the litigation process, and not wasting scarce genetic resources in litigation.

Domestic Relations

The use of genetic information in domestic relations substantially predates recent advances in genetics. Domestic relations law, as well as the law of estates and other areas, has long used a genetic or biological orientation for determining legal rights. But now genetic information is being used to predict future health, not merely to determine parentage.

In the context of child custody, a key issue is whether one parent's genetic predisposition to illness (including an untreatable disease) justifies giving custody of a child to the other parent. Parents determined to obtain custody have already petitioned courts to order genetic testing of the other parent to detect genetic risk factors. This argument raises the broader issue of when the current or future disability of a parent may be used as the basis of a child custody decision.

In the leading case of In re Carney, a mother challenged the initial award of custody of her two sons to her ex-husband after five years when an accident caused the father to become quadriplegic.[71] The trial court granted the mother's custody petition even though the mother had not seen her sons for five years because the father was presumed not to be able to maintain a normal relationship with his sons. In reversing this decision, the Supreme Court of California set out various factors for determining custody and stated that the "essence [of parenting] lies in the ethical, emotional, and intellectual guidance the parent gives to the child throughout the formative years and often beyond."[72]

The rationale of Carney, that a current or future physical disability should not necessarily be a determinative factor in custody decisions, should be used to prevent an ex-spouse from having to undergo genetic testing in a child custody case. The Carney court leaves unresolved the issue of mental disabilities, which would certainly be raised in a case involving Huntington disease or Alzheimer's disease. More generally, Carney stands for the proposition that custody decisions must consider a variety of factors and that when one of the parents has a current disability the court should consider, among other things, the age of the child, the nature of the parent's disability, and the effect of the disability on the parent's ability to care for the child.

Carney's reluctance to exclude from parental rights individuals with current (or future) disabilities should also be applied in evaluating whether individuals are fit to adopt a child. The possibility of prospective parents being subject to genetic testing to assess whether they have any alleles for aberrant mental or behavioral disorders, as well as alleles for debilitating physical illness, is disconcerting in light of the number of children waiting in foster care for permanent adoption.

A more difficult issue, as noted by Lori Andrews, involves whether it is permissible to test a child being placed for adoption.[73] In general, genetic testing of any child for adult-onset disorders is considered inappropriate because it impinges on the child's autonomy to decide whether to be tested on reaching maturity.[74] In contrast, genetic testing of children for childhood-onset genetic disorders is valuable because it permits parents, including adopting parents, to anticipate the health needs of their child and, in some instances, to take steps to reduce or ameliorate the effects of the disorder.

It has been asserted that the law should facilitate adopting parents to learn the adopted child's "health and genetic history."[75] I agree with the statement only in its narrowest sense. In my view, the timing is crucial. Genetic information should not be disclosed before adoption, and genetic testing of adoptive children should not take place until *after* the adoption.

The danger with preadoption genetic testing of asymptomatic children, even for childhood-onset genetic disorders, is that it can lead to treating children as if they were commodities. What chance for adoption does a child have after he or she tests positive for a severe or even a moderate genetic disorder? When parents "contract" with an adoption agency to adopt a "healthy child" and the child develops severe disabilities that were known (or perhaps only knowable) to the adoption agency but not disclosed to the adoptive parents, the parents have a legal right to rescind the contract and return the child.[76] Curiously, this is the same legal right afforded to any buyer or acquirer of defective merchandise.

It could be argued that adoption would be encouraged by medical and genetic testing that would provide adopting parents with a degree of assurance of the current and future health of the child. An argument also could be made that a couple seeking to adopt a child because they already had a child die in infancy or early childhood from a genetic disorder should be spared the emotional trauma of another tragedy by being allowed to adopt a child who had been tested and found not to have the gene mutation for a genetic disorder. Similar reasoning would apply where parents would be unable to care for an additional child with a severe disability. The issue of medical care for an adopted child could be resolved by amending the Federal Adoption Act to provide health care and related social services for all adopted children.

There are no guarantees when one becomes a parent, and once a state permits genetic testing to "certify" that a child is free of genetic disease, it will be extremely difficult to limit the scope of the genetic testing. Without question, adoptive parents should be informed before adoption if a child has a known severe illness, but predictive genetic screening seems imprudent. Inasmuch as adoption practices are regulated at the state level, the states should enact legislation limiting public and private adoption agencies from performing preadoption genetic testing. Without uniform state laws, couples desiring preadoption genetic information will be encouraged to adopt children in states where genetic testing is permitted. In addition, without laws limiting the ability of adopting parents to return the child shortly after adoption, adopting parents will simply perform their own genetic testing of the child.

FORENSICS

DNA-based technologies are powerful tools in forensics. Each year in the United States, more than 200,000 DNA tests are performed to determine paternity. DNA tests also have been used to determine heirship, sometimes even posthumously. In two areas, however, the use of DNA testing has been controversial. They are the use of DNA tests to identify remains and the use of DNA techniques in criminal investigations.

Although DNA tests have been used to identify the remains of airplane crash victims and other individuals killed in mass disasters, the military's use of DNA banks has received widespread publicity. In June 1992 the U.S. Department of Defense began collecting blood and buccal tissue samples of its 1.5 million active duty members. By 1996 nearly 1.5 million samples had been collected and stored at the Armed Forces Institute of Pathology in Gaithersburg, Maryland. The purpose of the program is to facilitate identification of the remains of war causalities, and DNA techniques were used for identification in the Gulf War.

In 1996, two marines, Lance Corporal John Mayfield III and Corporal Joseph Vlacovsky, were court-martialed when they independently refused to submit samples. They said they were "deeply uncomfortable about how the information might be used."[77] In particular, the marines were concerned that the genetic information might be used to discriminate against them in employment and insurance. Although the judge held that they had disobeyed an order, he merely ordered a reprimand placed in the marines' personnel files and confined them to base for a week. They were not required to give their samples.

Although the sole avowed purpose of the repository is to identify remains, Department of Defense regulations permit samples to be used by a donor or surviving next of kin, by judicial order, or for investigation of a crime punishable by a year or more in confinement. All samples are retained for 50 years, but according to amended regulations issued in 1996, a sample will be destroyed at the request of the donor when he or she leaves the military.

The controversy surrounding the military's use of DNA banks illustrates the interrelatedness of genetic privacy issues. The marines were not concerned about the taking of the samples per se but about the possible ways the genetic information could be used. In another case, Air Force Sergeant Warren J. Sinclair, an African American, also refused to provide a sample. "How do I know that someone won't get ahold of that information and use it to deny me a promotion or assign me to a job I don't want? You know, racism is still alive in this country."[78]

In implementing its DNA testing program, the military failed to recognize the depth of the concerns that collecting genetic data could arouse, and it simply expected its personnel to accept on faith that the information would be used only for humanitarian and other important purposes. At the least, more complete disclosure about the program is needed. Ideally, DNA samples should be used only to identify remains, and military personnel should have the right to opt out of the repository.

The technical issues surrounding the law enforcement uses of DNA information were discussed by Randall Murch and Bruce Budowle.[79] As they point out,

DNA data banks have been established for convicted offenders by most states as well as by the Federal Bureau of Investigation. Jean McEwen notes that a major threat to privacy raised by the existence of these data banks is that they could be used beyond their original purpose. Finally, research on samples could be used to draw group-based inferences on propensity to violent or antisocial behavior.

The use of DNA data banks has been challenged on various constitutional grounds, most significantly, that requiring the collection of genetic information violates the Fourth Amendment's prohibition on unreasonable searches and seizures. For example, in one case, inmates challenged a Virginia law requiring convicted felons to submit blood samples for DNA analysis.[80] The U.S. Court of Appeals for the Fourth Circuit, in accord with the unanimous judicial response to such challenges, upheld the law. The court stated that "the minor intrusion caused by the taking of a blood sample is outweighed by Virginia's interest, as stated in the statute, in determining inmates' 'identification characteristics specific to the person' for improved law enforcement."[81]

In a country increasingly frustrated by its inability to prevent violent crime, it is quite likely that there will be pressure to expand the scope of DNA data banks to cover, for example, arrestees, gang members, members of "crime families," known drug users, residents of high crime areas, or minors in youth detention or in violation of curfew laws. Would these expanded DNA collection requirements be constitutional? If so, can all U.S. residents be required to submit a blood sample? If not, what is the difference between a blood sample for DNA testing and a fingerprint? If it is the intrusiveness of drawing blood, would the result be different if the DNA were extracted from buccal swabs or hair? The inevitable line-drawing by the courts will be couched in constitutional terms, such as determining whether the particular individuals have a reasonable expectation of privacy, whether focusing on a certain group violates equal protection, and balancing the state's interest in law enforcement against the privacy rights of individuals. In a broader sense, however, it will be merely another variation on the familiar theme of identifying the extent of the right to physical and informational privacy as applied to genetics.

SCHOOLS

The possible increased use of genetic information in schools is often overlooked but nevertheless important. As Laura Rothstein points out, genetic information about students could be used for several educational purposes, such as educational programming, behavior management, provision of appropriate related services, and determining eligibility for special education.[82] Genetic information in schools also could be used for more general public health purposes. The use of genetic information for educational and noneducational purposes raises similar issues. These issues include obtaining informed consent, assuring the accuracy of the information, providing appropriate counseling for the students and their parents, protecting privacy and confidentiality, and preventing adverse social and economic consequences, such as stigmatization and discrimination.

Current federal and state laws are inadequate to protect the substantial privacy and confidentiality interests in genetic information. For example, the Family Educational Rights and Privacy Act (FERPA), which safeguards the privacy of "school records," applies only to recipients of federal financial assistance and provides for limited remedies.[83] In addition, it is not clear whether genetic information would be considered a "school record" subject to the act.

State school records laws are probably a better vehicle for protecting genetic privacy and confidentiality. These laws should be enacted or amended to limit the access of school personnel to genetic information in a student's record, grant parents a right to view and correct educational records, require that medical and other genetic information be stored in files separate from other educational records, and set time schedules and procedures for the destruction of the files.

The other appropriate area for legislative action concerns what in federal research would be regarded as the protection of human subjects. Parents often do not understand what genetic testing entails as well as the range of risks and benefits. Truly informed consent is necessary, especially when the testing involves commercial entities that may have an economic interest in providing the tests or other services. Before any school or school district initiates the use of any medical screening, including genetic testing or genetic assessment of groups of students, an independent, multidisciplinary panel including parents and community representatives, similar to an institutional review board, should review the proposal. Individualized assessments should be subject to an approved testing protocol. The panel should grant approval only if it determines that the testing is necessary for a valid educational purpose, that procedures are in place to ensure informed consent and appropriate counseling, and that the confidentiality of the information will be maintained.

COMMERCIAL USES

The use of genetic information for commercial purposes is also frequently overlooked, but it is another area in which genetic privacy and confidentiality may be challenged. As with employers and insurers, any entity with a financial stake in the likely future health of an individual could have an interest in using genetic information to make predictions about the individual's health. For example, a mortgage company might want to condition the granting of a mortgage on genetic test information indicating that the individual does not have one of several alleles that would cast doubt on whether the individual would be alive or be able to maintain a stable income in 15 or 30 years. Banks and other lenders also could start to require such information. Condominium owners and real estate interests in retirement communities might start to require ApoE-4 testing of applicants to screen out individuals who are likely to develop Alzheimer's disease[84] because these individuals would undermine the image of vigorous golden years that the real estate development is trying to promote.[85]

Genetic testing and the use of genetic information could also proliferate as individuals and businesses attempt to avoid possible legal liability for failing to detect a genetic propensity to violence and other behavioral problems. For example, a boarding school or summer camp might require genetic screening of its students or campers to exclude individuals who might be prone to aggression. Failing to do so, they may fear, would expose them to liability in the event that one of the children intentionally injures another child.

The possible widespread use of genetic test information as a condition of fully participating in society threatens to make rampant the inappropriate use of genetic explanations of health and behavior. To prevent the abuse of genetic information, it will be necessary to enact a wide range of substantive laws. As was suggested earlier, rather than a single antidiscrimination law, fair credit, fair housing, public accommodations, and other laws need to be amended or construed to contain a prohibition on the compilation and use of predictive medical, including genetic, information.[86] Without such legislation it will be increasingly difficult to preserve genetic privacy and confidentiality.

GOVERNMENT USES

In 1997 the American Psychiatric Association recommended that physicians should order their patients who have Alzheimer's disease not to drive because they can cause accidents even in the early stages of the disease.[87] It is a small step to imagine that there soon will be efforts to mandate the ApoE-4 testing of drivers to detect the allele thought to be responsible for a portion of Alzheimer's disease.

Genetic testing also may be used by the military and by government contractors in an effort to predict the future mental health of individuals who are given security clearances or who work in safety-sensitive jobs. Genetic test results could be used in Social Security disability and veterans' benefits claims to determine whether the claimant has met a statutory threshold of disability.

When federal and state government agencies obtain and possess genetic information, an additional concern is raised. Current laws regarding public records might actually require that certain information be made available to the public. Even if the information is not publicly available, there are problems in keeping highly sensitive information separate from other government agencies, inaccessible to computer hackers and snooping government employees, or otherwise maintaining confidentiality.

In a 1997 case, the Supreme Court struck down a Georgia law that required candidates for state office to take and pass a drug test.[88] The Court left open the question of whether a state could lawfully require "a medical examination designed to provide certification of a candidate's general health." How long will it be before candidates in federal, state, and local elections are required by law or public opinion to provide their detailed genetic profiles for public scrutiny? What effect would such governmental disclosures have on private sector uses of genetic information? As Justice Louis Brandeis observed, "Our Government is the potent, the omnipresent teacher. For good or ill, it teaches the whole people by example."[89]

CONCLUSION

Privacy is a central issue in determining whether American society will prove able to absorb the exponential increases in genetic information resulting from the Human Genome Project without experiencing deleterious or disastrous social consequences. It will not be easy to protect genetic secrets. Genetic information is deeply ingrained in medical information, and if there ever was a time when the two could be separated, that time has passed. Medical information is also highly marketable and has a substantial commercial value. Those who deal in medical information will not readily relinquish this asset.

As a society, we need to decide if or when we are going to permit third parties to condition commercial, contractual, educational, financial, and legal rights and opportunities on individuals disclosing or releasing medical information or agreeing to undergo a medical examination. On a political level, one option is to decide that privacy is an intrinsic good for which we are willing to pay more for health care and for which we are willing to forego some potential public health benefits. Another option, not necessarily inconsistent with the first one, is to decide that privacy is primarily a consequential good. In this event, we ought to focus on prohibiting a range of adverse consequences from the use of genetic and other medical information, such as discrimination, denial of opportunities, financial burdens, and social disadvantages.

Genetic secrets are powerful secrets. Thoughtful, direct, and specific measures are needed to protect them. These are secrets worth protecting. As Sissela Bok has written, "With no capacity for keeping secrets and for choosing when to reveal them, human beings would lose their sense of identity and every shred of autonomy."[90]

NOTES

1. See Leroy Hood and Lee Rowen, "Genes, Genomes, and Society," Chapter 1 in this volume.
2. Anita L. Allen, "Genetic Privacy: An Emerging Concept and Value," Chapter 2 in this volume.
3. Sonia Le Bris and Bartha Maria Knoppers, "International and Comparative Concepts of Privacy," Chapter 22 in this volume.
4. Paul M. Schwartz, "European Data Protection Law and Medical Privacy," Chapter 21 in this volume.
5. Scott Burris and Lawrence O. Gostin, "Genetic Screening from a Public Health Perspective: Some Lessons from the HIV Experience," Chapter 8 in this volume.
6. See generally Mark A. Rothstein and Bartha Maria Knoppers, "Legal Aspects of Genetics, Work and Insurance in North America and Europe," *European Journal of Health Law Health* 3 (1996): 143–61.
7. Madison Powers, "Justice and Genetics: Privacy Protection and the Moral Basis of Public Policy," Chapter 19 in this volume.
8. New State Ice Co. v. Liebman, 285 U.S. 262, 311 (1932) (Brandeis, J., dissenting).
9. See Mary Anne Bobinski, "Unhealthy Federalism: Barriers to Increasing Health Care Access for the Uninsured," *University of California–Davis Law Review* 24 (1990): 255.
10. See Maxwell J. Mehlman et al., "The Need for Anonymous Genetic Counseling and Testing," *American Journal of Human Genetics* 58 (1996): 393.
11. Ellen Wright Clayton, "Informed Consent and Genetic Research," Chapter 7 in this volume.
12. Thomas H. Murray, "Genetic Exceptionalism and 'Future Diaries': Is Genetic Information Different from Other Medical Information?" Chapter 3 in this volume.

13. See Daniel J. Kevles, *In the Name of Eugenics: Genetics and the Uses of Heredity* (New York: Alfred A. Knopf, 1985).

14. Mark A. Rothstein, "The Law of Medical and Genetic Privacy in the Workplace," Chapter 15 in this volume.

15. See Lori B. Andrews, "Genetic Privacy: From the Laboratory to the Legislature," *Genome Research* 5 (1995): 209.

16. George J. Annas, Leonard H. Glantz, and Patricia A. Roche, *The Genetic Privacy Act and Commentary* (Boston: Boston University School of Public Health, 1995).

17. Philip R. Reilly, "The Impact of the Genetic Privacy Act on Medicine," *Journal of Law Medicine and Ethics* 23 (1995): 378.

18. Wendy E. Parmet, "Legislating Privacy: The HIV Experience," *Journal of Law Medicine and Ethics* 23 (1995): 371, 373.

19. Powers, "Justice and Genetics."

20. Lori B. Andrews, "Gen-Etiquette: Genetic Information Family Relationships, and Adoption," Chapter 14 in this volume.

21. Institute of Medicine, Committee on Assessing Genetic Risks, *Assessing Genetic Risks: Implications for Health and Social Policy,* ed. Lori B. Andrews et al. (Washington, D.C.: National Academy Press, 1994), 278.

22. Ibid.

23. Pate v. Threlkel, 661 So. 2d 278 (Fla. 1995).

24. Safer v. Estate of Pack, 677 A.2d 1188 (N.J. Super. App. Div. 1996).

25. Ibid., 1192.

26. See Eugene Pergament, "A Clinical Geneticist Perspective of the Patient-Physician Relationship," Chapter 5 in this volume.

27. Barbara Bowles Biesecker, "Privacy in Genetic Counseling," Chapter 6 in this volume.

28. David Orentlicher, "Genetic Privacy in the Patient-Physician Relationship," Chapter 4 in this volume.

29. Neil A. Holtzman, *Proceed with Caution: Predicting Genetic Risks in the Recombinant DNA Era* (Baltimore: Johns Hopkins University Press, 1989), 158–64; Vincent M. Riccardi, "Educating Clinicians about Genetics," in Thomas H. Murray, Mark A. Rothstein, and Robert F. Murray, Jr., eds., *The Human Genome Project and the Future of Health Care* (Indianapolis: Indiana University Press, 1996).

30. See Lawrence O. Gostin, "Health Information Privacy," *Cornell Law Review* 80 (1995): 451.

31. See Sheri Alpert, "Smart Cards, Smarter Policy: Medical Records, Privacy, and Health Care Reform," *Hastings Center Report* 23, no. 6 (1993): 13. See also Paul M. Schwartz, "European Data Protection Law and Medical Privacy," Chapter 21 in this volume.

32. Clayton, "Informed Consent and Genetic Research."

33. Jonathan M. Samet and Linda A. Bailey, "Privacy and Confidentiality: Issues in Using New Genetic Technologies in Epidemiologic Studies," Chapter 11 in this volume.

34. 42 U.S.C. § 241(d) (1994).

35. Charles L. Easley and Louise C. Strong, "Certificates of Confidentiality: A Valuable Tool for Protecting Genetic Data," *American Journal of Human Genetics* 57 (1995): 727.

36. See Clayton, "Informed Consent and Genetic Research."

37. John Fanning, Senior Policy Analyst, Office of Protection from Research Risks, National Institutes of Health, personal communication, May 6, 1996.

38. Biesecker, "Privacy in Genetic Counseling"; Pergament, "Clinical Geneticist Perspective."

39. Robert M. Cook-Deegan, "Confidentiality, Collective Resources, and Commercial Genomics," Chapter 9 in this volume.

40. See U.S. Congress, Office of Technology Assessment, *Protecting Privacy in Computerized Medical Information* (Washington, D.C.: Government Printing Office, 1993), 96.

41. See Randolph C. Barrows, Jr., and Paul D. Clayton, "Privacy, Confidentiality, and Electronic Medical Records," *Journal of the American Medical Informatics Association* 3 (1996): 139.

42. Norman Daniels, "The Human Genome Project and the Distribution of Scarce Medical Resources," in Murray, Rothstein, and Murray, Jr., eds., *Human Genome Project;* Daniels, "Insurability and the HIV Epidemic: Ethical Issues in Underwriting," *Milbank Quarterly* 68 (1990): 497.

43. See Jean E. McEwen et al., "A Survey of Medical Directors of Life Insurance Companies Concerning Use of Genetic Information," *American Journal of Human Genetics* 53 (1993): 33.

44. See Deborah A. Stone, "The Implications of the Human Genome Project for Access to Health Insurance," in Murray, Rothstein, and Murray, Jr., eds., *Human Genome Project.*

45. See Nancy E. Kass, "The Implications of Genetic Testing for Health and Life Insurance," Chapter 16 of this volume.

46. Ohio Rev. Stat. Ann. § 3901, 49(3)(B)(4) (1996).

47. Ibid., § 3901, 49(F).

48. See Karen H. Rothenberg, "Genetic Information and Health Insurance: State Legislative Approaches," *Journal of Law, Medicine and Ethics* 23 (1995): 312.

49. See Kathy L. Hudson et al., "Genetic Discrimination and Health Insurance: An Urgent Need for Reform," *Science* 270 (1995): 391.

50. Colo. Rev. Stat. § 10–3–1104, 4(2)(b) (West Supp. 1996).

51. Deborah A. Stone, "The Implications of the Human Genome Project for Access to Health Insurance," in Murray, Rothstein, and Murray, Jr., eds., *Human Genome Project,* 150 (emphasis deleted).

52. See Mark Scherzer, "Insurance," in Harlon L. Dalton and Scott Burris, eds., *AIDS and the Law* (New Haven: Yale University Press, 1987); Deborah A. Stone, "The Implications of the Human Genome Project for Access to Health Insurance," in Murray, Rothstein, and Murray, Jr., eds., *Human Genome Project.*

53. 29 U.S.C. §§ 1001–1461 (1994).

54. Thomas H. Murray, "Genetics and the Moral Mission of Health Insurance," *Hastings Center Report* 22, no. 6 (1992), 12.

55. H.R. 3103, 104th Cong., 2d Sess. (1996).

56. Mark A. Rothstein, "Genetics, Insurance, and the Ethics of Genetic Counseling," in Theodore Friedmann, ed., *Molecular Genetic Medicine,* vol. 3 (San Diego: Academic Press, 1993), 159.

57. Personal communication from Professor Henriette Roscam Abbing, University of Utrecht, Aug. 26, 1996.

58. Stephen G. Post et al., "The Clinical Introduction of Genetic Testing for Alzheimer Disease," *Journal of the American Medical Association* 277 (1997): 832.

59. Paul W. Brandt-Rauf and Sherry I. Brandt-Rauf, "Biomarkers—Scientific Advances and Societal Implications," Chapter 10 in this volume.

60. See Karen Rothenberg et al., "Genetic Information and the Workplace: Legislative Approaches and Policy Challenges," *Science* 275 (1997): 1775.

61. 42 U.S.C. §§ 12101–213 (1994).

62. EEOC Compliance Manual, vol. 2, EEOC Order 915.002, Definition of the Term "Disability," at 902–45, reprinted in *Daily Labor Report* (Mar. 16, 1995), E–1, E–23.

63. Mark A. Rothstein, "Legal and Ethical Aspects of Medical Screening," *Occupational Medicine: State of the Art Reviews* 3, no. 1 (1996): 31.

64. Franklin M. Zweig, Joseph T. Walsh, and Daniel M. Freeman, "Courts and the Challenges of Adjudicating Genetic Testing's Secrets," Chapter 18 in this volume.

65. Skinner v. Oklahoma, 316 U.S. 535 (1942).

66. Ibid., 546 (Jackson, J., concurring).

67. Kansas v. Hendricks, 117 S. Ct. 2072 (1997).

68. See Dan W. Brock, "The Human Genome Project and Human Identity," *Houston Law Review* 29 (1992): 7, 13–17.

69. Personal communication with Bonnie S. Leroy, director of genetic counseling, Institute of Human Genetics, University of Minnesota Hospital, Apr. 1, 1997.

70. Mark A. Rothstein, "Preventing the Discovery of Plaintiff Genetic Profiles by Defendants Seeking to Limit Damages in Personal Injury Litigation," *Indiana Law Journal* 71 (1996): 877–910.

71. In re Carney, 598 P.2d 36 (Cal. 1979).

72. Ibid., 44.

73. Andrews, "Gen-Etiquette."

74. Diane E. Hoffmann and Eric A. Wulfsberg, "Testing Children for Genetic Predispositions: Is It in Their Best Interest?" *Journal of Law, Medicine and Ethics* 23 (1995): 331.

75. Demosthenes A. Lorandos, "Secrecy and Genetics in Adoption Law and Practice," *Loyola University Chicago Law Journal* 27 (1996): 277, 317.

76. See Cesnik v. Edgewood Baptist Church, 88 F.3d 902 (11th Cir. 1996).

77. Neil A. Lewis, "Two Marines Who Refused to Comply with Genetic-Testing Order Face a Court-Martial," *New York Times*, Apr. 13, 1996.

78. Darryl Van Duch, "DNA = Do Not Appropriate, Say Soldiers and Civilians," *National Law Journal*, May 27, 1996, B1.

79. Randall S. Murch and Bruce Budowle, "Are Developments in Forensic Applications of DNA Technology Consistent with Privacy Protections?" Chapter 12 in this volume.

80. Jones v. Murray, 962 F.2d 302 (4th Cir. 1992).

81. Ibid., p. 315.

82. Laura F. Rothstein, "Genetic Information in Schools," Chapter 17 in this volume.

83. 20 U.S.C. § 1232g (1994).

84. Cf. Ores v. Willow West Condominium Ass'n, 7 Nat'l Disab. L. Reptr. ¶ 440 (N.D. Ill. 1996) (denying motion to dismiss Fair Housing Act lawsuit brought by two brothers with fragile X syndrome against a bank, condominium association, and property management company).

85. Cf. Doukas v. Metropolitan Ins. Co., 950 F. Supp. 422 (D.N.H. 1996) (denying motion to dismiss ADA case in which applicant was denied mortgage disability insurance because she had a history of bipolar disorder).

86. See, e.g., Fair Credit Reporting Act, 15 U.S.C. §§ 1681–1681t (1994); Fair Housing Act, 42 U.S.C. § 3601 et seq. (1994); and Title III of the Americans with Disabilities Act, 42 U.S.C. §§ 12181–12189 (1994).

87. "Alzheimer's Driving Ban Is Advised," *New York Times,* May 1, 1997, A14.

88. Chandler v. Miller, 117 S.Ct. 1295 (1997).

89. Olmstead v. United States, 277 U.S. 438, 485 (1928) (Brandeis, J., dissenting).

90. Sissela Bok, *Secrets: On the Ethics of Concealment and Revelation* (New York: Pantheon, 1982), 282.

Contributors

Anita L. Allen, J.D., Ph.D., is Associate Dean for Research and Professor of Law and Philosophy, Georgetown University Law Center

Lori B. Andrews, J.D., is Professor of Law, Chicago-Kent College of Law, Illinois Institute of Technology

Linda A. Bailey, J.D., M.H.S., is Assistant Director, Center for Epidemiology and Policy, Department of Epidemiology, The Johns Hopkins University School of Hygiene and Public Health

Barbara Bowles Biesecker, M.S., is Co-Director, Genetic Counseling Research and Training Program, National Human Genome Research Institute, National Institutes of Health

Paul W. Brandt-Rauf, M.D., Sc.D., Dr.P.H., is Professor of Public Health and Director of Occupational and Environmental Medicine, Columbia University School of Public Health

Sherry I. Brandt-Rauf, M. Phil., J.D., is Assistant Professor of Social Medicine, Center for the Study of Society and Medicine, Columbia University College of Physicians and Surgeons

Bruce Budowle, Ph.D., is Chief, Forensic Science Research Unit, Federal Bureau of Investigation

Scott Burris, J.D., is Associate Professor of Law, Temple University School of Law

Ellen Wright Clayton, M.D., J.D., is Associate Professor of Pediatrics and Law, Vanderbilt University Schools of Medicine and Law

Robert M. Cook-Deegan, M.D., is Staff Director, National Cancer Policy Board, Institute of Medicine and Commission on Life Sciences, National Academy of Sciences

Daniel M. Freeman, J.D., is Counsel and Parliamentarian, Committee on the Judiciary, U.S. House of Representatives

Lawrence O. Gostin, J.D., is Professor of Law, Georgetown University Law Center

Leroy Hood, M.D., Ph.D., is William Gates III Professor and Chair of the Department of Molecular Biotechnology, University of Washington School of Medicine

Nancy E. Kass, Sc.D., is Associate Professor, Program in Law, Ethics and Health, Department of Health Policy and Management, The Johns Hopkins University School of Hygiene and Public Health

Bartha Maria Knoppers, LL.D., is Professor, Faculty of Law, University of Montreal

Sonia Le Bris, LL.M., is Researcher, Faculty of Law, University of Montreal

Jean E. McEwen, J.D., Ph.D., is Associate Professor, Boston College Law School

Randall S. Murch, Ph.D., is Chief, Scientific Analysis Section, Federal Bureau of Investigation

Thomas H. Murray, Ph.D., is Professor of Biomedical Ethics and Director of the Center for Biomedical Ethics, Case Western Reserve University School of Medicine

David Orentlicher, M.D., J.D., is Associate Professor of Law, Indiana University School of Law–Indianapolis

Eugene Pergament, M.D., Ph.D., FACMG, is Professor of Obstetrics and Gynecology, Northwestern University Medical School, Director, Graduate Program in Genetic Counseling, Northwestern University, and Head, Section of Reproductive Genetics, Northwestern Memorial Hospital

Madison Powers, J.D., Ph.D., is Senior Research Scholar, Kennedy Institute of Ethics and Associate Professor of Philosophy, Georgetown University

Philip R. Reilly, M.D., J.D., is Executive Director, Shriver Center for Mental Retardation

Laura F. Rothstein, J.D., is Law Foundation Professor of Law, University of Houston Law Center

Mark A. Rothstein, J.D., is Hugh Roy and Lillie Cranz Cullen Distinguished Professor of Law and Director, Health Law and Policy Institute, University of Houston Law Center

Lee Rowen, Ph.D., is Research Scientist, Department of Molecular Biotechnology, University of Washington School of Medicine

Jonathan M. Samet, M.D., M.S., is Professor and Chairman, Department of Epidemiology, The Johns Hopkins University School of Hygiene and Public Health

Paul M. Schwartz, J.D., is Professor of Law, University of Arkansas–Fayetteville School of Law

Arthur C. Upton, M.D., is Clinical Professor of Environmental and Community Medicine, Robert Wood Johnson School of Medicine

Joseph T. Walsh, LL.B., is Justice, Supreme Court of Delaware

Franklin M. Zweig, J.D., Ph.D., is President and Chief Executive Officer, Einstein Institute for Science, Health and the Courts

Index